The Lost Supper

TARAS GRESCOE

THE
LOST
SUPPER

SEARCHING
FOR THE
FUTURE OF FOOD
IN THE TASTES
OF THE PAST

DAVID SUZUKI INSTITUTE

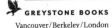 GREYSTONE BOOKS
Vancouver / Berkeley / London

Greystone Books Ltd.
greystonebooks.com

David Suzuki Institute
davidsuzukiinstitute.org

Cataloguing data available from Library and Archives Canada
ISBN 978-1-77840-212-8 (pbk)
ISBN 978-1-77164-763-2 (cloth)
ISBN 978-1-77164-764-9 (epub)

Editing by Paula Ayer
Copy editing by Crissy Calhoun
Proofreading by Jennifer Stewart
Indexing by Stephen Ullstrom
Cover design by Jessica Sullivan
Cover illustration ilbusca / iStock
Text design by Belle Wuthrich

Printed and bound in Canada on FSC® certified paper at Friesens.
The FSC® label means that materials used for the
product have been responsibly sourced.

Greystone Books thanks the Canada Council for the Arts,
the British Columbia Arts Council, the Province of British Columbia
through the Book Publishing Tax Credit, and the Government
of Canada for supporting our publishing activities.

Canada

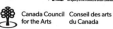

MIX
Paper | Supporting
responsible forestry
FSC® C016245

BRITISH COLUMBIA

BRITISH COLUMBIA
ARTS COUNCIL
An agency of the Province of British Columbia

Canada Council   Conseil des arts
for the Arts   du Canada

Greystone Books gratefully acknowledges the xʷməθkʷəy̓əm (Musqueam),
Sḵwx̱wú7mesh (Squamish), and səlilwətaɬ (Tsleil-Waututh) peoples on
whose land our Vancouver head office is located.

To my father, Paul Grescoe (1939–2023),
who taught me that to tell any story well, you need
curiosity, attentiveness, and compassion.

Homo sum, humani nihil a me alienum puto.
I am a human being, and consider
nothing human alien to me.
TERENCE, Roman-African playwright,
163 BCE

Contents

Prologue *1*

1 MONTREAL
Kitchen Dreams   *17*

2 MEXICO CITY
The Secret of Axayacatl   *23*

3 OSSABAW ISLAND
Some Pig   *55*

4 CÁDIZ
The Quintessence of Putrescence   *90*

5 YORKSHIRE DALES
Hard Cheese   *119*

6 PUGLIA
The Death of the Immortals   *151*

7 CAPPADOCIA
Lost and Found   *182*

8 SAINT-JEAN-SUR-RICHELIEU
Bread Alone   *209*

9 MI'WER'LA
The Cooked and the Raw   *244*

Epilogue   *280*
Acknowledgments   *297*
Selected Bibliography   *301*
Further Reading   *315*
Index   *317*

Prologue

HALF AN HOUR'S DRIVE SOUTHEAST OF KONYA, famous for being the city where the Persian mystic Rumi was laid to rest and Sufi dervishes whirl, a lone hill looms over the parched, pita-flat basin of a vast prehistoric lake.

For centuries, the oval-shaped rise, carpeted with grasses and Syrian rue, was known to local farmers as Çatalhöyük, Turkish for "the mound at the fork in the road." When archaeologists began to excavate the site in the early 1960s, they realized the mound concealed the remnants of an important prehistoric community. It would prove to be the most populous site ever discovered from the Neolithic, the period when our species began to domesticate plants and animals and gather in permanent settlements. Eight and a half thousand years ago, Çatalhöyük was home to as many as eight thousand people, making it the single largest concentration of humans that had ever lived on Earth. At its peak, Çatalhöyük covered about thirty-two acres, a little larger than Battery Park, at the tip of Manhattan, is today. It was also, judged by modern standards, a very odd place.

From the visitors' parking lot next to a teahouse and souvenir stand, a sinuous path leads to the top of an archaeological dig known as the East Mound, which is as tall as a seven-story building. A wooden frame stretched with translucent polymer—a structure that from a distance resembles the shell of an armadillo—keeps sixty years' worth of painstaking excavations protected from the elements. In the milky, filtered light of midday, walls of clay, marl, and plaster, buttressed by sandbags and wooden support beams, glow in warm, earthen hues. A gangway following the structure's inner perimeter offers a variety of viewpoints on the site, which reveals itself as an irregular gridwork of three-dimensional rectangles, rising in tiers. The jumble of buildings suggests a Spanish hill village, of the kind the Cubists liked to paint, albeit one whose houses have had their roofs sheared off. After a while, the attentive visitor might notice a few curious details: the presence of circular pits in many floors; the fact that there is virtually no space between the walls of neighboring houses; the complete absence of front doors.

At the base of the mound, four replica dwellings give visitors a sense of what daily life was like for Çatalhöyükans. Because the 150 or so flat-topped houses in the settlement were so tightly packed, the sidewalks were on the roofs, which is where people gathered and slept during the warmer months of the year. The narrow spaces between houses appear to have been reserved for tossing garbage. Homes were entered through ladders that leaned against rectangular holes in the ceilings, which doubled as skylights that provided the only source of natural illumination. Those circular pits in the floor were, in fact, tombs, where corpses were interred, probably after being left outdoors to be picked clean by vultures; the people of Çatalhöyük went to sleep each night on raised platforms over the skeletons of their dead. Homes were kept impeccably clean, their floors swept daily, with the walls, which were sometimes replastered monthly, providing surfaces for murals and sculptures. After seventy or eighty years, each building reached the end of its useful life-span, and was torn down. Rubble from the roofs and upper walls became the foundations of new dwellings, a process of stacking that explains the mound's vertical rise over the 1,200 years Çatalhöyük was inhabited.

For decades, archaeologists have asked themselves why humans crammed themselves into this settlement on the Konya Plain. *Homo sapiens* emerged as a separate species as much as 300,000 years ago. Between seventy thousand and fifty thousand years ago, a small band of behaviorally modern humans, identical in intellectual capacities to people living today, struck out from northeastern Africa. For the vast majority of our species' existence, descendants of this band spread themselves thinly over the landscape in search of food. Occasionally, we gathered at places like Göbekli Tepe—an 11,500-year-old arrangement of Stonehenge-like monoliths three hundred miles to the east of Çatalhöyük that is thought to be the world's first temple—before scattering to continue our fruitful existence of foraging and hunting. After the last ice age ended, though, some humans decided to stay put and adapt to changes in an ecosystem rather than pull up stakes and move on when the environment changed. Some speculate Çatalhöyükans chose to settle down in order to work with obsidian, a volcanic stone from nearby Cappadocia, useful for making blades, mirrors, and jewelry, which they may have traded with the people of the Levant. Others believe they were attracted by the local soil, which provided the clay to build permanent dwellings, as well as the lime-rich plaster with which they covered the walls and floors of their homes.

One thing is certain. There was no shortage of food in the area. From the top of the mound, you can make out the tops of the trees that grow along the Çarşamba River. Twelve thousand years ago, a huge lake that had covered much of the Konya Plain drained out, and a woodland of oak trees soon emerged. By the time settlement at Çatalhöyük began, the river regularly overflowed its banks in the spring, turning this semiarid area into a wetland, teeming with ducks, geese, and coots and such small edible fish as loaches and minnows. When the Çarşamba's waters receded, they left behind clay ideal for house-building, but also nutrient-rich fields on which the cereals that grew among the oaks could be sown for harvest in late summer. This may be the real reason why, for over a millennium, a total of 100,000 Çatalhöyükans lived their lives on this site. With relatively little work, they could benefit from a reliable supply of calories by harvesting grains, while still enjoying the challenge of the hunt and the nutritional variety offered by gathering wild plants.

The skeletons recovered from the in-home burial pits, each of which could contain the remains of up to fifty-two individuals, show remarkably few marks of violence. If they survived childhood and its attendant accidents and diseases, Çatalhöyükans tended to reach the age of seventy or eighty, living lives as long we do today. Women and men show similar levels of wear and tear on their bones, indicating that household tasks were shared, in a way they wouldn't be in later farming societies. There were no temples or administrative buildings, and no home was appreciably larger than any other, suggesting egalitarianism was held at a premium.

"Each household," archaeologist David Wengrow and the late anthropologist David Graeber observed of Çatalhöyük in their 2021 book *The Dawn of Everything*, "appears more or less a world unto itself—a discrete locus of storage, production and consumption... Despite the considerable size and density of the built-up area, there is no evidence for central authority." For them, the settlement provides a counterexample to the idea that settled farming life was our first fall from grace. "Agriculture did not mean the inception of private property, nor did it mark an irreversible step towards inequality."

According to the influential maxim of the English philosopher Thomas Hobbes, the life of humans in the absence of governing authority was "solitary, poor, nasty, brutish, and short." For the unoppressed agriculturalists of Çatalhöyük, life on the contrary appears to have been sociable, rich, pleasant, peaceful, and long.

In one of the structures in the East Mound, the building labeled B.108, a horseshoe-shaped ridge is clearly visible in the floor. This was a hearth, which functioned like a stovetop, where glowing coals and dung would have been used to keep food hot. Next to it, in the center of the house, is a circular indentation once occupied by an oven. An archaeologists' re-creation in the replica house shows it would have been positioned just beneath the sloping entry ladder, so smoke could escape through the hole in the ceiling. Beehive-shaped, with a rectangular slot in front, it resembles the ovens known as *firins* still used to bake flatbread in local villages.

Before coming to Turkey, I talked to an archaeobotanist who has studied tens of thousands of charred remains recovered from Çatalhöyük. Using a scanning electron microscope, she confirmed that naturally leavened bread was regularly baked in the site's ovens. Seeds from stands of grasses, the wild ancestors of wheat, which thrived in the oak and juniper woodlands about seven miles from the site, were likely gathered and brought to the settlement, where some would have fallen to the ground and sprouted. This domesticated wheat growing on the floodplain of the Çarşamba River was harvested with sickles, which were made from animal horns set with blades of flint or obsidian, and then ground into flour.

Fresh-baked bread, in other words, provided the long-lived people of Çatalhöyük with a large percentage of the calories in their diet. It was made with a kind of wheat the ancient Babylonians called *ziz*, the Egyptians called *zeia*, the Hebrews referred to as *kassemet*, and contemporary Turks know as *kavilca*. In English, we call it emmer. Along with barley, it was the first wild grass ever domesticated, putting it among the most ancient of the ancient grains.

According to an argument that has lately become widespread, all of the world's problems began when small bands of hunter-gatherers gave up their nomadic existence and embraced farming and the settled, community-based existence that went with it. Inequality, war, oppression of women, rule by zealots and tyrants, epidemics, slavery, environmental degradation, and individual ill-health—all are a direct result of agriculture.

Yet Çatalhöyükans seem to have enjoyed their daily bread without sacrificing good health, longevity, or the challenges of gathering varied foodstuffs from the natural world. Rather than being a problem, farming was a solution. Admittedly, eight thousand years and a couple of other revolutions—industrial and "green"—later, we humans have made a mess of agriculture and, with it, the planet. Yet agriculture continues to remain the best hope for *Homo sapiens*. (Not to mention *your* only hope of getting something to eat later today.) What we still haven't figured out is how to do it right.

This book makes the case that the future of food lies in the past, including such lost, forgotten, or nearly vanished foods as emmer wheat. The fact that bread, the age-old staff of life, has lately come to stand for all the ills of civilization is a basic mistake and an indication of how much we need to learn—or relearn.

Don't blame the grain, in other words. Blame what we've done with it.

"THE GREATEST MISTAKE in the history of the human race," according to American geographer Jared Diamond, was farming. "With agriculture came the gross social and sexual inequality, the disease and despotism, that curse our existence."

The notion of farming-as-disaster has been reiterated in such works of popular history as Spencer Wells's *Pandora's Seed*, Richard Manning's *Against the Grain*, and Yuval Noah Harari's *Sapiens*. Some anthropologists, conservationists, and environmentalists have turned the idea into a basis for activism, most famously George Monbiot. The British journalist argues that the world would be a better place if protein were synthesized by scientists in a lab and if the land currently devoted to raising crops and livestock were "rewilded," allowed to return to a state of nature that would allow salmon, wolves, and ospreys to repopulate a reemergent wilderness.

As I left Çatalhöyük, driving north across the Anatolian plain, I felt a twinge of sympathy for these new anti-agriculturalists. Turkey was where some of the first crop and animal domestications occurred, and farming seemed to be turning the place into a shambles. It was late October, and the river whose annual floods once provided a lush habitat for people on the Konya Plain was a sinuous trickle of dirty water, confined, as it has been for the last half century, between the high walls of a concrete channel. Farmers' fields were linked to the

Çarşamba River by raised aqueducts, all of which were bone-dry; in some places they had simply toppled over. Our car raced past fields filled with rows of dead cornstalks, their husks caked with a fine layer of salt. At one point, a dramatic plume rose from the plain parallel to the highway. At first I thought it was an isolated bushfire, but as we passed, I saw a shepherd leading his troop of sheep down a path so parched that it sent up an opaque cloud that lingered malevolently in the air.

"It's the dust bowl," muttered the Turkish scientist in the driver's seat beside me. "Everything is dry. There is no water." A lack of rainfall had contributed to an ongoing drought, one that would reduce the year's wheat crop by a staggering two million tons.

The GPS said our route was taking us near the western shore of Turkey's second-largest lake, a vast expanse of hypersaline water that provides the nation with half its refined salt. Twenty years ago, its shores had started to retreat, and this would turn out to be the year Lake Tuz completely disappeared. Pink flamingoes migrating from Africa have long used the lakeshore to lay their eggs. A few months after my visit, a photographer would document the skeletons of thousands of flamingo chicks against a bleak background of salt crystals.

Turkey is believed to be one of the "centers of origin" of domesticated wheat, and the greatest global diversity of landraces of wheat—distinct seed-propagated populations adapted to local conditions—is still found in the eastern part of the country. Since the 1960s, local varieties have been replaced with semidwarf hybrids, and today eighteen million acres are planted with bread wheat and durum for pasta. Emmer and einkorn are grown on fewer than ten thousand acres, mostly on marginal lands in a few northern villages.

As we continued north, high-sided trucks, their beds piled with beets, thundered past. Some swerved off the road into sugar refineries, vast complexes of stainless-steel pipes and belching chimney stacks. In recent years, many farmers on the Konya Plain have replaced wheat with more valuable—but also far thirstier—crops of corn, clover, and sugar beet. Desperate to irrigate their crops, they've taken to drilling into underground aquifers. We could see the illegal wells on either side of the highway, jerry-rigged lengths of black pipe plunged into orifices of poured concrete, 180,000 of them by some counts. Their incessant pumping has already lowered the water table by sixty-five feet. Much of the plain is karst, or water-soluble limestone, and the vanishing groundwater has pockmarked the landscape with sinkholes, which can open suddenly, swallowing flocks of sheep whole. In many places, they have made it impossible to operate tractors, forcing farmers to abandon their ancestral fields.

Twelve thousand years after the world's first agricultural revolution began in the Fertile Crescent, it was clear that farming had brought this part of Turkey to a desperate pass. The same can be said for much of the rest of the world. When Çatalhöyük was founded, just two or three million humans may have lived on the entire planet, no more than live in Brooklyn today. Today we number eight billion, and this prodigal growth can be attributed to the most recent agricultural revolutions. To meet the dietary needs of a global population on course to top ten billion, economists say we'll have to increase food production by 50 percent by midcentury.

Çatalhöyük existed for just over a millennium. The Roman Empire also lasted for about one thousand years, as did the civilizations of the Greeks and of the Maya. Though the causes of civilizational decline are complex, one of the simplest may lie in a failure to tend to the foundation of farming, the dirt under our feet. As geomorphologist David R. Montgomery puts it, "Soil erosion that outpaced soil formation limited the longevity of civilizations that failed to safeguard the foundation of their prosperity—their soil." On that count, modern Turkey seems to be on the verge of catastrophic failure. It is not alone.

for novel, distinctive, and pleasant flavors has been neglected as one of the drivers of human evolution—and that is a mistake. One of the most convincing explanations for why we learned to master fire was that meat tasted so much better roasted than raw. (The smoke from fire was also useful for tranquilizing bees, giving us access to the sweetest substance in nature, honey.) Intensity of flavor is often an indication of the presence of polyphenols and other micronutrients, many of which fight disease and increase stamina. Hunger and famine certainly called the shots at many points in our story, but I'm pretty certain that often the reason we bothered going over a hilltop, or to the far side of the river, was to discover how things tasted over there.

Among the cases of artifacts in the Museum of Anatolian Civilizations, there was a mock-up of the interior of a Çatalhöyük house, more detailed than the one I'd seen at the archaeological site. It gave me the answer to a question that had been nagging at me. A pair of ceramic pots sat on a raised platform in one corner of the room. Beside it was a dome-shaped oven made of clay. And between them was a rectangular stone, about twenty inches long; the curators had spread a thin layer of grain over its slightly concave surface, and a round muller, or grindstone, sat amid the seeds.

This, I realized, was how the Çatalhöyükans made their bread. They'd take a few handfuls of emmer wheat from the storage pots, scatter them on the stone, and crush them into flour with the grindstone. After adding water to the flour, and letting the mixture collect natural yeasts for a few hours, they'd slap the dough onto the oven's inner surface. Before my journey was over, I resolved to learn how to bake my own loaf of Neolithic bread.

I had no idea how it was going to taste. But I was dying of curiosity to find out.

IF THIS BOOK HAS ONE MESSAGE, it's this: diversity is resiliency. It's a message that applies to human cultures, natural ecosystems, and even the microorganisms in our bodies. And where can we find the most culinary and nutritional diversity? Not in the food we eat today. And probably not in the future, which, if we choose to pursue lab-grown meat, patented transgenic produce, or some as-yet-undeveloped version of Soylent Green, is bound to be even less varied than what we eat today. We need to look to the past, to the huge variety of foods we've eaten through the course of our species' existence, a diversity that we are now at risk of losing.

It's been half a million years since our venturesome, adaptable primate ancestors left their home in the African treetops, seeking ways to thrive and survive in new habitats. And now we've come to the point in our story where the way *forward* involves looking *backward*, to the forgotten or near-vanished diversity of our ancestral diets—to all our lost suppers.

1

MONTREAL
Kitchen Dreams

WHAT AM I GOING TO EAT?

I don't know about you, but that's something I've been asking myself several times a day, for as long as I can remember. Lately the question has become: What are *we* going to eat? When I'm at home in Montreal, finding plausible answers seems to occupy a fair chunk of my day.

My wife, Erin, and I have two elementary-school-aged boys, and when it's my turn to make supper, I take a lot of pleasure in the process. As best I can, I try to make our meals varied, nutritious, and flavorful—a challenge, because Victor, our youngest son, who is the pickiest of eaters, prefers to subsist on cherry tomatoes, cucumbers, cubes of mild Cheddar, and sauce-free pasta. Desmond is more open to trying new things, and I often go to extravagant lengths to put together an interesting meal, hopping on my bicycle to ride across the city to the markets where I know I can forage for zucchini flowers, salt-packed capers, this spring's harvest of maple syrup, or a bottle of extra-virgin olive oil from Puglia or Crete.

That said, I'm no horticulturalist. Montreal is a wintry city, and we live in a third-floor apartment, so not much more than herbs and tomatoes grow in the boxes on our back balcony. But I've gotten pretty good at some of the lower-hanging fruit of urban home economics. There's usually a wet lump of dough made with some obscure wheat variety bubbling away in a bowl atop the washing machine, mason jars of hand-rubbed napa cabbage perfuming the air with their kimchi burps, and symbiotic communities of bacteria and yeast industriously turning whole milk into kefir and black tea into kombucha. True, all of this is a long way from self-sufficiency. Yet every time we sit down to a meal of slow-cooked lentils or homemade fettucine—hold the alfredo sauce for Victor—I'm conscious that we've taken a step, if only a small one, away from industrial agriculture.

I also know that avoiding processed food takes effort. The time I devote to seeking out ingredients and preparing a meal is time I could be spending at work—being economically productive. But I'm all right with that. Engaging with the slow routines of home cooking feels like a way of coming to terms with the ecological and demographic crises that have been boiling up for my entire life.

Half a century ago, concern about population growth and the consequences of the green revolution began to inspire warnings and calls for change. The landmark bestseller *Limits to Growth*, published by the Club of Rome, a group of European industrialists and scientists who met in the Italian capital in 1968, predicted that if nations continued to pursue unlimited economic and population growth, the world would face ecological collapse by 2050. E. F. Schumacher, who set out a theory of "Buddhist economics" in his 1974 book *Small Is Beautiful*, encouraged readers to look at the soil, water, and atmosphere as nonrenewable natural capital—rather than expendable income to be squandered—while championing smaller farms over industrial-scale agriculture. Influential voices such as Aldo Leopold and Wendell Berry questioned the dubious morality of patenting the products of nature, which began with the ill-considered U.S. Plant Patent Act of 1930 and has led to multinationals suing small farmers for daring to replant their seeds. The Slow Food organization,

2

MEXICO CITY
The Secret of Axayacatl

AS THE FIRST LIGHTS of Mexico City became visible from the port-side window of the Airbus A319, I was thinking about the prophecies of overpopulation that had haunted my childhood.

A slender paperback, whose cover featured the alarming image of a sparking fuse burning down toward a diapered baby, was a fixture on book racks in the 1970s. *The Population Bomb* opened with the lapidary declaration "The battle to feed all of humanity is over." Humanity had already lost. In the decades to come, "hundreds of millions of people are going to starve to death." The author described a taxi ride through Delhi, where the streets swarmed with desperate people who "thrust their hands through the taxi window, begging. People defecating and urinating, people clinging to buses ... people, people, people, people ..." The population of India, according to the book, was doomed to extinction. Thanks to impending food shortages, the chances were also good that "England will not exist in the year 2000."

Paul R. Ehrlich's hastily written screed would prove to be one of the most influential books of the twentieth century. Appearances on *The Tonight Show*, in which the gaunt pundit traded rueful wisecracks with host Johnny Carson, made Ehrlich a household name.

Advocates for ZPG—zero population growth—argued that diapers, cribs, and toys should be subject to a luxury tax, with "responsibility prizes" awarded to childless couples. The more zealous supporters of ZPG wore lapel buttons that read "Two Is Enough." The movement saw birth control pills being scattered from helicopters in the Philippines, Indian men being rewarded with transistor radios for submitting to vasectomies, and the forced sterilizations of tens of thousands of impoverished women in Indonesia, Peru, Bangladesh, and Mexico.

Sensitive to the zeitgeist, my parents decided it would be more ethical to adopt than bring another child into the world. But when my mother went to an agency in her hometown of Hamilton, she was told she should try to have a kid of her own first. If it weren't for that rebuff, I probably wouldn't exist. Two years after I was born, my parents moved west to Vancouver, where they adopted a six-week-old baby, my sister, Lara. After that, they called it quits. Two, for my parents, was enough.

The nightmarish taxi ride Ehrlich described had taken place the year I was born, when fewer than three million people lived in Delhi. (The Indian capital's population, which has since multiplied tenfold, is now exceeded only by Tokyo's.) Yet at the time, Mexico City was more populous and well on its way to becoming one of the world's first megacities; it would hit the defining ten-million mark eight years later, in 1974. By the beginning of the new millennium, when Mexico City's population had nearly doubled again, it was being trotted out as a case study in cancerous urban growth, a dysfunctional dystopia where smog-choked birds dropped from the sky.

Thanks to the city's sheer vastness, I had plenty of time to think before we landed. Even at jet speeds, it takes a decent chunk of time to circle into the Valley of Mexico. For at least the last two thousand years, the mountain-ringed basin, fifty miles from east to west, seventy from north to south, has been one of the largest population centers in the Americas. From my vantage point in the night sky,

What had allowed the conquistadors to vanquish fatigue and fear was their lust for riches. After arriving from Cuba, on the shore near what is now Veracruz, Cortés told an Aztec emissary, in one of the most naked giveaways of true intent in the history of colonialism, "I and my companions suffer from a disease of the heart which can be cured only with gold."

Their march had taken them past well-irrigated fields of corn and plantations of prickly pear cactus. But the Spaniards scorned agriculture, partly because they associated it with the Moors, who had undertaken impressive feats of irrigation that made parts of the arid Iberian Peninsula into a garden. Cortés himself was the son of a minor nobleman from Extremadura, a landscape dominated by the oak forest of the *dehesa*, which over five hundred years had been grazed to the roots by sheep and the region's celebrated *pata negra* pigs. Though Cortés had learned to ride horses while herding swine, the pigs required few people to tend them, and still fewer owners. Born too late to profit from the domestic crusade against Islam, the young hidalgo sailed for the island of Hispaniola at the age of nineteen to seek his fortune.

As they rode along the five-mile-long causeway of hewn stone that led to Tenochtitlán, Cortés and his men saw cobbled streets lined with willow trees, aqueducts that brought fresh drinking water to the whitewashed villas of the rich, and steep pyramidal temples that rose fifteen stories—taller even than the cathedral of Seville—above a plaza that measured a quarter mile on each side. With a population of 200,000, the island-city was larger than any settlement in Spain. The Aztecs boasted accurate calendars, state-run education, zoos and botanical gardens, efficient waste-management systems, and a network of relay runners who transmitted messages from as far as present-day Guatemala at the rate of two hundred miles a day.

On their side, the Spaniards had arms, auspicious timing, and antibodies. From their ships, they unleashed iron-clad mastiffs that had been fed on the flesh of the Indigenous people of Cuba. They rode atop "hornless stags"—sixteen Spanish warhorses—a species of megafauna that vanished from the New World after the Ice Age. They carried swords with blades of fire-hardened Toledo steel and deployed wheeled cannons whose balls could shatter trees into splinters and make hillsides explode. The Aztecs had formidable weapons of their own, including the *macuahuitl*, a massive club edged with razor-sharp obsidian, which could disembowel a horse with a single blow—provided they could get close enough to use it.

When Cortés and Montezuma met in the sacred heart of Tenochtitlán that day, the emperor could have ordered the four hundred or so Spaniards who had survived the march exterminated with a wave of his hand. They were surrounded, after all, by the fifteen million subjects of the greatest empire Mesoamerica had ever known. It was the Spaniards' good fortune to have made landfall at the exact point in the fifty-two-year Aztec century when Quetzalcóatl was prophesied to return from the east. The portent-obsessed Montezuma decided it prudent to welcome the newcomers, and he invited them to bivouac in the palace of his late father, Axayacatl.

Looking for a spot to build an altar to the Virgin Mary, the Spaniards discovered a walled-off entrance to a hidden chamber filled with gold, silver, and intricate turquoise inlay. This was the secret treasure of Axayacatl, surplus tribute that had been delivered from the corners of the empire, and just as promptly sealed up and forgotten. They set about stripping gems from shields and bracelets and melting the gold from finely wrought jewelry into ingots; anything deemed unworthy of plunder was burned.

The Spaniards, who remained in Tenochtitlán for eight months, were clearly impressed by its great market, Tlatelolco, which could welcome sixty thousand buyers and sellers at a time.

"They will eat virtually anything that lives," Cortés marveled. "Snakes without head or tail; little barkless dogs, castrated and fattened; moles, dormice, mice, worms, lice; and they even eat earth which they gather with fine nets, at certain times of year, from the surface of the lake . . . it is made into cakes resembling bricks [and] eaten as we eat cheese; it has a somewhat salty taste, and, when taken with *chilmole* [seasoning], is delicious." The "earth" Cortés described may have been the protein-rich blue-green algae known as spirulina. But some historians think he was referring to the eggs of the *axayacatl*, a Nahuatl word that means "water-face" and describes the bulbous, transparent eyes of an insect known as the water boatman.

It turns out the real secret of Axayacatl—son of the first Montezuma, father of the second—was not his hidden troves of gold and silver. It was the fact that he was named after a bug. The same lowly insect that, along with a few other protein-rich aquatic resources in the Valley of Mexico, allowed an obscure tribe of nomads to rise to the hegemony of one of the most impressive civilizations the New World has ever seen.

From atop their warhorses, the treasure-obsessed Spaniards kept their gazes fixed on the pyramids. But one of the most astonishing things in this new land was right under their noses: a plant-eating insect of the *Corixidae* family, known for sculling along the surface of freshwater lakes with its oarlike legs and singing with its penis.

ON A TUESDAY MORNING—it happened to be five hundred years and one month to the day after Cortés and Montezuma's first meeting—I rode the metro to one of the southeastern barrios in Mexico City's historic center. The Mercado San Juan Pugibet is the direct inheritor of Tlatelolco. After the conquest, the great Aztec market was relocated to the barrio of San Juan Moyotlan, where its stalls eventually occupied the buildings of a nineteenth-century cigar factory. Pugibet is where Mexico City's top chefs now come to scare up a choice cut of acorn-fed ham from Spain, a jar of Argentinian chimichurri, or an unpasteurized Camembert from France.

It quickly became obvious to me that Pugibet also targeted tourists in search of the exotic. Menus and handwritten signs advertised grilled ostrich, crocodile, llama, zebra, and lion burgers. On a stool in one of the aisles, a slender biker with a well-trimmed gray beard froze for a selfie as he worked his way through a plate of deep-fried scorpions. Plaster statues of Jesus and Mary shared space on the walls with the taxidermied heads of deer and antelopes. At one stall, I sampled *cocopaches*, which live in mesquite trees and spit iodine when attacked; ground into a salsa with sesame seeds and dried cranberries, they had a smoky crunch that suggested mesquite-flavored potato chips. The biodiversity on offer, which surpassed what I've seen even in Cantonese wet markets, would have given the most unflappable of epidemiologists palpitations.

I stopped at El Gran Cazador, a stall notorious for retailing giraffe, antelope, and zebra. Alongside such ethically questionable big game, "The Great Hunter" sells prey at the other end of the terrestrial food chain. Behind the counter, a tour guide in a low-cut zebra-print blouse was handing out samples to a group of American tourists, conspicuous in this urban market for their beach-resort attire. "In Mexico, we've been eating insects for all our history," she said, as she offered a plastic scoop of *chicatanas*, the winged form of the leaf-cutter ant, to a young woman in cut-off jeans. "For Mexicans, the ant is just like an M&M—except it's got much more protein!"

Beneath the maw of a snarling stuffed lion, I talked to manager Pepe Díaz, who told me his mother had founded the business almost half a century earlier. He looked a little surprised when I asked him if he had any water boatman eggs for sale.

"Not many people are interested in *ahuautle* anymore," said Díaz. "The species has diminished a lot. The people who collect the eggs still come here, every once in a while, and when they do we'll buy twenty-five kilograms from them. The collectors aren't fishermen— they don't use boats—they wade in the water and gather the leaves they spread out on the lake so the *axayacatl* can lay its eggs. It's like fishing for leaves, instead of fish. Then they let the eggs dry on the shore." When I asked Díaz if he could put me in touch with his suppliers, he looked away. "I don't know their names. They come to the market during the rainy season. They live on Lake Texcoco." He suggested I try calling the State of Mexico's tourism department.

I'd been warned that the stallholders in the markets were unlikely to share their sources, particularly with a gringo they'd never seen before. At El Gran Cazador's tiny snack bar, I consoled myself with a bottle of beer and some *volcanes*, crisp corn tortillas curled at the edges, each covered with a layer of *chicatanas*, whose bulbous black bodies were blanketed in a layer of melted cheese. Their savory crunch, nicely complemented by the bite of Manchego, left a peppery aftertaste of formic acid on my tongue; it reminded me of the thrilling mouth-numbing tingle of tetrodotoxin, the residual poison in puffer fish I'd once tried at Tokyo's old Tsukiji Market. As I worked on my breakfast, I watched the tourists I'd seen earlier daring each other to eat chocolate-covered tarantulas between shots of tequila. My light meal cost over four times the price of a street vendor's tacos, and almost as much as the stall was charging for a plate of crocodile or ostrich meat.

The high price reflects the challenge of collecting edible insects, but also something more disturbing. Recent reports of a global "insect apocalypse," while exaggerated by the media—it's very difficult to drive any insect species to complete extinction—aren't without foundation. Bee colonies are indeed collapsing, monarch butterfly numbers are in freefall, and pesticides and herbicides have driven down many ant and grasshopper populations in North America and Europe. In many nations, bugs are seen as a form of bushmeat, and as their prestige and price rise, so does evidence of destructive overharvesting in the wild.

The edible insect whose abundance on Lake Texcoco had been responsible for the rise of the Aztec Empire, I was learning, was lately proving as hard to find as the lake itself.

WHEN HUMANS FIRST ARRIVED in what is now Mexico City, some time after the glaciers retreated at the end of the last ice age, they found the happiest of hunting grounds.

Three-quarters of the oval-shaped plateau, 7,500 feet above sea level, was occupied by a chain of salty and freshwater lakes. (Because it lacks any natural drainage, the "Valley" of Mexico is in reality a closed basin.) The shallow waters of the largest of them, the ancient Lake Texcoco, attracted wild boar, rabbits, deer, waterbirds, and such now-extinct species as mastodons, camelids, and giant sloths. Recent excavations have uncovered the world's largest known cache of mammoth bones, some of which show signs of being transformed into tools by human hands fifteen thousand years ago.

The fact that this immense watering hole was hemmed in by mountains made it easy for human hunters to ambush prehistoric megafauna with rocks and spears. Too easy, as it turned out: they drove archaic oxen, humpless camels, and a species of horse that had survived the Ice Age to extinction. In so doing, they also wiped out animals that could have become beasts of burden or livestock, and provided manure to fertilize agricultural land.

The lack of large domesticated herbivores (apart from llamas and alpacas in the Andean empire of the Incas) put the Indigenous Peoples of the Americas at a fatal disadvantage when invaders from overseas arrived. Since the days of Çatalhöyük, the people of the Old World had been living alongside their cows, sheep, horses, pigs, and goats, being sickened by, and adapting to, zoonotic microbes. As bearers of the pathogens for influenza, smallpox, measles, yellow fever, cholera, and malaria—diseases unknown in the western hemisphere before 1492—the filthy, bearded invaders initiated a hecatomb.

In only a century after Cortés's arrival, the Indigenous population of the Valley of Mexico was reduced from well over a million to a mere seventy thousand—and this was just one of the episodes in the microbial genocide that would kill 90 percent of the Indigenous Peoples of the Americas in a little over three generations. Observing the effect of smallpox on the Aztecs, a Franciscan monk wrote, "They died in heaps, like bedbugs."

Bugs, as it happened, were on my mind as I walked out of the Chapultepec metro station. Signs all over the platforms bore the silhouette of a giant *chapulín de milpa*, or cornfield grasshopper. Three stations on the metro system's map, I'd noticed, were represented by stylized insects. In Nahuatl, the language of the Aztecs, Chapultepec means the "hill of grasshoppers." It is now the city's largest park, and walking along the tree-shaded Paseo de la Reforma took me past rows of monumental stone statues of big-eyed *chapulines*.

When the Aztecs arrived in the basin, after journeying from their northern homeland of Aztlán, Chapultepec was a bug-infested patch of wooded high ground west of Lake Texcoco. It was here that they were allowed to settle in 1280, in an area where all the good lakefront property had already been spoken for. They offered themselves as mercenaries to the Tepanecas, the strongest of the area's tribes. By 1325, they had taken possession of one of the lake's uninhabited islands—guided, it was said, by an eagle atop a prickly pear cactus devouring a serpent, an image now found on the Mexican flag—which they called Tenochtitlán. It took the Aztecs a little over a century to transition from scorned outsiders to absolute rulers of the basin. As leaders of the Triple Alliance of Tenochtitlán, Texcoco, and Tlacopan, they established an empire that stretched from the Atlantic to the Pacific.

It's a story well told in the Museo Nacional de Antropología, at the north end of Chapultepec. Sprawling buildings of rainwater-stained concrete, in a style that might be described as midcentury Aztec brutalist, convey some of the horror and wonder that was Tenochtitlán. In the hall devoted to the Aztecs, I circumambulated a room-sized model of the temples and palaces in the sacred heart of the city, and gazed at a twenty-seven-ton disc of basalt carved with images of vultures, lizards, and death's heads, which was discovered buried beneath the paving stones of the Zócalo, Mexico City's main plaza. The Aztec Sun Stone is not a calendar, as scholars once believed, but a temalacatl, a sacrificial altar for gladiators. In the center of the monolith, a knife-tongued monster holds forth human hearts in outstretched hands.

The Aztec elite, some anthropologists argue, were a parasitic class on long-established communities of farmers, hunters, and fisherpeople, who lived in egalitarian settlements, much like the inhabitants of Neolithic Çatalhöyük. Geneticists have found evidence that, as early as nine thousand years ago, people in the highlands of southwest Mexico were selecting the most promising stalks of a scrawny wild grass known as teosinte,* which they eventually domesticated into plump ears of corn (known outside the Americas as maize). Easier to cultivate than wheat or rice, corn grew quickly, typically requiring only fifty days of labor a year to bring to harvest. Farmers used an alkaline bath of limewater or wood ash to remove the thin, translucent skins of the kernels. Nixtamalization, as the process is known, made niacin and essential amino acids more bioavailable, turning corn gruel and tortillas into something truly nutritious.

Cornstalks could also be intercropped with, or grown between, rows of squash and beans, a practice that continually replenishes the soil's nitrogen. Such fields, still common in highland areas, are known as milpas. ("Three Sisters" farming, in which climbing beans are allowed to twine around cornstalks planted in piled soil, with squash planted between the mounds, spread as far north as modern-day Quebec and Ontario, where it's still practiced in traditionally Iroquoian-speaking Nations.) Unlike fields of wheat and other Old World cereals, milpas don't have to go through fallow seasons to restore their fertility. Up to a dozen crops, including chiles, avocados, tomatoes, and melons, are typically grown at once. While industrial

---

* Teosinte is so scrawny that an entire ear has as much nutritional value as a single kernel of corn, which has led some biologists to argue that corn couldn't have been its direct descendant. Instead they propose that corn was a hybrid of two other grasses.

agriculture can degrade topsoil in a matter of decades, some milpas have been continuously farmed for four millennia.

The seasonal camps that hunter-gatherers established in such fertile zones as Oaxaca and the Valley of Mexico, initially to harvest wild grains, became the year-round settlements of sedentary farmers. Corn in the Valley of Mexico, like wheat and barley in the Fertile Crescent, brought food surpluses, booms in population, and cities. An hour's drive northeast of Mexico City, the spectacular, flat-topped pyramids of Teotihuacán, which predated the Aztec pyramids of Tenochtitlán by 1,100 years, rise out of the basin's floor. At its height, the city, whose existence overlapped with imperial Rome, had 100,000 inhabitants. Some scholars believe that, early in its history, this cosmopolitan urban republic rejected rule from the top, turning away from the era of pyramid-building and human sacrifice. The Teotihuacános instead set about building two thousand rectangular, single-story multifamily apartment complexes, which were all about the same size. Ecological factors may have led to the city's collapse. Forests on the surrounding hills had been cut down to make way for farmland; shorn of their trees, the hills no longer absorbed the rain that fed the underground springs that allowed corn to grow.

The successors of the Teotihuacános were the Toltec people, whose two-century reign came to a similar end: droughts and frosts led to a failure of the corn crop, leaving the state susceptible to raids. The Aztec adventurers who arrived from the north set about occupying the ruins of the Teotihuacános and the Toltecs, like Ostrogoths among the crumbling monuments of a fallen Rome. It was the misfortune of the farmers of the Valley of Mexico to come under the domination of the Aztecs, a tribe whose long ordeal had left them quick to resort to force.

"The fifteenth century in Mexico was an age of competition for shrinking resources," author Ronald Wright argues in *Stolen Continents*. Human sacrifice was "not the persistence of an old 'savage' practice among civilized people who should have known better but rather a hypertrophy of sinister elements in their culture, which in more gracious times would have been kept in check."

That's not to minimize some of the darker aspects of Aztec culture, whose gastronomic traditions stretched to cannibalism. Today's pozole, that savory stew of hominy, chile peppers, and pork, may have originally been made with chunks of human flesh. This was probably an elite practice rather than a matter of necessity. Despite the lack of livestock, Tenochtitlán was amply supplied with protein. From the moment the Aztecs took possession of their island home in Lake Texcoco, they made the most of its aquatic resources.

Farmers boosted the productivity of the basin's lakes by driving stakes into the lake bottoms, weaving them together with reeds, and piling them with aquatic vegetation and soil gathered from higher ground. Seedlings germinated on land were planted on these artificial islands, with the capillary action of the roots providing all the necessary irrigation. The practice of fertilizing the fields with human manure solved the city's potentially crippling waste disposal problems.

The conquistadors believed these chinampas, as they are known, were floating gardens, which farmers paddled to market. In reality, the Aztecs had turned their island headquarters into a spider's web of fields, separated by dirt paths, irrigation ditches, and canals filled with canoes and barges. About 25,000 acres, an area twice the size of Manhattan, were under constant cultivation. It is estimated that, at the time of contact, the chinampa system provided two-thirds of the caloric needs of the population of the Valley of Mexico, which was home to as many as 1.2 million people. Modern megacities survive by exploiting distant farmlands. The Aztecs had solved the problem that had led to Teotihuacán's collapse by turning their imperial capital into a massive, self-sustaining urban farm.

Back in the museum's Aztec hall, I was drawn to the display cases filled with the mundane artifacts of everyday life: a communal bowl, shaped like a rabbit, for sharing pulque, the pleasantly intoxicating fermented sap of the cactus-like maguey plant; tiny figurines, carved from clay, shell, and jade, of the frogs, turtles, and other aquatic animals that inhabited Lake Texcoco; and countless images and sculptures of *chapulines*, ants, and even fleas.

Like a gringo Gulliver, I peered through glass at a detailed diorama of the teeming market of Tlatelolco, a sprawling rectangular plaza filled with the Lilliputian buyers and sellers of turkeys and caged dogs, silver and gold jewelry, serpents and cacti. It was a reminder that the real wealth of the Valley of Mexico—the reason Mexico City was here at all—had always been the land, water, and plant and animal life whose diversity had allowed its human population to multiply and thrive.

THOUGH THE CHINAMPAS HAVE SHRUNK to a quarter of their former acreage, they are still under cultivation a dozen miles south of the Zócalo. Early one afternoon, I jumped onto the deck of one of the hundreds of wooden canal boats moored side by side on the wharves of the neighborhood known as Xochimilco. These *trajineras* serve as moving party platforms for people celebrating weddings or birthdays with leisurely, and usually drunken, weekend cruises. Painted bright yellow and orange, my *trajinera* bore the name *Conchita* in block capitals on its sun canopy. After inviting me to take a seat on one of fourteen wooden-and-wicker chairs, my *ramero*, a teenager in tight jeans named Dylan, set me up with a beer. ("My mother," he explained, "was a big Bob Dylan fan.")

"Déjame pasar!" cried Dylan from the rear deck as he shouldered *Conchita* through a logjam of haphazardly moored boats. Leaning diagonally into his punting pole, he propelled us beneath a footbridge decorated with murals of bleeding hearts and sombrero-wearing death's heads. It was a sunny Sunday, and the canal was a slow-moving highway of fully loaded, fiesta-hued *trajineras*, trailed by smaller boats loaded with mariachi musicians and tamale vendors jostling for pesos.

On either side of us were the chinampas, raised platforms of soil, some occupied by run-down shacks, others with picnic-table-filled cantinas, still others with gardens for ornamental flowers, carnivorous plants, and chile peppers. Banners invited punters to come ashore to look at aquaria full of baby alligators and specimens of the axolotl, the endearing, feathery-eared salamander that has become an unofficial mascot of Mexico City.

In spite of their touristy toppings, the chinampas were built the same way they had been for thousands of years. Branches and logs protruded from the water's surface, forming the supports for solid underwater fences that surrounded and retained the soil atop each plot. The corners, I noticed, were secured with slender willows, whose branches seemed to grow straight up.

"They're called *ahuejotes*," said Dylan. "Their branches don't stick out, so they don't make as many shadows. You can grow more food that way."

Dylan directed us into one of the quieter side canals, where chickens and pigs roamed free on miniature islands that bristled with tomatoes, spinach, lettuce, chiles, and radishes. The self-irrigating chinampas are impressively productive: each plot can yield a half dozen or more harvests a year. They also bring down the air temperature during heat waves, boost biodiversity by attracting birds and insects, and serve as carbon sinks while their root systems filter and clean water. The potential for chinampas to provide fresh produce to the world's megacities is enormous, and experiments with such raised-field systems, as they're known, are being carried out in Bangladesh, Bali, Indonesia, and Poland.

Yet it's something of a miracle that there are still any chinampas left at all. The drying up of the basin's water bodies accelerated when the Aztecs built a nine-mile-long dike that cut Lake Texcoco in two. The barrier prevented floods and kept salty water from reaching the chinampas, but it also subdivided the original lakes, hastening evaporation and further reducing their surface area. When the Spaniards raised a new capital on the ruins of Tenochtitlán, they completed the deforestation of the surrounding mountainsides. The massive tunnels they dug to channel away excess rainwater failed to stem flooding, which caused repeated outbreaks of cholera and typhoid.

The cattle, goats, and sheep brought from Europe were allowed to wander free, fattening themselves on Indigenous farmers' fields. What native vegetation remained was ground between their flat teeth, preventing regrowth of shrubs and trees, which encouraged erosion and further flooding. The Spanish conquerors changed Mexico City from a city built *within* a lake to a city built *on top* of a lake, with consequences that persist to this day. Much of the city's water now has to be drawn from deep aquifers, a process that undermines the clay, gravel, and sand on which its foundations are built. In some places, the city is being swallowed into the earth at the rate of eight inches a year; dramatic evidence of this subsidence can be seen in the cracked and listing facade of the Zócalo's sixteenth-century cathedral.

As Dylan turned *Conchita* back toward the dock, he cursed the water plants—buoyed to the surface by tomatillo-like bulbs—whose thick fronds curled around his bamboo punt. *"Lirio acúatico,"* he growled. "It makes life hard for a *ramero*." Water hyacinth, an invasive species that chokes out native plants, is just one of the problems plaguing the canals of Xochimilco. By the middle of the last century, they had run completely dry. The opaque water we were gliding through was supplied by a nearby sewage treatment plant, and local residents used the canals as cesspools. In the 1970s, the federal government began to stock the canals with carp and tilapia. These voracious bottom-feeders thrived on the local vegetation, but they also gobbled up the eggs of the critically threatened axolotl. At one time, there were as many as fifteen thousand axolotls per square mile; now there may be as few as seven hundred left in the wild. Axolotls are trapped for research purposes: the tiny amphibian boasts the largest genome of any animal and is being studied for its ability to regenerate lost limbs, heart tissue, and even parts of its brain.

Laconically, Dylan added, "I tried axolotl once, when I was a kid. We fried it like a fish fillet. It tasted a bit like salmon."

The Aztecs believed the axolotl was the mischievous brother of the god Quetzalcóatl, but, oddly enough, that didn't stop them from eating it either. When they arrived on their island home, they had survived by fishing and hunting waterfowl, turtles, and snakes. One of their best sources of nutrients was a quinoa-like plant called amaranth, whose leaves are full of vitamins and whose seeds can be ground into a flour that provides all the essential amino acids.

Amaranth seeds are almost exactly the same size and color as the eggs of the water boatman. In Nahuatl, the word *ahuautle* means "amaranth of the water." The Aztecs are said to have harvested 3,900 tons a year; special runners were employed to fetch fresh eggs from the lakeshores in time for Montezuma's breakfast. As late as the end of the nineteenth century, it's estimated that 3.6 trillion water boatmen could be found gliding over the surface of Lake Texcoco. Their eggs, which are 57 percent protein, are good sources of iron and vitamin B. Together with amaranth, spirulina, fish, and waterfowl, they likely provided the Aztecs with all the protein they needed when they arrived in the Valley of Mexico. One of the greatest warrior cultures of the New World, in other words, was nourished by bugs.

Back on the dock, as I settled the bill for my excursion and beer, I asked Dylan if he'd ever seen people skimming the waters of Xochimilco for *ahuautle*, or heard the adult insects' mating call.

He shook his head, a little sadly. "No, I think there is too much pollution for anything like that to survive here."

I WAS BEGINNING TO DESPAIR. In modern Mexico City, *ahuautle* was nowhere to be found. The lakes that had served as the water boatmen's habitat seemed to have been fouled by pollutants, lost to evaporation, or covered with asphalt.

I'd had some luck in a little restaurant near Pugibet Market, where I'd found the adult insects on the menu. Shorn of its oar-like legs, each *axayacatl* was the size of a large caraway seed; close-up, they looked like tiny brown torpedoes with big black eyes.* I spooned a few dozen over two slices of avocado on a soft corn tortilla and topped them with a dollop of *salsa roja*. The cook said they reminded him of *charales*, small freshwater fish traditionally served dried and cooked into *tortitas*. They tasted a little like cooked crabmeat, but left me with a dry mouth, a scratchy throat, and an unsatisfied belly. If this was what a boatman-infested quesadilla was supposed to taste like, I'd take roasted grasshoppers as a filling every time.

I rode the metro to Pino Suárez Station, where commuters rushed past the glassed-in foundations of a small circular Aztec temple, believed by some to be the spot where Montezuma first met Cortés. A short walk along the cobbled Calle Regina led me to the tangerine-toned facade of the Restaurante Bar Chon. Within, the gaudy decor suggested the quinceañera party of a natural-history-obsessed teenager. A table near the entrance had been set with small statues of an eagle, an armadillo, and a leopard; handwritten posters extolled the medicinal virtues of pulque; and wall murals depicted scenes of life in ancient Tenochtitlán. I flipped through an encyclopedic menu that listed iguana, wild boar, frogs' legs, rattlesnake, crocodile steak with rice, armadillo in mango sauce, and *rata de campo*, until I came to a page labeled "*Entradas Prehispánicas.*" I'd finally found it: *ahuautle*. A trio of *tortitas*, topped with a choice of *salsa verde* or *mole poblano*, would set me back 160 pesos.

As I sipped from a stein of honey-sweetened pulque, a waiter offered to give me a quick look at the kitchen. Behind a swinging door, a stocky gray-haired man with a wispy moustache in a stained

---

* I couldn't make out the penis, which the water boatman rubs against the ridged surface of its abdomen to make its piercing mating call. Some members of the *Corixidae* family have been recorded at 99.2 decibels—the equivalent of standing fifteen yards from a passing freight train—which makes these water striders the loudest animals relative to their size known to science.

T-shirt was sitting on a stool next to a stainless-steel grill, atop which three circular grayish-brown patties were being heated. The *tortitas* arrived at my table shortly thereafter. I took a bite: greenish inside, the savory pancake, given bite by serrano peppers, was slightly crunchy, as though the batter had been mixed with marshy-tasting poppy seeds. An interesting texture, certainly, but I wasn't sure *ahuautle*, at least the way it was prepared at Chon, merited the name "Mexican caviar."

As I was finishing, the man I'd seen on the stool—"Don" Chon himself—emerged from the kitchen. While I'd been eating, Fortino Rojas had put on chef's whites and a cylindrical toque with a small Mexican flag sewn over the rim. I invited him to sit down, and he told me his life story. Rojas had come to Mexico City from Puebla in 1947 and, at the age of four, started selling tomatoes in the local streets. He began to work as a dishwasher at the restaurant, which had been catering to local workers since 1924, and was known as "Chon" after the original chef. When Mexico City's new wholesale market, the Centro de Abastos, opened, business dropped off, and the restaurant added exotic foods to the menu in an effort to attract clients from all over the city.

"Everything that crawls, walks, or flies," Rojas told me, "goes into the pan. I've cooked lion, elephant, scorpion, monkey, boa constrictor." He explained that his predecessor, Chon, had a special interest in Aztec cuisine. When Rojas took over, he went on to master the art of cooking with insects.

He told me how he made the *tortitas*: "You heat the mosquito eggs slightly over a comal, putting them on some paper, because they are very delicate. Then you take finely chopped onions, cilantro, and add them to the toasted *ahuautle*. You add a spoonful of flour, and then eggs. Before, we used duck eggs, because you could find ducks in nearby lagoons, but now we use chicken eggs. A little vegetable oil, then you spoon the *tortita* onto the grill. They're done in a couple of minutes." The taste, he said, reminded him of powdered shrimp. "It's crunchy, rich, unique. Also very nutritious, full of fats, protein, and phosphorous. Eating a *tortita* is like taking a multivitamin!"

When Rojas was younger, peasant women would gather eggs from the ponds and lagoons then found in the streets around the restaurant. "There were peddlers who would walk around shouting, '*¿Compran ahuautle?*' You could buy a kilogram for twenty centavos." Today, he said, a single kilogram can cost a thousand pesos at Pugibet Market. "It's getting harder to find the environment that nourishes the *ahuautle*. All the little lakes and ponds have evaporated." I asked him if pollution was a problem. "The real problem is *man*. Man has overexploited it. The harvesters today are very voracious. They take the *ahuautle* before the season starts, and after it ends."

Rojas told me he bought his *ahuautle* at La Merced. "But the woman I get it from will never tell you who she buys it from. Otherwise you could bypass her and buy directly from the collectors. You can try to ask her, though. Go to door number two, in the section where they sell nopales."

The following morning I plunged into the labyrinth of La Merced, the capital's largest retail market. There are four thousand stalls in the Nave Mayor—just one of the market's eight buildings—but Rojas had told me to go to the receiving area, where corn is husked and spines are removed from the paddles of prickly pear cacti. There, at stall eighty-two, I found Hilda Bardines, standing behind a glistening white pyramid of tangled chicken intestines and piles of well-blackened fish tamales. Chubby-cheeked and amiable, Bardines handed me free samples—of *acociles*, tiny river shrimp that turn maraschino-red when boiled, and of *chicatanas*, flying ants—while showing me her selection of scorpions, Madagascar cockroaches, and *cocopaches*.

Bardines also stocked *ahuautle*. She filled a sardine can to overflowing with the eggs, which she then transferred to a plastic bag. I paid her 180 pesos for a quarter of a kilogram. The eggs were black and white, midway between the size of ground pepper and poppy seeds.

When I asked if she could introduce me to her supplier, though, her smile disappeared.

"He only comes once a year, from Texcoco. People don't consume it a lot, so the batch he brings me might last a whole year. I never ask him for his name, Señor." By then, Bardines was looking away, trying to catch the eye of another paying customer—presumably one who wouldn't ask so many questions.

As I carried my plastic bag of insect eggs back to the metro, I had mixed feelings. I'd managed to track down the legendary *ahuautle*. But I was still no closer to the shores of Texcoco, a lake whose existence I was beginning to doubt.

THE SOURCE OF *AHUAUTLE* was proving elusive, but my dining experiences were showing me that edible insects were still part of the nation's gastronomy. Shortly after the Conquest, Franciscan friar Bernardino de Sahagún put together an encyclopedia of Aztec culture, compiled with the help of Nahuatl-speaking informants; in it, he cataloged ninety-six kinds of insects used as food. All continue to be consumed in some part of Mexico, and many are still fixtures on the capital's menus.

One afternoon I stopped at El Cardenal, a half-century-old restaurant that occupies three floors of a Parisian-style townhouse near the Zócalo. I watched with trepidation as a frock-coated waiter set down a stack of handmade corn tortillas and my order: a clay casserole dish of segmented white worms, the kind you find sloshing around the bottom of a bottle of mezcal. Each was as large as the pinky finger of a well-fed toddler.

A *champoloco*, or maguey worm, is actually a caterpillar, the larva of a butterfly—the tequila giant skipper—that feeds on the stems and roots of the agave or maguey plant. In half a year, a single agave can produce 250 gallons of the sap known as aguamiel—"honey water"— which is then fermented into pulque or distilled into mezcal. Rather than resorting to pesticides, farmers have turned the pests into a bonus crop, and a profitable one at that. At El Cardenal, an order of *champolocos* fried in vegetable oil cost 380 pesos, over twice as much as the next most expensive appetizer on the menu.

They were also, I was happy to discover after rolling a half dozen into a guacamole-smeared tortilla, delicious. Because of their high volume-to-surface-area ratio, many insects are excellent candidates for the Maillard reaction—the browning that occurs when free sugar molecules and amino acids combine at high heat—sought after by cooks when they baste a rotisserie chicken or sear a steak. Between the teeth, the *champolocos*' silky skin yielded a burst of beefy nutti-ness, as if each caterpillar were a tiny well-browned sausage stuffed with almond butter.

The rise of bugs to star billing on the menus of Mexico City's white-tablecloth restaurants turns out to be a recent phenomenon. Entomophagy, it's true, goes deep into Mexico's prehistory; archae-ologists have analyzed coprolites—fossilized feces—and found evidence that people here were supplementing their diets with a sub-stantial input of insect protein 8,700 years ago. But by the twentieth century, many in the Mexican middle and upper classes had come to see bug-eating as backward-looking. In recent decades, reclaiming pre-Hispanic roots has become a matter of pride: pulque bars, once reviled as sawdust-floored dives, now cater to the hipsters of Roma Norte and La Condesa, and the capital's top chefs pride themselves on serving edible insects.

On the second-floor terrace of Azul, a restaurant in La Condesa, I ordered *escamoles*, a dish that vies with *ahuautle* for the title of the "caviar of Mexico." The chef, Ricardo Muñoz Zurita, is the author of Larousse's encyclopedia of Mexican cuisine. He plated the *escamoles* in a casserole dish, alongside a wooden spoon for transferring them to corn tortillas that had been imprinted with images of eagles, cacti, and other Aztec motifs. Lightly sautéed in butter with finely chopped onions, green serrano chiles, and epazote—a herb that straddles a fine olfactory line between sage and turpentine—each glistening beige *escamol* resembled a dimpled pearl. A mouthful made me feel like tiny well-larded baked beans with delicate skins were gamboling over my tongue.

Escamoles are the eggs of a species of leaf-cutter ant, *Liometopum apiculatum*. The 3.5-ounce appetizer at Azul cost 325 pesos, a price that reflects their scarcity and the challenges of harvesting them. Each *escamol* has the potential to develop into a queen, capable of founding her own colony. Competition to supply Mexico City's restaurants has led to destructive overharvesting.

"The problem with *escamoles*," José Carlos Redon told me, "is the black market. The prices are so high that people gather them before enough ants have reached adulthood. They don't think about the fact that the population has been decreasing for the last few years."

I'd met Redon in the office of his delicatessen, Camilla, which specializes in traditional foods and liquors from the state of Hidalgo. His mother's family still owns a farm-estate in the Valle de Mezquital ("Valley of Mesquite Trees"), just north of Mexico City.

"We have this little patch of land," said Redon, "less than an acre, which is basically useless for farming. It's semidesert, kind of like the outback in Australia: everything there has spikes or can bite you. But for collecting insects, it's great." After training as a chef in Australia, Italy, and the United States, Redon returned to Mexico to set up one of the capital's first food trucks, where he topped *sopes*, soft circles of fried corn dough with pinched-up sides, with insects from the family's property, including *cocopaches* plucked from mesquite trees. "Younger people weren't that attracted to the insects. But the older generations, you didn't have to convince them. They knew we were selling them cheaper than any restaurant." Though he no longer runs the food truck, his family still lets villagers harvest insects on their property.

"If you do it the pre-Hispanic way," continued Redon, "it's sustainable. The harvesters leave their home at five in the morning, walk seven miles, following marks on different plants that lead them to

the nest. There's no water, no shelter; it's a very hot area. The ants
live in the ground, usually next to maguey plants. Then they have to
open the nest carefully to get to the larvae, without damaging it, or
killing the plants." For every one hundred larvae a queen ant lays, only
one will become a princess. "After it rains, the soil gets softer, and the
princesses hatch. They fly up into the air, and then lose their wings.
Where they drop to earth is where they start a new colony." Each
colony works on the principle of a dairy farm: leaf-cutter ants "milk"
aphids, which excrete a kind of royal jelly they use to nourish the
queen. If the colony is attacked or damaged, the workers actually pick
up the aphids, along with the eggs, and move them to a safer location.

"You can only take a certain percentage of the eggs, though, or the
population goes into decline." Redon said his family has been trying
to boost awareness of the issue in the communities surrounding their
property, but the demand from restaurants has encouraged amateur
poachers. "For local people, *escamoles* can be a big part of their annual
income." A nest can be harvested three times a year and continue
producing larvae for up to forty years. Destructive poaching, though,
can destroy a fifty-thousand-member colony in a single afternoon.

Redon is a founding member of the Mexican branch of Slow Food,
and has traveled the world with the team from the Future Consumer
Lab, cofounded by René Redzepi, the chef at Copenhagen's Noma,
advocating for eating insects.

"A lot of chefs have realized that insects add these peculiar, exclusive flavors. But if we only take insects from specific areas of the
world, like Mexico, we're going to have a shortage. And if we bring
it up to an industrial level, we begin to destroy ecosystems." Many
edible insects in Mexico have become unaffordable to those people—
most of them Indigenous—who traditionally benefited from them.

I figured Mexican chefs were doing well to elevate insects, once
maligned by middle-class diners, into the choicest items on the
menu. I realized I'd gone beyond simply overcoming my disgust long
enough to choke down a few roasted crickets. *Escamoles* and maguey

worms had awakened a craving, and I was curious to discover what else was out there.

It's unfortunate that the most delicious, wild-caught bugs tended to be the ones most vulnerable to overharvesting. Redon agreed this was a problem, but added it wouldn't stop him from encouraging visitors—gringos like me—from sampling ant eggs and *ahuautle*. These were the gateway bugs, the indulgences that could encourage people to look at sustainably harvested and farmed species as food to be enjoyed rather than pests to be exterminated.

"Don't be scared," he advised, with a smile. "Eat more bugs. If you don't like them, that's fine. But you have to try." I told him that when I got home, that was exactly the approach I was going to take with my son Desmond.

ACCORDING TO THE CITY MAPS, there is still a place called Texcoco, so I decided to go there myself to see what was left of the vast lake that had once been the heart of Tenochtitlán. Redon remembered buying olive oil from a woman who also sold *ahuautle*, which he thought she'd harvested herself. He thought she lived close to the shores of Lake Texcoco. Using Facebook, I made an appointment to come by Kasbah, in the rough-and-tumble neighborhood of Chimalhuacán.

I took a long taxi ride, along traffic-choked roads that followed the course of ancient canals that had once been filled with Aztec canoes and barges, to the eastern part of the State of Mexico. Samuel Buendía Peralta was waiting for me in a hole-in-the-wall shop that retailed the products of his family's business: plastic jars of table olives, bottles of olive oil and red wine, tamales stuffed with green olives, and soap and hand cream made with olive leaves. He led me up a narrow lane to the family home, whose garden was an agreeable jumble of carboys for oil and wine and bonsai-like olive tree saplings. Samuel introduced me to his father, Rosario Buendía, who invited me into an open-sided workshop area on the house's ground floor, which was partly occupied by a boulder projecting from the hillside.

A table had been set for a light morning meal: olive paste spiced with za'atar, green and black table olives, pita bread, and a bottle of sweet red wine, made from the family's own grapes.

The table olives we were snacking on were from 450-year-old trees, which may have been among the first to be planted in Mexico, if not North America. Rosario pointed out that the road my driver had taken to get to Chimalhuacán was once the causeway the conquistadors had taken on their march into Tenochtitlán. In the sixteenth century, Franciscan monks from Spain had planted olive groves along the ancient Aztec road. There were over a thousand trees in the area—Rosario and his family had planted a hundred of their own—and the oldest still yielded rich harvests of Empeltre, Mission, and a large, meaty cultivar called Sevillana. The family paid local landowners to allow them to gather olives from their trees and press them into oil, which was snatched up by Mexico City's Lebanese and Palestinian communities.

As we talked, Rosario's wife, who had been making food in the kitchen, brought us a plate of *tortitas*, similar to the ones I'd had at Chon. I used a spoon to cut off a piece, and the marshy taste and crunchy texture were unmistakable: we were eating *ahuautle*, traditionally and expertly prepared.

Margarita Peralta Gonzalez removed her apron and joined us at the table. "My grandfather, on my mother's side, made his living off Lake Texcoco. And before that, my great-grandfather. They would fish the mosquito, and its eggs, off the surface of the lake. They called the mosquito *requeson*. They would ship it to Veracruz, and the Europeans would buy it." The dried adult water boatmen went to make food for pet fish and birds in Europe. She remembered her father going down to the lake to hunt ducks and gather *ahuautle*. "He would take leaves from the *tule* plant [a species of sedge] off the surface of the lake and shake them, and the eggs would fall off." The eggs had to be harvested while they were still fatty enough to form into *tortitas* but before they hatched, typically twenty-two days after being laid. The trade in water boatmen, she said, had made the Gonzalez family one of the two or three richest in Chimalhuacán.

"But nobody makes a living off *ahuautle* these days. A few people still gather it, sporadically. The tradition has gone, because the lake is shrinking." She pointed down the hill. "Before, the waters of the lake would have come all the way up to the foot of this mountain. But there's no free access anymore. It's surrounded by a fence." A few locals gathered the eggs from small ponds that formed on parts of the former lake bed during the rainy season, from June to September; that's where Margarita had gotten the *ahuautle* for our *tortitas*. This time of year, she told me, I wouldn't find anyone gathering eggs.

I looked back down the hillside, in the direction of the family's olive-oil shop. Over the rooftops of single-story homes and shops, I could make out the bluish smudge of a stretch of shorefront, two and a half miles distant. This was Lake Nabor Carrillo, a nine-hundred-acre reservoir, which, because it's at the lowest point of the basin, receives much of the city's wastewater. This, then, was all that remained of the mighty Lake Texcoco. Its waters, which drew the first hunters to the Valley of Mexico and nourished the Aztecs, are the only reason there is a city here at all. And it is the management of these life-giving lakes, rivers, and aquifers that will determine whether Mexico City will have a future to look forward to.

It was a melancholy realization, but I had to remind myself that the Aztecs themselves had never really disappeared. In Mexico, first meeting point of the Old and New Worlds, the sophistication and vigor of Indigenous society had permanently transformed the invaders, in a way that didn't happen in New France, colonial America, or Patagonia. Far from wiping out Aztec culture, the conquistadors themselves had been conquered by it; their genes, languages, cuisines, and worldviews had mingled, producing a *mestizo* nation unique in the world. *Cem Anahuac*, the one world of the Aztecs, was all around me: in the bold colors of graffitied murals on barrio walls; in the words used by the 1.7 million people in central Mexico who still identify Nahuatl as their main language; in the cantinas where gluey pulque is sipped from clay bowls; in the profiles of the vendors in the *tianguis* and on street corners; and in the chinampas that continue to nourish the residents of the megacity.

Which was why the *almuerzo* prepared for me by Margarita and her family was unmistakably Mexican. Five hundred years after the first meeting of the Spanish and the Aztecs, olives, tapenade, and red wine, a meal that Cortés would have relished, could still share the same table with pre-Hispanic *ahuautle*—a delicacy fit for Montezuma.

A FEW DAYS LATER, as I left Mexico City, I understood why my quest to reach the shores of Texcoco had failed. My flight path home happened to take me back over Chimalhuacán. The white roofs of the megacity stopped abruptly at the Circuito Exterior, a city-girdling highway. Beyond that, the former lake bed was parched, white, and barren; the runways for the aborted international airport were clearly sketched out over the salt flats. There was no Lake Texcoco left to see. The only standing water was in the rectangular, man-made reservoirs that received the capital's treated sewage. It was not an attractive sight.

It turns out that Ehrlich had been wrong when he predicted that the teeming cities of the twenty-first century would doom our species to famine and extinction. When *The Population Bomb* was published, Mexico's fertility rate was 5.3 children per woman. Today it has reached 2.1, replacement level, a decline largely driven by urbanization. Women who move from rural areas to cities, where education and contraception are more readily available, almost always have smaller families. On bad days, when the air is caustic with pollution and the smell of sewage, Mexico City can suggest an urban hellscape. But as it grows, the rate of population growth is slowing—a process that could eventually reduce the impact of human numbers on the environment. Mesoamerican history may be marked by tales of civilizational collapse, but out of catastrophe came the stores of human ingenuity that created the milpas and the chinampas and found a way to skim sustenance off the surface of shallow waters.

I saw that a word had been inscribed, in huge white letters, on the top of a hill: "*PROMESAS*." I chose to read it as a message, one that hinted at the bitterness of promises unkept but also looked to the promises, and challenges, of the future. Part of me relished the ambiguity.

As for myself, I was leaving Mexico with a suitcase full of *chicatanas*, *ahuautle*, *chapulines*, and other tasty creepy-crawlies. (I hasten to add, should any customs agents be reading these words, that this is a work of creative nonfiction.) At home, I'd be facing a challenge of my own: convincing my children that insects, far from being disgusting, are a plausible source of nutrition for the future.

3

OSSABAW ISLAND
Some Pig

I WAS WALKING DOWN CANE PATCH ROAD, senses alert for my prey, when I began to get the feeling something was tracking me. For the second time, there was a dry rustling in the tangles of fallen palm fronds alongside the dirt road. Yet when I stilled my footfalls, all I could hear was the whistling of the wind tousling the dreadlocks of the cabbage palms. Then I saw the fan of a saw palmetto a few steps from me twitch. Suddenly I was all attention: something deep in the reptilian core of my brain had been activated. The maritime forest, bewitching at first, had turned spooky and menacing.

I'd come to this uninhabited island off the coast of Georgia with a couple of dozen other day-trippers. It was a rare opportunity to set foot on Ossabaw, which is unlinked to the mainland by any causeway or public ferry. This semitropical island is overseen by a founda-tion that allows a limited number of visitors a year. As the *Island Explorer* left the dock at Butternut Beach, a twenty-minute drive south of Savannah, we were escorted down the Moon River—the one immortalized in the song by Johnny Mercer, a native son—by an honor guard of dolphins. In the channel of the Little Ogeechee River, we motored past osprey nests and blue herons wading for frogs. But when we approached the island's lone dock, Captain Bob gave us some bad news. A big blow was expected in off the Atlantic that afternoon, and we'd have to head back earlier than planned.

We moored alongside a motor launch that had overtaken us as we crossed Ossabaw Sound. Its occupants had already hopped in the back of a pickup truck, which jounced down a dirt road bordered by palms. The foundation's tour guide, Robin Gunn, had told us over the PA that today happened to be the memorial service for Eleanor "Sandy" Torrey West; her friends and loved ones were gathering in her former home, a pink stucco Spanish revival mansion where Sandy had lived for almost a century.

Sandy's family had acquired the island in 1924. It was a time when industrialists from the north paid bargain-basement prices for Georgia's barrier islands, the chain of fourteen marshy, low-lying islands that buffer the mainland from storms. Howard Earle Coffin (Hudson Motors) purchased most of neighboring St. Catherines Island; R. J. Reynolds, Jr. (Pall Mall, Lucky Strike, Camel) got all of Sapelo; the Carnegies (U.S. Steel) built a castle on Cumberland; and Nell Torrey (heiress to the Pittsburgh Plate Glass Co.) bought Ossabaw—all forty square miles of it—for $150,000. After Nell died in 1959, making her daughter the sole owner of an island larger than Bermuda, Sandy married an oil painter and set about happily dilapidating the family fortune. For two decades she bankrolled the Genesis Project, inviting geologists, writers, astronomers, composers, and ecologists to reside in her sixteen-bedroom mansion, stroll on Ossabaw's beaches, and reimagine the world. When the money ran out, she sold the island to Georgia for half its assessed value, on the condition that it be left in a state of nature. Sandy made sure to hive off thirty acres for herself, which allowed her to live in her pink palace until 2016.

I wish I'd met Sandy. She was said to be a real pistol, as feral and free-ranging as the menagerie of Brahmin bulls, peacocks, and Sicilian donkeys she'd surrounded herself with. I'd been invited to stay at her mansion for a writers' festival, and a former participant in the Genesis Project suggested I visit her in Savannah, but the coronavirus pandemic closed the border before I could head south. Though Sandy had died a year later, at the age of 108, her legacy lived on all around us, in this magnificent enclave she had spared from the empire of asphalt. Because of the incoming storm, though, it looked like my opportunity to explore Ossabaw would be limited to a few hours.

The tour group had gathered next to the porch of a two-story house, a mile from the mansion. It was a prefabricated catalog job that had been shipped to the island, nails and all, a century ago, and now served as quarters for visiting archaeologists. Gunn, our guide, walked us through the human history of the island. She explained the word *Ossabaw* came from the language of the Guale, Indigenous ancestors of the Creek, and meant "the place where the yaupon holly grows."* As many as two thousand Creek had once lived on the island, in a village called Asapo, where traces of their presence remained in an enormous shorefront midden of oyster shells.

I noticed a patch of brilliant green next to the porch, a few clusters of pinnate leaves that looked like they might have been planted as a border of ornamental shrubs. Gunn said that the plant, which was found growing wild, had been identified as Sea Island indigo. In 1760, the island was sold to a Savannah merchant who turned it into a plantation. Until the Civil War, enslaved African Americans toiled on Ossabaw over steaming vats of indigo leaves. The liquid took several days to boil down to small bricks, which were shipped to England, where they were rehydrated to dye fabrics a rich and durable blue.

---

* Yaupon holly, or *Ilex vomitoria*, is the only native North American plant that delivers an appreciable punch of caffeine; it also contains theophylline and theobromine, present in cacao. Native Americans brewed it into what they called the "black drink," which in high doses induced vomiting and visions. Yaupon iced tea, which can be bought in stores in Savannah, makes for a sudden wake-up.

Processing indigo was a death sentence for the enslaved workers: the toxic fumes emitted by the fermenting leaves were said to reduce life expectancy to between five and seven years.

Gunn walked us past a fenced pasture where the last of a herd of Sicilian donkeys, the breed said to have carried Jesus to Jerusalem, were being allowed to live out their lives. We stopped in front of a row of low bone-white buildings, where she explained how the enslaved workers had built their homes from tabby, a cement made of equal parts lime, ash, water, and shells. As Gunn spoke, something in the placid gaze of the donkeys reminded me my time on Ossabaw was running out. Sidling around the oyster-shell-studded wall of one of the cabins, I detached myself from the group and headed for a twin-rutted path that curved into a sun-dappled tunnel of forest.

Immediately, I was in another world. Overhead, the limbs of live oaks—so-called because they are evergreens, remaining "live" year-round—were rigged with tattered sails of Spanish moss, like the yards of just-dredged pirates' galleons slimed with seaweed. Pushing into the forest, I ran into the first mate of the *Island Explorer*. There was a black rattlesnake in the middle of the path up ahead, and she'd taken it as a sign to turn back toward the dock.

I kept on walking. Wild gusts had started to throttle the palms, creating an uncanny aural environment. An oak branch would crack, two loblolly pines would slam together, and a shriek would issue from the brush. Earlier, a pair of whitetail deer had bounded across the trail. I knew the island was rife with alligators—one of the other day-trippers had spotted a big one next to the dock—and that they regularly surged from the salt marshes to grab an unwary raccoon or a visitor's dog. If a giant sloth, a gomphothere, or some other specimen of Pleistocene megafauna had loomed over me, it wouldn't have seemed entirely out of place.

As wild as Georgia's barrier islands seemed, I knew they were far from pristine. Invasive species, almost all introduced by humans in the last five hundred years, have transformed the environment. Up until twenty years ago, neighboring St. Catherines was managed by the Bronx Zoo, which used it as a living ark for Arabian oryx, Grevy's zebras, and other exotic and endangered species. Because Ossabaw joins St. Catherines at low tide, it was likely the klaxon-like shrieks I was hearing were coming from a colony of ring-tailed lemurs, originally from Madagascar, who continue to leap through the treetops.

Holding my breath, I crept toward where I'd seen the palmetto twitch. Beneath a log, something was hard at work, digging energetically with pointed claws. It must have heard me, because suddenly two pointed ears pricked up over a long snout and beady eyes. I jumped back, heart pounding. A roly-poly rocket with a striped lizard-like tail shot off in the direction of the shore. I'd just been spooked by a nine-banded armadillo, which I'd surprised as it was rooting for grubs.

An armadillo, an animal that probably came to Georgia from Central America in the nineteenth century, was definitely *not* the invasive species I'd come searching for. I was hunting for Ossabaw Island hogs, feral descendants of pigs dumped by the Spanish, a breed that has been fattening itself on forest mast for the last five hundred years. In culinary circles, Ossabaws are considered the closest thing to the acorn-fed pigs of western Spain, whose ham is counted among the treasures of European gastronomy. Thirteen-pound legs of *pata negra* pigs, black hoof included, sell in the markets of Madrid for upward of €650. I'd been told there were a couple of thousand feral hogs on Ossabaw, decimating native plants and animals. A pig could snarfle up an entire nest of hundreds of endangered loggerhead sea turtle eggs in a single meal.

To the consternation of Georgia's Department of Natural Resources, Sandy West had insisted on treating the feral hogs as pets. She had named her favorites Paul Mitchell and Sassoon, in homage to their bristly coiffures, and given them the run of her mansion. The state now employed a hunter who lived on the island year-round to keep the population in check.

The path emerged from the forest, cutting through a salt marsh picketed with smooth cordgrass, which binds together the marsh's quicksand-like mud. Just before a wooden bridge, I came upon a cadaver in the middle of the trail. It was in a grisly state, reduced to a skull and a tangle of matted fur. But there was enough of it left—rows of flat molars on the mandibles, prominent canines, forward-facing incisors, and all-black bristles—to make a positive identification. I removed the lens cap from my camera and took my shot. I'd bagged my first Ossabaw Island hog.

It didn't take me long to see my second. The trail ran out after the marsh, on a stretch of higher ground called Cane Patch Island, where the scorched trunks of trees and the lack of forest-floor brush hinted at a recent fire. By then, the wind was blowing steady from the northeast, and as I walked back to the boat, I saw movement in the understory. A wake of vultures had gathered on the edge of a pond the color of long-steeped tea, and took flight with languorous flaps, like undertakers cheated of a client. They'd left behind a pudding of gore and black fur, barely recognizable as a recently deceased pig.

Back near the boarding house, I stopped to chat with Elizabeth DuBose, the foundation's director. She told me the resident pig-hunter was responsible for the fire-marked trunks I'd seen at Cane Patch. He'd started a controlled burn to clear out the underbrush so he could have a clearer shot at the pigs. He was pretty good at his job, she added. Visitors used to see pigs all the time. Now entire days could go by without a single sighting—at least of a live hog.

As the *Island Explorer* was nudged back to the mainland by the obliging tailwind, I thought about what I'd seen. I remembered something Anthony Martin, a specialist in ichnology (the study of animal traces) at the University of Georgia, had written: "The post-Pleistocene ecosystems of the southeastern United States, and especially of the Georgia barrier islands, have never encountered anything like feral hogs." Martin, who has seen evidence of hogs beating the defenses of even heavily armored horseshoe crabs, believed the swine had returned to their prehistoric roots. In going feral, they had become a menace to just about everything remotely edible on the islands. Martin was of the opinion that reintroducing bobcats and red wolves might be the most ecologically sound way of controlling the hog population.

I wasn't so sure. There are often unintended consequences when we humans plug apex predators back into an ecosystem. And after five hundred years, I figured that those little black hogs might have a pretty good claim to being naturalized residents of Ossabaw Island. That said, endangered sea turtles have a right to live too.

As I was about to learn, when it came to any preconceived notions I had about the cuisine, agriculture, and culture of the American Southeast, it was best to keep a supple mind. Native, exotic, or invasive. Black, red, or white. Purebred, hybrid, or feral. In these steamy parts, categories tend to get real fuzzy, real fast.

That was something I'm pretty sure Sandy West knew too. Before leaving, I made sure to mutter my thanks to her for letting me experience, even for a few hours, the magic of the island she'd loved best.

"THE OSSABAW HAM is the most extraordinary delicacy in American porcine cuisine," in the opinion of author David S. Shields.

That's saying a mouthful, because the gastronomy of the pig in the United States ranges from humble chitterlings (boiled or deep-fried intestines, served with cornbread, collard greens, and hot sauce) to the rarified Southern Louisiana tasso (a highly spiced lean pork cut smoked over a pecan-wood fire). Before leaving for Georgia, I'd asked Shields, a University of South Carolina literature professor who is also one of the Southern Foodways Alliance's most dogged culinary detectives, about the experience of eating Ossabaw.

"I've had it several different ways," he told me. "Ossabaw is not an ideal barbecuing pig, because there's not much meat. If you do cook it, you should treat it like a highly marbled slice of Wagyu at a teppanyaki restaurant. It's excellent quick-fried in a skillet with salt and pepper." Shields believes it's better to salt, cure, and age the meat, as you would an Italian or Spanish ham. "I've had Ossabaw cured, as a kind of *lardo*, and there's a creaminess to the fat that makes it respond physically to the heat in your mouth, so it just slips down your throat. One of the things that's really interesting is the way Ossabaw takes salt. A lot of cured pork just excretes salt onto your tongue, meaning there's a kind of salt-forward sharpness to it. With Ossabaw, the salt is veiled, muted, and somehow organic."

About fifteen years ago, chefs in the Southeast fell in love with the breed. It helped that the waitstaff at such high-end Charleston restaurants as Cypress and Husk had a great story to tell. Centuries ago, they explained to patrons, the conquistadors dropped off a load of pigs on a barrier island, creating a kind of living larder, a fast-multiplying source of food for future expeditions. These were nothing like the tame, pink pigs you remember from *Charlotte's Web*. These were black hogs from Spain, hairy and tusked, like wild boars, though smaller and plumper. They lived in the forest, fattening up on mast—acorns, chestnuts, and the other fallen fruit of shrubs and trees—which left them marbled with fat so rich in oleic acid that it was as healthy as eating extra-virgin olive oil. Lately, farmers had started raising them on the mainland. The cured meat was as rich as Spanish ham, but the beauty of it was that it was all-American. So, who wanted a plate of Ossabaw as a starter?

Me, for one. The problem was culinary fashions had changed, and the pandemic had shaken up the restaurant scene in Georgia and the Carolinas. Sean Brock, the hard-driven wunderkind of Southern molecular gastronomy, who was once shown barbecuing a whole Ossabaw on the documentary series *The Mind of a Chef*, had recently moved from Charleston to Nashville, closer to his roots in Appalachian coal country. Another Ossabaw fan, charcuterie master Craig Deihl, had shuttered Artisan Meat Share, Charleston's leading source of high-quality meat, and moved on to a seafood restaurant in Charlotte.

The morning after my visit to Ossabaw Island, I bid adieu to Savannah—with regret, for it is a cultured, slow-moving, magical kind of place. Driving north along Highway 170, I crossed country roads with such names as Bulltomb, Heffalump, and Crippled Oak, skirting the former plantations where enslaved workers had waded through marsh to harvest rice. On St. Helena Island, I pulled up next to the post office at the crossroads of Sea Island Parkway and Dr. Martin Luther King Jr. Drive.

I was in Frogmore, a community in the heartland of the Gullah/ Geechee Nation, which encompasses the coastal sea islands that stretch between Jacksonville, Florida, and Jacksonville, North Carolina. By their own count, the Gullah/Geechee number 200,000, and speak a Creole peppered with loanwords from fifty African languages. Many are descendants of enslaved plantation workers, who toiled growing African rice. Unlike its Asian counterpart, *Oryza glaberrima* thrived in the lowcountry of the Carolinas because it had developed a resistance to pests and pathogens in the similar climate of West Africa. After the Civil War, the Gullah/Geechee, freed from enslavement, were among the first African Americans to own large swaths of property. They remain deeply rooted in their lowcountry homeland, and their "rations," which include yams, okra, peanuts, hot peppers, fish and game, and benne, a kind of sesame seed, have produced a cuisine that is among the richest in North America. As I walked up to a two-story clapboard house, I was conscious of being in a very special place.

My timing was good, because Gullah Grub, where I planned to grab lunch, had just opened. This being Sunday, many people were still making their way home from church. On other days, the rocking chairs on the shaded porch would have been occupied by women working on sweetgrass baskets, made from a marsh grass, which are woven so tightly they can be used to carry water. The old corner store's interior had been painted French's Mustard yellow, its shelves packed with jars of locally made preserves, barbecue sauce, and seafood seasoning.

Taking a seat at a Formica table, I told a teenaged server in a black hoodie that as tempted as I was by the seafood on the menu—fried strips of shark, and big bowls of shrimp gumbo—I'd come here for the hog. He smiled, and in no time I was working on a half pound of barbecue pork ribs, served with rice, collard greens, a scoop of potato salad, and a square of cornbread on a separate plate. The ribs were sweet and sticky; the rice crimson with tomatoes and sweet with brown sugar; the collards marshy and nicely bitter; the potato salad cool and vinegary; and the cornbread light and spongy, with just the right amount of grit. After washing it all down with swigs from a mason jar filled with Swamp Water—a mix of sweet iced tea and lemonade—and chasing it with a mess of peach cobbler, I had to fight a strong urge to head for one of those chairs out front and spend the afternoon rocking in the shade.

Instead, I went out back to meet chef Bill Green, who was sitting on the porch of the community center behind the restaurant. Green, who sported a windbreaker, a well-worn fedora, and a white beard, has long been an ambassador for Gullah cuisine; for years he'd hosted a cooking show that taught viewers how to make such staples as Frogmore stew, a lowcountry boil of corn on the cob, new potatoes, shrimp, and smoked sausage. I asked the chef how pigs fit into Gullah culture.

"I was raised up south of here," Green said, in a rolling baritone, "on a little island called James Island. In the Gullah neighborhoods, some people got pigs, some got chickens, some got cows. We had a couple of cows, but we raised them for the market. I was an old man before I really started eating beef!" Early in his cooking career, he found work at a former plantation north of Charleston, where he oversaw the barbecue for parties of hunters. "The thing about the Gullah people is that they eat what grows in the season. Summer, it was seafood and fresh vegetables. Come September and October, a lot of dry beans. Back when I was raised up, we'd only do a pig kill in the dead of winter."

It was a ritual, he explained. "Everybody would get together. One of the older gentlemens would shoot the pig in the head, or hit him with a hammer, then cut his throat and hang it up to bleed. While he's hanging, you'd clean out the insides." They'd put a barrel of water over an open fire until it was hot, but not boiling. "You drop the pig in the scalding water for a while, then pull him out on a board. Everybody gets to scraping all the hair off him, until he's clean and white." There were two distinct ways of preserving the meat: curing and smoking. "If you're salting him for cure, you put on your pepper, curing salt, stuff like that, and let him hang for a day or two. Then you pack it in a wooden box. After seven days, you pull it out, and if everything looks good, all the seasonings are penetrating, you pack it down again, and wrap it in a brown bag"—vital for keeping the bugs away—"somewhere where the air can get around it."

Eight or ten hours in a smoker, over a slow-burning fire, would add flavor. With or without smoke, Gullah tradition called for soaking the ham in cane-sugar syrup. "You put some syrup on top, let it drip dry, that will *lock* all the flavor in, make it hard as a rock, so nothing can get in." It was possible to be enjoying meat from a December-killed pig as early as the spring, but Green thought it best to wait nine months. "The longer you wait, the better it tastes."

What Green was describing was a classic dry cure; the addition of cane syrup was one way to make that Southern classic, the country ham. Wet cures, which produce a moist ham, involve pickling the meat in brine for up to a week, with the option of smoking it after. Unsmoked pickled ham was traditionally considered a food of the poor.

"Meat never spoiled in a jug of brine," wrote novelist Harry Crews in *A Childhood*, his memoir of his hardscrabble early years in rural Georgia in the 1940s, but "it took real courage and a certain desperation to eat through all that salt."

A dry-cured country ham is probably the closest thing in the Americas to *jamón ibérico*—the kind you see mounted on those wood-and-metal frames known as *jamoneras*. But Spanish ham, like prosciutto, is never smoked; conditions in southern Europe are dry enough that hams can be hung to ferment for two years without risk of spoilage. In the steamy American Southeast, smoking, usually over smoldering hickory—"the sweetest smoke a man was ever to smell," according to Crews—afforded additional protection against bacteria, mold, and the depredations of ham beetles and skippers, flies whose eggs can survive a bath of human stomach acid.

Green couldn't recall the breeds of the hogs his neighbors used to keep. He did remember they were on the small side, no more than three hundred pounds. As a hunter, his favorite were the wild boars. "Man, the difference in the meat is night and day. They're a lot sweeter. They don't have the fat line, because they exercise a lot. They eat acorns, grubs, roots. Lot better for you. But they're mean if you corner them." When I asked Green what kind of pork he liked best, his answer surprised me.

"Since I found my religion, I don't eat ham. I follow the Hebrew law. We have some Ethiopian in us, and some of my family has Jewish blood. I show other people how to cook pigs, but I don't come into contact with the pig. I wear gloves." That explained why Gullah Grub was closed on Saturdays; Green was Ethiopian Orthodox Christian and kept the Sabbath. "Nobody ate more pork than I used to! But I backed off from eating it thirty years ago." I mentioned that almost all the churches I'd seen driving up were Baptist, and asked if there were a lot of other people in his local faith community. "Not many, but a good handful." He seemed to want to leave it at that.

A reminder, I thought as I walked back to the car, not only of how often people will surprise you, but also of the fact that for a good portion of humanity, pork is simply not on the menu. Islam is clear on the matter. "Prohibited to you are carrion, blood, the flesh of swine" is how the fifth sura of the Quran expresses it. The followers of Moses are permitted to eat cows, goats, and sheep, but a fine distinction is made in Leviticus: "The swine, though he divide the hoof, and be clovenfooted, yet he cheweth not the cud; he is unclean to you." Some anthropologists have speculated the prohibition derived from a quite rational fear of foodborne illness. Symptoms of trichinosis, however, take a while to appear after eating an infected animal, and people in the ancient Middle East are unlikely to have made the connection; the *Trichinella* roundworm was only formally identified in 1835.

Archaeologists have discovered pork consumption in the region went into sharp decline about three thousand years ago, well before the prohibitions in the Torah and Quran. For the earliest Neolithic farmers, keeping pigs had conferred several advantages. You could let them run free, and they would fatten themselves on scraps and mast until it was time for the slaughter. A pig provided food security and autonomy to a household and, like the potato hidden in an Irish field, tended to be invisible to state authorities. When tax collectors showed up, your porker could always be shooed away from the village, and all ownership denied. The disadvantage was that, unlike grass-feeding cattle and sheep, omnivorous pigs ate pretty much the same things we humans do. An ill-controlled herd of swine could easily gobble up a season's stockpile of wheat and barley.

Pig remains disappear from the archaeological record around 1000 BCE, a time when the Middle East was becoming more arid and the size of settlements was growing. As the marshes and forests fit for foraging shrank, pigs would have been increasingly underfoot in villages, gobbling up grain and ravaging vegetable gardens. As early states and their priestly elites were finding creative ways to tax households in order to fill storehouses with grain, devising a metaphysical justification for not eating pigs would have made good political and economic sense.

Besides, another tasty farm animal had recently filled the gap. The chicken, first domesticated in China eight thousand years ago, was brought to the Middle East by nomads or seafaring peoples and became a fixture in the region around 1200 BCE, at the end of the Bronze Age.

"The chicken duplicated the role of the pig," wrote anthropologist Richard Redding. "The chicken, however, was a more efficient producer of proteins for human consumption than the pig and came in a smaller package. It also produced eggs that could be consumed without damaging the breeding stock." Poultry also has a smaller ecological impact: it takes 750 gallons of water to produce a pound of pork, but just 440 to yield a pound of chicken, and water has long been a scarce resource in the Middle East.

The coming of chickens—I imagine them arriving from the eastern steppes, lashed alive by the feet to the backs of nomads' donkeys—doesn't fully account for the pork prohibition. But, as Redding points out, the availability of chickens may have *permitted* the pig taboo to evolve. Banning pork, he argues, would have been a way to codify optimal economic behavior. Especially, it seems to me, for the ruling elite, who must have viewed every pig loose in the streets or fields as a maddeningly untaxable affront to priestly authority.

The amazing thing is that, while two billion people—among them Muslims, Jews, Seventh-Day Adventists, Rastafarians, and Ethiopian Orthodox Christians like chef Bill Green—won't touch pork, and consumption in India is negligible, pigs somehow manage to be the single most eaten species of animal in the world. The global average is thirty-three pounds of pork per person a year, with Americans eating sixty pounds, and the Spanish, the world champions, just over twice that. But the real growth market is among the 1.4 billion people of China, who are lately averaging eighty-four pounds per person a year, and climbing.

I should add that my own consumption of pork, and all other forms of animal flesh, is closer to Hindu than Iberian norms. I will eat meat proffered out of sincere hospitality, and I will sample meat, especially if it's in a form new to me, in the course of research. As for *jamón ibérico*, that I eat enthusiastically, because it's healthy, ethically raised, and absolutely delicious. But it's something I do on special occasions—as a treat.

So far, though, I hadn't even had a taste of *ibérico*'s closest American equivalent: locally raised, acorn-fed Ossabaw Island ham, which was the whole point of my coming to the South.

As I drove across the soaring cantilever bridge that leads to downtown Charleston, I was already thinking about dinner. I was going to experience one of the glories of southern cuisine, whole-hog barbecue, prepared by one of the great living pitmasters, in the gastronomic capital of the Southeast.

For a whole number of reasons, the plan was making me feel pretty uneasy.

I STEPPED LIGHTLY AS I ENTERED RODNEY SCOTT'S BBQ in North Charleston. I was aware that I was in a temple, and my presence might be seen as a profanation. Though I'd had a few pulled-pork sandwiches in my time, at heart I was a whole-hog-barbecue know-nothing. To make matters worse, I'm a Canadian, which is somewhere beyond Yankee. That said, I figured I could make a spirited case for my home province of Quebec, whose cuisine includes *cretons* (spiced pork spread) and *oreilles de crisse* ("Christ's ears," or deep-fried fatback), being the center of its own devoted pork cult.

Fortunately, I'd shown up on a Sunday night, near closing time, so there weren't enough people around for me to make a fool of myself. I went up to the counter, where it became pretty obvious that the ordering process had been tourist-proofed. I was there for one thing: Rod's Original Whole Hog Pork Sandwich. The young woman at the counter took my order without raising an eyebrow. I carried my tray, loaded with a cardboard container of collard greens and a glass of Unsweet Tea, to a booth to have my first proper plate of whole-hog barbecue.

I can't lie. It was fantastic. A rectangle of untoasted white bread was topped with half a pound of pork, cut from a hog that had been barbecued overnight, and then sprinkled with salty cracklings—pig skin fried in lard until it's curly and seriously crunchy. Twelve hours of cooking at a low temperature had worked its magic: the collagen that bound the muscle fibers had turned into gelatin, while the back fat had melted, further tenderizing and moisturizing the meat. The thin strands of juicy pork parted easily under fork and tooth. Beneath the straightforward smoky savoriness, the meat itself reminded me of chicken breast—more a triumph of texture than flavor—but a squeeze of Rod's vinegar-based sauce banished any thought of blandness. This was a great American meal, cooked by the James Beard Award–winning Scott, an African American who is one of the great barbecue pitmasters and also one of the great American chefs.

I highlight Scott's cultural background because in the last few years, many Black-owned barbecue joints have shut down, and Black barbecuers have found themselves shouldered off the stage of American culinary history.

"Influential food media platforms," wrote historian Adrian Miller in *Black Smoke: African Americans and the United States of Barbecue*, "have fallen deeply in love with four types of White Guys Who Barbecue." These are "fine dining chefs," "the Urban Hipster who sports interesting tattoos," the "Rural Bubba, who is an overalls-and-ball-cap-wearing guy that one might see on the television shows *Duck Dynasty* or *Dukes of Hazzard*," and, finally, some combination of all of the above.

As Miller points out, the history of barbecue begins with a bunch of white guys stealing things. The first record dates to a 1513 account of Columbus's second voyage. At what is now Guantánamo Bay in Cuba, a landing party found fish and meat slow-cooking over an unattended fire. Columbus's men grabbed the fish and rabbits, which they found delicious, leaving behind the iguanas, which they considered pretty disgusting. The feast was being cooked on a wooden lattice that in the language of the Arawak natives was known as a *barbacrot*, a word that became *barbacoa* in Spanish. In its original sense, *barbecue*, which entered the English language in the sixteenth century, referred not to a cooking process but to any kind of platform, table, or grill for preparing food. It was African Americans who carried on the tradition, tending the outdoor fires for generations—until the Bubbas and the rest decided it looked like fun.

I was glad my first whole-hog experience was at a place as good as Rodney Scott's, because I wouldn't be seeking out barbecue again. My decision had nothing to do with the quality of the cooking.

"Is there anything more ludicrous than the present day barbeque contests in which contestants are prohibited from supplying meat that might be more sapid than those of their fellows?" David S. Shields has asked. "The organizers give everyone the same hybrid pink pig. It's all about the sauce, the rub, the heat—it has nothing to do with the meat."

And in the end, of course, it should be *all* about the meat. And, just as importantly, where the meat comes from.

THE SILVER DODGE WAS WAITING FOR ME outside Williamsburg Packing, a slaughterhouse in Kingstree, a town an hour and a half's drive due north of Charleston. I tailed the pickup as it made a turn off the pavement. For a second, I wondered about the advisability of following a pig farmer named Tank down a dirt road in rural South Carolina.

I'd met Tank Jackson the day before, when he was grilling the pork he markets under the name Holy City Hogs in the loading bay of a Charleston microbrewery. With hair that flowed from under his ball cap to past his shoulders and his ZZ Top beard, Tank was a recognizable mash-up of the Rural Bubba and the Hipster. He explained he'd just now gotten back from Manhattan, where he'd personally delivered some hogs to Lodi, a high-end restaurant on Rockefeller Plaza. Over platefuls of sausages at a picnic table, talk turned to how pig farms were meant to be good places to dispose of a corpse.

"No, dude," he said, in a southwest Georgia drawl, "pigs'll leave the bones and shit out the teeth. That's *evidence*. Better way is to dump it in the ocean wrapped in chain-link fence. That way it won't float."

Really, though, I wasn't too worried. Not only was Tank funny and smart, with a kind-eyed smile, but he also had the good sense to keep pure-bred Ossabaws. Besides, by then I'd been hearing about the breed for so long, I might have driven through a minefield for an up-close look.

On his leased acreage, Tank raises old-line Durocs, a bacon hog called the Sowega King, and a lard hog known as the Carolina Black Hoof. The pigs seemed overjoyed to see him, jostling as he emptied a line of corn-based feed from a sack. In a separate enclosure, fenced off behind electric wire, was Tank's herd of Ossabaws. They were small pigs, about half the size of the Durocs, which could reach 650 pounds. Tank had seven sows, two gilts—pigs that haven't had their first litter—and a boar hog, with white tusks, the biggest of the herd. He'd named him Ponce de León, after the Spanish explorer. I could see why people found Ossabaws endearing: Tank's hogs were round, long-legged, and almost comically plump.

"They're walking-around bowling balls of fat," said Tank, with a chuckle. "Their bodies are almost like a camel's hump." Tank pointed out the features that he figured had helped them survive for centuries on Ossabaw Island. "You see those huge elephant-style ears? They're like a baseball cap. They gave their eyes protection from the sun, dust, and heat." Black furry coats kept them warm in the cold months and shielded them from the sun's rays when it was hot. Their delicate high-heeled hooves suggested a flamenco dancer's shoes. Modern domesticated breeds, in contrast, have large splayed feet, suited for supporting heavy frames and a life standing on the concrete floor of a factory farm.

The Ossabaws' toes were unusually long, as were their snouts, which made them excellent at scenting and digging up grubs and roots (and, unfortunately, sea turtle eggs). Any time Tank needed to remove a stump, he would use a steel bar to dig a cone shape around its base, and fill it with feed. In a Tom Sawyer–like arrangement, the pigs would do all the hard work of excavating by using their snouts and hooves to get every last grain of corn. "It's diesel-free land clearing!" Tank drawled.

"What does this look like to you?" he asked, pointing to a balloon-shaped indentation in a metal fence. "The head of an Ossabaw, possibly? That fence is made of fucking steel." One morning he'd made the mistake of sneaking up on a sow. "The fight-or-flight kicked in. She came running at me and hit the fence at full speed. Your regular domesticated breed wouldn't even have looked up." Tank appreciated the wildness the Ossabaws have in them. "They're actually one of the easiest pigs to raise, as long as you have the proper infrastructure and plenty of space for them."

I asked if, like Spanish pigs, his Ossabaws were finished on forest mast. "One hundred percent! That line of trees you see there are all acorn-producing oak trees. We're going in and planting native grasses, heirloom grains, and clovers. We're trying to make this as close to the *dehesa* in Spain as possible."

He admitted they took longer to bring to market weight than other hogs. "Ten months for an Ossabaw, while an indoor hog takes four months." It was worth it, though, for the meat they produced.

"We call it redneck prosciutto. The only difference from European ham is that we cold-smoke it with hickory for a brief period. It's a country ham, but once you age it for nine months, you can slice it paper thin, eat it just like you would a Spanish-style cured ham."

Tank was making a good living catering to chefs in New Orleans, Charleston, and New York. But he was aware that producers of heritage breeds provided an infinitesimal percentage of all the pork consumed in the United States. "I'll sell less than three hundred pigs a year," he said. "A single slaughterhouse around here will kill three thousand in a *day*. I can appreciate what they offer to the world. They're making cheap pork fast; they feed a lot of people. But I prefer to do it this way."

Tank seemed preoccupied; one of his Ossabaws was missing. He told me to hop on the running board of the pickup, and we bumped over a few hundred yards of ruts to a shaded grove. Beneath one of the oaks, a sow had built herself a nest out of leaves, twigs, and underbrush, and was suckling nine squirming pigs, who were busy jostling for teats. While Tank had been up north, Stella Rose had gone and had a litter.

"They farrow in the woods, wild and free," whispered Tank, careful not to alarm her. There was a little shine in his eyes as he watched the squirming newborns. "I think, let the pig be a pig, let it express its true nature. That's how you're going to have the best pork." The wildness in the Ossabaws that makes them liable to buckle a steel fence is exactly what gives them their flavor. Because they lead active outdoor lives, their flesh is high in myoglobin, which helps muscles store oxygen and produces a ruby-red ham streaky with intramuscular fat.

But there's more to the Ossabaws than their deliciousness. The real story is more complicated, and a lot weirder, than the one the waiters in the fine-dining restaurants like to tell.

HUMANS HAVE BEEN HUNTING AND EATING PIGS for a long time. *Sus scrofa*, or wild boar, which is closely related to hippos and peccaries, is native to Europe, Asia, and North Africa. At a site in northern Spain, wild boar bones, with cut marks that suggest butchering, have been found alongside the remains of one of our hominin forerunners, *Homo antecessor*, dated to a million years ago.

Sus domesticus, as the common pig is known, is the first animal modern humans domesticated for food.* The earliest evidence of pig husbandry dates to eleven thousand years ago; remains found in Hallan Çemi, in what is now Turkey, actually predate the domestication of grains. Pigs made the leap across the Bosphorus Strait into Europe with Neolithic farmers around 7,500 years ago. The environmental

---

* *Canis lupus*, wolves, had been domesticated into *Canis lupus familiaris*, dogs, five thousand years earlier than that, but humans, most of us anyway, tend not to eat dogs.

issues that led to the pork prohibitions in the urbanized Middle East weren't a factor in heavily forested Europe, where pigs didn't have to compete with humans for food. Pannage, the practice of allowing animals to range widely into forests to feed on windfall fruits, acorns, and other mast, also allowed pigs to interbreed with wild boar. European pigs eventually lost almost all traces of their domesticated Middle Eastern genetics and became lean, agile, slab-sided, and long of snout and leg, sporting bristles and fearsome tusks. On the continuum from savage to tame, the forest-raised pigs of medieval Europe were definitely on the wild side.

The *pata negra* pigs of Spain are living examples of this fierce strain. DNA extracted from a pig killed around 1550, recently discovered at a castle in Girona, revealed a genome very similar to a contemporary species used to make *jamón ibérico*. About the same time, the practice of fattening pigs on forest mast was formalized in the *dehesa*, a territory that now covers 1,700 square miles in the Extremadura region of western Spain.

This mythologized landscape, the source of Spain's most prized black-label acorn-finished ham, is often portrayed as an untouched, primeval savannah of cork and holm oaks. But the word *dehesa* is a variant of *defensa,* in reference to the fact that this was the territory that noble hidalgos could defend, or fence off, from outsiders. Within the boundary of the *dehesa*, grapevines and grains were forbidden. The only other livestock allowed were sheep sheared for merino wool, which were allowed to graze on the grass the pigs had left behind. The pigs' relentless munching allowed oaks to outcompete shade-tolerant plants in the understory, creating a parklike landscape. As sustainable and productive as this human- and pig-controlled ecosystem is, the *dehesa* tended to benefit only the lucky landowners who could reap the profits from cork, wool, and ham.

As chef and pig breeder Peter Kaminsky emphasizes in his fascinating book *Pig Perfect*, the landscape the first Spanish explorers encountered on the American mainland, a classic oak park of shaded grove, grassland, and scrub, was eerily similar to the *dehesa*. Columbus had offloaded eight pigs on Cuba in 1493, and Hernando de Soto released thirteen of their descendants on the mainland after landing south of what is now Tampa Bay. By 1543, just four years later, thousands of feral swine roamed the Southeast, and Europeans reported that the Choctaw, Shawnee, Miami, and other Indigenous Americans had taken to keeping pigs. In Virginia, the colonists' feral pigs rooted up tuckahoe, the bulb-like root of a semiaquatic plant that the Powhatan people ground into flour and which served as a primary food source when the corn harvest failed.

The character of New World forests had been formed by mammoths, giant sloths, and other gargantuan mammals, which, like elephants in Africa, left in their paths swaths of broken and uprooted trees. With the coming of humans, armed with flint spearheads, the megafauna that had crashed through the forest, making it a dynamic, species-rich environment, were driven to extinction. Two factors prevented a closed-canopy climax forest from dominating eastern North America: the Indigenous practice of controlled burns, in many areas meant to clear the land for the raising of corn, and the presence of bison, which partially occupied the niche of the megafauna, grazing on species that would have otherwise prevented oak from becoming established. The deep dark woods feared by the Pilgrims turned out to be a phenomenon of the Europeans' own making: their guns killed off the forest-dwelling bison, and their germs killed the Indigenous people whose controlled burns made the forest more of a parklike *dehesa* than an ominous *Urwald*.

The conquistadors' swine, Kaminsky believes, played a role similar to aurochs in Europe and bison in the New World: "Pigs, in rotation with cattle and sheep, are proxies for the now extinct large animals of Europe ... The closer husbandry is to the wild model, the more sustainable it will be." Many ecologists advocate returning bison to the Great Plains—creating a naturally manured "buffalo commons"—as a way of restoring the impoverished soils of the Midwest. Kaminsky believes that "pigs help preserve a savannah-and-woodland ecology from which we humans first evolved and where, psychologically, we feel most at home."

Unchecked, though, pigs are voracious consumers of just about anything remotely edible. In Spain, the *dehesa* is delimited by fences. This is not the case in the United States, where five million feral hogs roam free in thirty-nine states, and have recently crossed the northern border into Saskatchewan. Most are descendants of escaped domestic pigs, which, after a few generations off the farm, become the fearsome scavengers whose bristle-covered spines have earned them the name razorbacks. (Tank Jackson told me that the owners of White Oak Pastures, a large farm in southwest Georgia, are forced to shoot feral hogs, up to twenty a night, to stop them breeding with their heritage pigs.) In the last decade, *American Hoggers*, *Lady Hoggers*, *Boss Hog*, and other reality shows have documented hunters with machine guns, often fired from helicopters, bagging their prey. All told, feral hogs are thought to cause $1.5 billion in damage a year.

The pigs of Ossabaw are their own brand of feral. Historians guess they were brought to the barrier islands by Lucas Vázquez de Ayllón, a Spanish explorer and magistrate, who in 1526 set up the first European settlement in what's now the United States, on St. Catherines Island, which was as far north as the Spanish ever settled on the Atlantic coast. Zooarchaeological analyses of the Spanish sites have turned up extensive evidence of cattle, chickens, and domesticated pigs. Whether originally brought by colonists or missionaries, the pigs could easily have trotted over to neighboring Ossabaw when the tide was at its lowest.

A recent sequencing of the Ossabaw genome shows they are less closely related to contemporary Spanish *pata negra* pigs than to a breed known as the Canary Island Black pig. From Columbus on, Spanish explorers had made it a habit to pick up pigs on the archipelago off the coast of Morocco before heading to the New World. Most of them ended up on the American mainland, where they crossbred with wild and domestic pigs, losing the qualities that made them true *patas negras*.

While the Ossabaw bloodline remained more or less pure, over the centuries the pigs underwent a sea change—a sea-island change, to be precise—becoming something rich, strange, and new. Life on Ossabaw tends to be feast or famine; oaks might drop abundant acorns one year but none the next, while freshwater ponds can dry up for months on end. The pigs possessed a thrifty gene, which allowed them to gorge themselves when times were good and lay on fat for the lean years. They also developed a high tolerance for drinking salt water, and eventually underwent insular dwarfism, in which animals living on an island become smaller than their mainland counterparts. A fully grown Ossabaw sow carrying a full-term litter of fetuses can weigh less than one hundred pounds.

Dr. Lehr Brisbin first got to know the breed as a young man, in the 1970s, when Sandy West invited him to live on the island as part of the Genesis Project. He went on to become a research scientist at the University of Georgia and a leading authority on the genetics of wild pigs. The little black hogs he'd seen dashing through the palmetto on the Georgia barrier island always stuck in his head. I'd had a few conversations with the genial septuagenarian ("Call me Bris!") before coming south, and he'd explained just how unique, and important, the Ossabaws were.

"Feral pigs in general might be a scourge, only a pest, to most ecologists, but these pigs in particular represent a biomedical treasure," Brisbin told me. Ossabaws turn out to be the fattest terrestrial wild mammal on Earth. They're so plump, in fact, that they're prediabetic; in the lab, given access to abundant food, they develop full-blown type 2 diabetes. In the wild, though, they remain healthy and active, while humans similarly afflicted tend to become morbidly obese, to the extent that they go blind or have to have a foot amputated. Theorizing that the pigs must have unique enzymes and hormones that allow them to mobilize body fat reserves in ways humans can't, he decided they were eminently worthy of study. Brisbin was of the opinion that the hunters of Georgia's Department of Natural Resources were doing the world a disservice by shooting the pigs.

"Loggerhead turtles nest on a lot of different islands," he pointed out, "but only Ossabaw has Ossabaw Island hogs."

Deciding to do an end run around the state of Georgia, twenty years ago Brisbin oversaw the loading of twenty-six Ossabaw pigs onto a barge headed for the mainland. From there, they were taken by tractor-trailer to a lab at the University of Missouri, where they would provide a core population for diabetes researchers to study. Brisbin believes that since then the gene pool on the island has become tainted: he accuses "good ol' boys" of dumping boars onto Ossabaw to mate with the local sows, so there will be more animals to shoot when the island is opened to the public for semiannual hunts.

For Brisbin, the deliciousness of Ossabaws was a detail. What got him excited was their potential to help treat a disease that affects hundreds of millions of people around the world. It was an example of a beautiful concordance between cuisine and science. The diversity of the past—preserved through the passion of farmers, chefs, ecologists, and medical researchers—was providing hope for the future, not only of cherished foodways but also of human health.

It was fitting that it was happening in the South, because it is here, in a dramatic way, that the richness of the past is being erased. The culprit is Big Hog, as the industrial pork industry is known, and its efforts to churn out ever cheaper, ever blander, ever crueler versions of the "other white meat."

TRY AS I MIGHT, I still hadn't found a proper plate of Ossabaw ham. I'd sat down at the counter of FIG, one of Charleston's most esteemed restaurants, with chef-owner Mike Lata. He'd first served the breed twenty years earlier. He'd gotten his Ossabaws from farmer Emile de Felice—no longer in the pig business—who in turn got his herd directly from the load of pure-bloods Brisbin had rescued from the island.

"Here I am breaking them down in the kitchen," Lata recalled. "The yield was terrible, the muscles were tiny compared to what I was expecting. But the meat was delicious, with nice intramuscular fat, and it had this fat cap on the exterior that was just remarkable. I was like, how can I use this thing?" Ossabaw was too fatty to grill, but too expensive to be right for barbecue. "Turns out it's great for charcuterie. You can extract the lean meat and make your own blends."

Lata's restaurant is local and market-driven, and since pig, rather than cattle, is what's available in the coastal Carolinas, he makes sure it's on FIG's menu. That night, though, the only Ossabaw available was in the chicken-liver pâté. Lata served it in the form of a small loaf, the liver whipped with Ossabaw fat and accompanied by cornichons, pickled cauliflower, and Dijon. Spread on toast, it was silky and surprisingly delicate in flavor. As a consolation, Lata brought out ham from another heritage breed, Lady Edison, sliced Spanish-style, drizzled with olive oil, and served with a dollop of cultured *fromage blanc*.

All excellent, though the check made me wince. As a corrective, the following morning I paid a visit to Daps, a casual breakfast joint that gets its pork from Tank Jackson. Co-owner Jeremiah Schenzel agreed that Ossabaws were the closest American breed to Spanish ham. I ordered a melted-Brie-and-egg sandwich, served on sourdough toast, that included triangles of maple-glazed ham from Holy City Hogs. Most of the items were just over ten bucks—cheaper, in fact, than the barbecue at Rodney Scott's. Ham that came from ethically raised heritage breeds, in other words, wasn't something you could only find at high-end restaurants like FIG.

I was glad to have a big breakfast, because I had a long drive ahead of me that day. I was headed for North Carolina, the place where, when it comes to the pork industry, everything started to go south.

IN THE FAR EAST, pig domestication began eight thousand years ago, on the shores of the Mekong and Yangtze Rivers. In a region where sheep, goats, and cattle were scarce, pig manure served as a useful fertilizer. Raised in sties and fed on table scraps, pigs became home garbage-disposal units; to this day, the Chinese character *jia*, which means "home," is composed of the symbol for a pig written under the symbol for roof. Unlike Europe, there were few forests where pigs could fatten on acorns; the increasing population density that came with intensive rice cultivation in the first millennium CE had led to the wholesale felling of trees. And unlike the Middle East, China has never turned its back on pork, a protein that continues to figure prominently in each of its eight major regional cuisines.

Over the millennia, pigs in East Asia evolved into round, pale, short-legged, pot-bellied creatures—think of the piggy bank, a toy whose origins lie in China—notable for their ability to quickly transform organic waste into fatty edible meat. The first Chinese pigs seem to have arrived in Europe around 1700. Farmers in Leicestershire, who supplied salt pork to markets in London and to the Royal Navy, found that Chinese breeds crossed with native stock could be brought to slaughter in nine months rather than two or three years. By the 1850s, Yorkshire, Berkshire, Hampshire, and Suffolk hogs had emerged as the most prized of these crosses. They would soon be joined by Durocs, Large Whites, Welsh, and Poland Chinas.

While the Spanish had little interest in their bland white meat—to this day, the prestige Iberian breeds contain no Chinese pig DNA—the fast-growing breeds from the Far East became popular in the United States. Late in the eighteenth century, a Philadelphia firm began shipping a breed called Big Chinas to farmers in Ohio, and in the 1830s a group of Kentucky farmers imported Hampshires from England. By the nineteenth century, the pig had become the most important source of meat in the United States, Canada, and Australia. While the slaughter and transport of the meat were industrialized, pigs were mostly raised on small farms. As late as 1950, there were 2.1 million hog farmers in the United States, with an average of just 31 pigs per farm. Today, only 60,000 remain, and they average 1,900 pigs per farm.

Family farms have been almost completely replaced by "confined animal feeding operations," the porcine version of the factory farm.

As I drove up Interstate 95 into North Carolina, the presence of these CAFOs became impossible to ignore. Turning off onto NC 41, I drove west to Tar Heel, and then followed the Cape Fear River north until I reached the Smithfield Foods facility. This is the largest slaughterhouse in the world, a place where 32,000 pigs can be reduced to their component parts in a single day.

I had no intention of going inside. I've visited abattoirs before; some have been humane, others hellish. This was on another scale; at almost a million square feet, distributed through a complex of low gray buildings, it took some time to drive its length. In his book *The Chain*, journalist Ted Genoways vividly describes the conditions in such mega-slaughterhouses, where employees, a large number of them undocumented, work through injuries, mysterious ailments, and grueling line speeds in order to touch their paychecks.

Turning back toward Interstate 95, I took a detour up Chicken Foot Road. Just past Plainview Primary School, I saw the gleaming roofs of CAFOs visible behind screening rows of trees. Each consisted of a complex of up to a dozen rectangular sheds; most such sheds house a thousand or more pigs. Conceived by artificial insemination, the pigs inside would have been born to sows at another site. They then would have been trucked to these "wean-to-finish" facilities, where they are fattened on genetically modified soybeans and corn from automatic feeders. To survive in the hot, crowded sheds, the pigs have to be injected with vaccines and antibiotics and treated with insecticides. They defecate through slatted floors, and their waste is flushed into clay-lined, open-air "lagoons" as big as Olympic-sized swimming pools. When these cesspools reach capacity, pumps are deployed and the manure, laden with antibiotic-resistant pathogens, is shot with giant spray guns into nearby fields.

I couldn't see the cesspools—I later confirmed on Google Earth that they were well hidden behind the sheds—but I could smell them. It was a cool day in March, but something acrid in the air made my nose twitch, and I started to feel an acidic burn deep in my throat, as if I had just retched. I wondered about the children in the elementary school, whose playground was a couple of hundred yards from the nearest cesspool, and about the air they would have to breathe on a hot day.

There are five million hogs in Bladen and the surrounding counties; in Duplin County, the center of the industry, there are now thirty-five hogs for every human resident. When cesspools rupture, or overflow after storms, the toxic sludge that pours into rivers provokes massive fish kills. Most of the residents of coastal North Carolina are Latinos, Native Americans, or African Americans; many of the latter have been property owners since the abolition of slavery. Since the 1980s, they've watched as multigenerational tobacco farms have been replaced by toxic industrial sites. Their suffering—which includes brain fog, headaches, burning eyes, and breathing problems—and their legal battle against Smithfield Foods, the world's largest pork producer, are recounted in Corban Addison's nonfiction book *Wastelands*. He describes a once idyllic rural geography turned into "a farrago of forested wastelands" by the greed of the pork industry.

A decade ago, Smithfield Foods, which contracts with two thousand CAFOs in the United States, was purchased by WH Group, or Wanzhou Guoji, the Hong Kong–based multinational, of which it's now a wholly owned subsidiary. The $7 billion takeover, the largest-ever acquisition of an American company by Chinese buyers, met a pressing need: China, which holds only 7 percent of the world's farmland, now consumes half of the world's pork.

The triumph of fast-growing, garbage-eating Chinese pig breeds is now complete: the world's largest producer, source of most of the pork eaten by Americans, is now Chinese. The CAFOs of Duplin County produce as much waste as Guangzhou, a megacity with eighteen million residents. In China, where the majority of pigs are still raised outside on small farms, cesspools are strictly forbidden, as is the practice of spraying manure on fields. American hog farmers supply the middle class of China—who, like Americans, have come to expect meat at every meal—while fouling the environment and ruining the lives of their neighbors.

That is the irony of eating barbecue, pulled pork, and ribs. In the South, barbecue is almost always made with cheap commodity pork, bought at a Sam's Club or a Piggly Wiggly supermarket, with no thought given to the breed or its provenance.

That's why I believe seeking out good meat, from heritage breeds, isn't a niche pursuit for the privileged few. It's the decent, healthy, and *just* thing to do. And because it's costlier, eating quality pork is something I can't afford to do often—and eating less meat is certainly better for my well-being and the planet's.

Factory-made meat is cruel from start to finish. It's cruel to the animals, cruel to the workers in the slaughterhouses. It's cruel to the farmers who own the CAFOS, who assume all the risk, and often end up clearing less than minimum wage. It's cruel to the people whose lives are poisoned by their proximity to factory farms. If such cruelty is to end, people will have to stop using and glorifying factory pork.

That includes every food-television star, celebrity chef, and cookbook writer who raves about a slice of ham without acknowledging that what their viewers or readers consume is almost certainly commodity pork, 97 percent of which comes from large commercial operations. For barbecue pitmasters, that will mean making the effort—and passing on the cost—of grilling pigs raised not in CAFOS but on diversified family farms.

Author Harry Crews wrote unforgettably of the pig kills he'd attended in rural Georgia; as a child, he'd suffered serious burns after falling into a boiling vat of water used to scald the pigs. "Animals were killed but seldom hurt," he recalled in *A Childhood*. "Farmers took tremendous cautions about pain at slaughter... As brutal as they sometimes are with farm animals and with themselves, no farmer would ever eat an animal he had willingly made suffer." That is no longer the case. Everybody who eats cheap, factory-made meat is eating suffering.

By then I'd had about all I could take of the stench. I rolled up the windows, though it only helped a little. Turning the car around, I started driving west.

THAT NIGHT, I slept in a rusted-out school bus in Snow Camp, North Carolina, which the owner of Cane Creek Farm rented out on Airbnb. I'd finally tracked down my cured Ossabaw ham. Eliza MacLean promised she'd hook me up the following morning.

My arrival coincided with a gathering of some of MacLean's fifty cousins, who had come from all over the United States, filling the farmhouse kitchen with laughter late into the night. The next morning, a somewhat bleary MacLean showed me around her property. She had bought Cane Creek from an inventor and tinkerer who had let his sixty-five acres go to seed. Her property included a Quaker-built barn, an old general store, and a stretch of Cane Creek whose banks were lined with towering ash and poplar trees. MacLean had worked hard to bring it back to life.

"I raise seven species of animals and poultry," she said as we crossed a field. "I use every inch of my land, rotating multiple species." I'd already been charged by her geese, which acted like great honking watchdogs, and patted a lamb snuggling against a puppy. "I've got Guinea hens, heritage-breed turkeys, chickens, sheep." She also kept a cattle breed known as Red Devon, descendants of animals brought to Plymouth Colony, which could be used for milk, meat, and as draft animals. "They've been running around the southern states for four hundred years, and they've got all their stuff figured out. They don't get hoof rot; they don't really get parasites. They've developed natural resistance to everything in the environment." Rotating the animals from field to field solved a lot of MacLean's problems. She didn't have to buy expensive fertilizer, because the animals themselves were portable manure-dispensing machines. And she didn't treat her animals with pesticides and antibiotics, because the chickens and geese pecked the bugs out of the dung before they could parasitize her livestock.

This is something opponents of animal husbandry tend to forget. Since the beginning of the Neolithic, livestock has been an integral part of agriculture. When pigs, cattle, goats, and sheep are allowed to roam, as they are on mixed farms, their manure is churned into the soil. Records kept continuously at a study farm in Britain since 1843 show that plots treated with manure tripled in soil nitrogen and carbon content. Those plowed and treated with chemical fertilizers, meanwhile, lost nitrogen, which was dissolved in runoff. Factory farms and CAFOS have completely removed the livestock from the land, and with them, the manure they put into the soil. Industrial agriculture, like so many products of reductionist thinking, has torn an ancient system asunder, reducing it to its component parts in the name of greater efficiency. In so doing, it has inflicted enduring damage on the land, the water, and the air we breathe.

"Mother earth never attempts to farm without live stock," Sir Albert Howard wrote in *An Agricultural Testament*, the founding text of the organic farming movement, in 1940. "The mixed vegetable and animal wastes are converted into humus; there is no waste; the processes of growth and the processes of decay balance one another." With the ancient techniques of crop rotation, no-till farming, and manuring, as well as such Indigenous techniques as intercropping of beans, corn, and squash, a plot of soil can retain its fertility indefinitely. Being on MacLean's farm was like traveling back to the 1820s, a time generally considered the heyday of mixed farms and soil fertility in the United States.

We walked up to the area where fifty Ossabaws were kept enclosed in temporary fencing. These were descendants of the small herd Lehr Brisbin had removed from Ossabaw Island. After the pigs had undergone a half-year quarantine at the University of Missouri, MacLean was one of two farmers to receive a small herd. Tank Jackson of Holy City Hogs would later get his pigs directly from her.

"They're the epitome of slow food," said MacLean. "I don't even take these guys to slaughter until two years." She looked fondly at a sow standing next to a small wooden Quonset hut that served as a sty. "Look at the curly coat. Some of them are smooth; some are naked. But all the blubber they've got keeps them warm through the winter." In the cold months, she feeds her hogs on corn, whole-roasted soybeans, and barley. "In the warm season, which is long here, they're out under the trees, around the creek, eating acorns."

MacLean sold her meat at the Carrboro Farmers' Market and made ends meet by hosting weddings in the barn. MacLean had raised her two children, now in their twenties, as a single mother; a rotating cast of young cousins pitched in on the farm. The work was hard, but it clearly fulfilled her.

Cane Creek was a corrective to the CAFOS I'd seen in the eastern part of North Carolina. It was a truly diversified farm and a real-life example of regenerative agriculture, which seeks to rehabilitate land by improving the water cycle, sequestering carbon, and increasing biodiversity. Rather than impoverishing the soil, MacLean was reviving it. Nor was she poisoning the water and the air of her neighbors. Her farm was an ark, a living gene bank of breed diversity. By keeping Ossabaws alive, in an environment close to the one in which they'd evolved, MacLean was providing living backup for an industrial food system on shakier ground than most people realize. Seventy years ago, a staggering variety of pigs were raised by two million farmers in the United States. Now, only eight breeds dominate the CAFOS, led by Berkshires, Chester Whites, and Durocs, infused with the genes of fast-growing breeds from China.

In 2009, a new strain of the H1N1 influenza virus spread around the world. Russia and China temporarily banned pork imports, and hundreds of thousands of animals around the world were slaughtered. This outbreak of swine flu may have killed 284,000 people globally. It began in the Mexican village of La Gloria, where the virus made the leap to humans from a crowded factory farm—a CAFO—owned by a subsidiary of Smithfield Foods.

"THE INDUSTRIAL EATER," wrote the American poet and essayist Wendell Berry, "is one who no longer knows that eating is an agricultural act, who no longer knows or imagines the connections between eating and the land, and who is therefore necessarily passive and uncritical—in short, a victim."

It was because I didn't want to be a victim that, decades ago, I cut meat and poultry out of my everyday diet. According to the Food and Agriculture Organization of the United Nations, a female of average weight needs forty-five grams of protein a day, and a male needs fifty-five grams. (Athletes and people over the age of sixty-five require slightly more.) Almost all of that amount can easily be provided by vegetables and legumes. The average European consumes eighty-five grams, and an American gets more like one hundred. It's estimated that to meet the growing demand, global protein production will have to increase by 50 percent by 2050. If the global model of factory-farm production continues, that will mean a lot more pollution, and a lot more cruelty.

In my ten days in the South, I ate more meat than I normally would at home in a year. It was a strain on my wallet and on my digestion. But I didn't regret it. With the exception of the ribs and the barbecue, all the pork came from small farmers who gave their animals good lives. After years of noncarnivory, I've come to a place where I think it's ethical, and healthy, to eat meat raised this way. It's not a foundational part of my diet, but something I enjoy every now and then. For that reason, I'm willing to go out of my way for good meat and pay the true price for it when I find it.

In the end, I found what I was looking for. I flew back home with two packages of cured Ossabaw Island ham from Cane Creek in my bags. I've been promising it to myself for a while now, as a treat for finishing this chapter.

Eight pieces of thinly sliced ruby-red ham, each shot through with a snow-white layer of fat, circle the plate on the desk next to me. I've let them come to room temperature over a couple of hours, at the same time as a bottle of Rioja. I put the slice on my tongue, like a communion wafer. Not too salty, just a little bit sweet, and as the fat melts, and I take a mouthful of Spanish red, I feel a little shiver of pleasure go deep into my spine. It has been worth the wait.

4

CÁDIZ

The Quintessence
of Putrescence

FIFTEEN OR SO YEARS AGO, I had a culinary epiphany, one that changed the way I think about food. I lived alone at the time, and spaghetti tossed in the pan with puttanesca, the offensively named "whore-style" sauce of Italy, had become one of my stay-at-home staples, a reliably delicious way to make the most of the contents of my reliably ill-stocked pantry. I'd lightly sauté a clove or two of garlic, mash in whole tomatoes, then add plump black kalamata olives, capers that had been packed in coarse salt, and a handful of parsley or basil leaves. The secret, I soon discovered, was to wait until the last minute to throw in some finely chopped anchovies, and let them deliquesce in a pool of olive oil. The liquefied fillets seemed to enhance the sweetness of the tomatoes, while drawing the herbal and savory ingredients into a unified whole.

At the time, I was working on a book about the collapse of global fisheries, and my research was making it clear that rather than grinding up anchovies—and other small fish, like herring, anchoveta, and sardines—to make animal feed, we'd be better off using them to feed humans. Low in toxins, rich in omega-3 fatty acids, minerals, and B vitamins, and still abundant in the oceans, humble anchovies could also transform a hastily thrown-together sauce of canned tomatoes into a deeply flavored ragù worthy of an Italian *nonna*. For a little fish, that was a lot of things to love. It helped that the woman I was then courting—and whom I later married—liked my sauce, and the prospect of a deeply flavored puttanesca (that and a tub of caramel-cone ice cream) was often enough to lure her to my apartment for the evening.

I was already familiar with the century-old Japanese word *umami*. The idea that, along with sweet, sour, salty, and bitter, our mouths have receptors for a fifth taste—the yeasty, fishy, meaty flavor of foods rich in glutamic acid—made a lot of sense to me. I'd come to think that a turn of the pepper mill, a shake of smoked paprika, or a dash of Tabasco functioned like a piccolo or a clarinet, bringing the high notes to a dish. The savoriness of grated Parmesan, stewed mushrooms, or aged tamari, all umami flavors, were like the bass line undergirding the whole composition. It seemed fitting that the most potent imparters of umami—the ones that brought a big cello or double bass throb to cooking—were among the smallest fish in the sea.

There's a lesser-known Japanese term that describes the role flavorful small fish can play in cooking. *Kakushi-aji*, or "hidden taste," refers to something added to a dish to enhance the flavor of the main ingredients. Examples include the diaphanous bonito flakes that get shaved into miso broth, a bit of coffee or chocolate added to a curry sauce, or the splash of mirin—sweet wine made from glutinous rice—in a salad dressing. *Kakushi-aji* is the secret ingredient that brings harmony to the whole; its absence can reduce a complex stew, sauce, or soup to a gallimaufry of ill-annealed components. Omit the *kakushi-aji*—which is often, but not always, umami—and certain recipes just don't make sense.

The concept of *kakushi-aji* can also be applied to entire cuisines. Future anthropologists, should they be unfamiliar with the semisolid mammary secretions of domesticated ungulates, or the fruit of plants from the genus *Capsicum*, would puzzle over recipes by Escoffier or Prudhomme. Subtract butter and chile peppers, after all, and French Cordon Bleu and Cajun cooking become closed books.

I figured something similar was at work in our attitude toward ancient Roman cuisine, which, thanks to the tales of elite excess recounted by the satirists, has a reputation for being bizarre and unappetizing. The demented third-century emperor Heliogabalus was notorious for dining on camel's feet, rice sprinkled with pearls, and the coxcombs cut from living birds. Over the years, many historians have come to the conclusion that Roman palates were radically different from ours. Perhaps, the reasoning goes, living in crowded cities with open sewers, smoky kitchens, and spotty garbage collection left their palates so jaded they had to seek out extreme sensations. In the absence of evidence to the contrary, culinary historians have too often echoed the judgment of early Christian moralists. At best, Roman cuisine was off-puttingly alien; at worst, it was unhealthy, disgusting, and—like the pagans themselves—impossibly decadent.

Exhibit A was the mysterious sauce known as *garum*. Accounts of its manufacture describe mackerel, anchovies, sardines, or tuna being left to rot—blood, guts, and all—in open vats under the Mediterranean sun for up to three months. The contemporary scholarly consensus was summed up by the Italian classicist Ugo Paoli, who concluded, "Our stomachs would probably revolt at a dish prepared with *garum*." (One modern commentator has even made the tortuous argument that Romans used *garum* in spite of its rotten taste, as a way of being accepted into some elite "bad food club.") The near ubiquity of *garum* in recipes was offered as further proof of the unknowable foreignness of ancient palates.

I had a hunch that, far from being revolting, *garum* was actually pretty tasty. After all, nobody, not even the Romans, would spend close to a millennium choking down a sauce if they didn't like it. What if a few drops of *garum* was the *kakushi-aji* of ancient Roman cookbooks, the ingredient—like the pat of butter sizzling in a French saucepan—whose presence unlocked the secret of an entire cuisine?

Which is why, when I learned that a team at the University of Cádiz had used organic remains discovered at sites in Spain and Italy to make what they claimed was the first modern archaeological re-creation of *garum*, I decided that, one way or another, I was going to get my hands on a bottle of Flor de Garum.

The quickest way to do so, it turned out, was to go to Spain.

I KNEW RIGHT AWAY that I was going to like Cádiz. The Andalucían city was a paradise for what Plutarch or Xenophon would have called an *opsophagos*,* a person who—like me—prizes fish and seafood above all other foods.

Founded as Gadir at the beginning of the first millennium BCE, and considered the oldest continuously inhabited city in western Europe, Cádiz's character seemed entirely determined by the waters that surround and sustain it. Over a hundred *miradores*—domestic lookout towers—rise above flat white roofs, as if the neoclassical merchants' homes were craning their necks above the city walls for a glimpse of caravels returning laden with New World treasure. The bollards that protect the corners of buildings from the impacts of traffic are actually the upended barrels of cannons, salvaged from sunken ships. The heart of the city is occupied by the Mercado Central, built in what were once the gardens of a convent. At the market's gates, sunburned old men shucked flat-shelled oysters on card tables, while

---

* "*Opson* together with its diminutive *opsarion*," wrote James Davidson in *Courtesans and Fishcakes*, his study of the gastronomic culture of classical Athens, "were perfectly commonplace words for fish, not smoked, and not necessarily cooked, but certainly in dire danger of being, since they corresponded to *ichtus* as pork does to pig, referring to fish as food." I prefer *opsophagos* to the cod-Latinate *piscivore*, or the sniffy-sounding *pescatarian*.

the vendors within shouted over displays of mottled cuttlefish and ruby-red pyramids of tuna flesh; beneath the arcades, people sat on stools washing down the roe of freshly cracked sea urchins with swigs of sweet vermouth. Paving stones are made from *piedra ostionera*, a porous locally quarried sandstone studded with the shells of ancient oysters. There were times I had the feeling the entire city had been hoisted, still wet and gleaming, from the bottom of the ocean.

In Roman times, Cádiz was a series of islands, and though the old city is now linked to the mainland by a man-made causeway, every street still ends in water. The water in question belongs not to the Mediterranean but the Atlantic. The Bay of Cádiz is located just west of Gibraltar, where the mandibles of the Iberian Peninsula and North Africa clamp together, a geographic fact that forces shoals of fish close to shore. Extensive saltwater marshes made the Cádiz region a natural site for the development of salterns, the gleaming white flats where seawater has been sun-dried into edible salt flakes since pre-Roman times.

The first to exploit this happy confluence of calm haven, near-shore fish stocks, and abundant salt were the Phoenicians, who preferred to build their cities on promontories, reefs, and offshore islands. The Phoenicians get second billing to the more warlike Spartans and Romans, and that is a shame, because for almost three millennia they projected a different kind of power, one based on adaptability and commerce rather than brute force. From their early Neolithic origins in Byblos, a coastal village sheltered by the Mount Lebanon range from land-based marauders, they made themselves masters of the sea. Originally fishermen, the Phoenicians learned to fell and shape the massive cedars of Lebanon, trading them to the timber-hungry Egyptians for precious metals, and helped the Hebrews raise Solomon's Temple. Rather than masculine war gods, they worshipped a pantheon topped by Baalat Gebal—"Our Lady of Byblos," or Mother Nature—and seem to have decided early on that adaptability, tolerance, and open-mindedness, rather than conquest, would be their road to prosperity.*

More focused on accumulating wealth than territory, the Phoenicians used their forests to build cargo ships capable of carrying fifty-ton payloads, eventually filling, in the words of one writer, a "crucial niche role as the logistics experts of the Near Eastern luxury-goods market." They transformed the olives and grapes on the coast of the Levant into oil and wine that was minutely subdivided into brands, vintages, and terroirs. It was the Phoenicians of Tyre who founded Carthage, near modern-day Tunis, a culture Roman writers referred to, disparagingly, as "Punic." And it was the Carthaginian general Hannibal who led his elephants across the Alps, one of the more memorable episodes in the series of wars Carthage waged, and lost, with the Romans for mastery of the Mediterranean. According to the Greco-Roman geographer Strabo, Gadir, the future Cádiz, was founded by settlers from Tyre in 1104 BCE, though firm archaeological evidence of Phoenician presence doesn't appear until three centuries later.

I paid a visit to the Museo de Cádiz, located in a former convent in the Plaza de Mina. The centerpiece of the museum's archaeological collections is a pair of funerary marbles, a female figure sculpted with a perfume vessel in her left hand, lying next to a bearded male clutching a pomegranate-like fruit. The Phoenicians, who spoke a Semitic language related to Hebrew, were a product of the eastern Mediterranean, and it was striking to see these massive Egyptian-style sarcophagi so far west, on Atlantic shores. The collection's display cases were filled with terracotta fragments covered with inscriptions;

---

* The Phoenicians also have a dire reputation for being decadent child murderers. The Carthaginians in particular stand accused of placing living children into the extended arms of the statue of Baal, from which they plunged into a fiery furnace below. Such sacrifices appear to have occurred over a couple of hundred years of their three-millennia-long history and were largely limited to Carthage. The Phoenicians' penchant for secrecy, motivated by their need to avoid risky displays of their considerable wealth, probably contributed to their ill repute.

the Phoenicians invented most of the letters that served as the basis for the Greek and Roman alphabets. They set about trading olive oil, wine, ivory, and their purple-dyed textiles with the indigenous Iberians, who they also taught to extract, process, and refine silver.

By the sixth century BCE, a new industry had supplanted the trade in precious metals. Phoenician fishermen had always used salt to preserve their catch. In addition to shipyards, saltworks, and kilns for firing amphorae, excavations of Punic-Phoenician sites around Cádiz have uncovered one-story buildings with basins that were used to marinate fish in brine. Fifth-century BCE pottery from Cádiz containing tuna vertebrae has been discovered in faraway Corinth, Greece, and is considered the earliest evidence for a Mediterranean-wide trade in salted fish.

Did the Phoenicians invent *garum*? There would have been ample opportunities to salt small fish in rock pools on the sweltering shorefronts of the Levant. But there is no solid archaeological evidence they manufactured fermented fish sauce on a large scale. The Phoenicians themselves remain frustratingly silent on this, as on almost all subjects; they left thousands of temple inscriptions but no literature to speak of. The history of *garum* would be written by the victors—in this case the Romans, whose defeat of an army of Punic soldiers and elephants near Seville, inland from Cádiz, cleared the way for the occupation of Spain. By 146 BCE, the Punic-Phoenician city of Carthage had been razed by the Romans. No longer dominated by the ocean-loving "princes of the sea," the Mediterranean became the *mare nostrum* of the inheritors of Romulus and Remus. Spain became the Roman province of Hispania Baetica, and Gadir was renamed Gades.

Oddly enough, it was not the seafaring people from Byblos who would create an empire-wide trade in fish sauce, but the bellicose agriculturalists of Rome.

TWO THOUSAND YEARS LATER, *garum* was once more being made in Cádiz, and I was eager to get a taste. Outside a modern building, the permanent home of the city's celebrated Tía Norica puppet theater, I met Victor Palacios, the chemical engineer at the University of Cádiz responsible for manufacturing Flor de Garum, and Manuel Béjar, the director of Majuelo, the company that bottles the sauce. I followed them down flights of stairs to an archaeological site excavated as the building was rising in the 1990s. A rehearsal was taking place in the amphitheater above, and the echo of muffled voices brought an otherworldly touch to the gloomy cellars. At the lowest level, thirty feet beneath the cobblestones, were the stone walls of eight Phoenician homes, dating from the eighth century BCE. Béjar pointed out the foundations of a beehive-shaped clay oven, like the ones I'd seen in Çatalhöyük, and the saddle querns that would have been used to grind grain. In one of the passages between the homes, the footprints of oxen were visible, as was a tiny skeleton: the bones of a 2,800-year-old alley cat. When the new Roman rulers moved in after the fall of Carthage, this Phoenician residential district became an industrial zone for salting fish. From a gangplank, we gazed down at two rows of vats that had served as the heart of a *garum*-producing complex until the second century CE. Each of the eight vats was large enough to hold 2,750 gallons of salted fish.

"The tanks were lined with *opus signinum*," explained Béjar. Broken bits of ceramic were mixed with mortar, compacted with a ramrod, and allowed to harden, producing a waterproof lining. "They would alternate layers of fish with salt and aromatic Mediterranean herbs, at a ratio of about three parts fish to one part salt."

Outside the theater, the pair led me past the central market through the Plaza de las Flores, a municipal square whose air was perfumed by the flowers sold from outdoor kiosks. Two thousand years ago, Béjar pointed out, the odor would have been unbearable, especially in hot weather.

"This whole area, twenty-five acres approximately, was an immense factory for salting fish. We've discovered the remains of bonfires of pine branches, which were used to burn the remains of tuna, but also to cover up the smell of rotting fish." We paused next to a statue of a toga-wearing man with a sickle in his right hand. This was Columella, whose twelve-volume *De re rustica* ("On all things rural") is one of the most complete surviving works on Roman agriculture.

"Columella was born in Cádiz," said Béjar. "He may have been of Phoenician background. His work was so influential that European systems for producing wine and olive oil hardly changed from the time of Augustus until the nineteenth century."

We walked for a few more minutes, and Béjar unlocked a door to a storefront that was used as an event space for tastings of what his company called "Arqueofood." Balbo et Columela offered visitors a menu that included a Neolithic Iberian beer made from wheat and sagebrush, tapas-sized portions of sausages cured following Columella's recipes, and a goat cheese fermented with the Roman honey-wine known as *mulsum*. Béjar pulled a rubber stopper from a 3.5-ounce glass bottle of Flor de Garum and poured a few drops of the amber liquid into a plastic spoon. I took a sniff—it was a little fishy, like the oil from a freshly opened can of sardines, but certainly not rotten-smelling—then put some on my tongue and rolled it around in my mouth.

There it was: that umami taste I recognized from melting anchovies in sauce. But this seemed even more concentrated, with the kind of herbal undertone you get from throwing a bouquet garni into broth. It was also very salty, in a way that overwhelmed my palate. Béjar opened another bottle and poured out a trickle of *oxygarum*, a product based on ancient recipes that blended *garum* and vinegar. The sweet acidity of the sherry vinegar balanced the salty *garum*; *oxygarum* would have made a perfect ready-made dressing for a Caesar salad. Béjar laid out some appetizers, and we spooned up a tapenade made with dark Manzanilla olives mashed with Flor de Garum, then tried a dollop of *atún en manteca*—a Cádiz specialty that combines chunks of yellowfin tuna with lard—topped with little transparent spheres resembling fish eggs, each filled with a drop of *oxygarum.* I told them the *garum* seemed to supercharge these already savory dishes.

"Our *garum* is very salty, very concentrated, very powerful," Palacios agreed. "But the aromatic herbs, which Romans loved to cook with, make it distinct from other fish sauces. When Japanese clients try our *garum*, they call it the 'umami of the Mediterranean.'"

Béjar explained that while remains of *garum* factories, like the one we visited beneath the theater, have been found from Turkey to northwest France, intact organic remains were harder to come by. The breakthrough occurred in 2011, when Italian researchers examined sealed dolia (large clay storage containers) in a structure long known as the Bottega del Garum of Pompeii. Mount Vesuvius's eruption buried the villa under six feet of volcanic ash, perfectly preserving a small urban factory just as it was salting down a late-summer catch of locally fished picarels.

The following day, I rode a bus to the University of Cádiz. In the campus's food technology lab, Palacios showed me a petri dish filled with gritty grayish-brown powder, a sample of the charred fish bones sent by Italian researchers from Pompeii. Using a gas chromatograph and a scanning electron microscope, his team was able to identify the species of fish—a mix of anchovies, sardines, and picarels—and, through pollen analysis, the families of aromatic herbs that had been found in the dolia. The signatures seemed to correspond to the mint, sage, thyme, and oregano listed in a Latin text by Gargilius Martialis, one of the handful of fish-sauce recipes in the classical literature. Gargilius calls for small oily fish—their heads and viscera intact—to be layered between herbs and salt. Palacios showed me the large glass vessels used to ferment the fish. This was a concession to modernity, he explained, that allowed them to avoid fluctuations in temperature, which was kept between 94 and 105 degrees Fahrenheit.

"We bought the anchovies fresh, from fishing boats at a local pier," Palacios explained. "We used three parts fish for one part salt. The conditions were very stable."

When small fish start to decay, the bacterial flora in their guts burst through cell walls, initiating a process known as autolysis. The fish essentially digest themselves, as the proteins in muscle tissue liquefy into oligopeptides and amino acids. Salt slows down this fermentation process, promoting lactic acid bacteria that defeat pathogens and such foul-smelling toxins as cadaverine and putrescine. (Too much salt stops autolysis altogether; too little invites botulism.) Palacios's team monitored the nitrogen content, which correlates to the proportion of protein in the final sauce; after twenty-five days, the fish had become a paste of dissolved bones and flesh topped by a salty amber-hued liquid. The sauce proved to be especially rich in glutamic acid, the amino acid that stimulates the mouth's umami receptors.

"The first time we made it," Palacios recalled, "it came out perfectly. We saw that there was almost a complete fermentation, similar to the levels of organic nitrogen you get in Asian fish sauces."

The real test, Palacios knew, would come in the kitchen. Fortunately, as I was about to discover, Cádiz was full of chefs who were delighted by the idea of cooking with *garum*.

I'D SPENT A FEW DAYS WANDERING CÁDIZ in a happy, jet-lagged daze, remembering how much I loved the no-fuss approach to eating and drinking that prevails in Spain. You belly up to the bar, order a *caña* of beer or a glass of sherry, and then the tapas start to arrive, with the total recorded on the counter in front of you with a chunk of white chalk. I became a regular at the Casa Manteca ("House of Lard"), whose walls were covered with black-and-white photos of matadors—as well as a portrait of the Fascist dictator Franco, hung upside down—where clients peeled *chicharrones*, translucent cuts of fat-marbled pork, from rectangles of wax paper and washed them down with swigs of Cruzcampo beer.

To see how *garum* was being used by local chefs, I knew I'd have to visit Cádiz's more formal restaurants. I called up El Faro, famous for its authoritative takes on Andalucían seafood classics, and explained what I was doing. The young chef, Mario Jiménez, greeted me at the door; he admitted that, inspired by the challenge, he'd lain awake the night before planning an entire tasting menu built around *garum*.

Jiménez explained that El Faro was a Cádiz institution; he was the third generation to cook there. He wasn't allowed to change the recipe for the house specialty, *tortellita de camarones*—a lacy fritter of tiny translucent shrimp that resembles an omelet with eyes—which his grandfather had made when El Faro opened as a waterfront tavern in 1964. Jiménez's training at the Culinary Institute of America, where he'd gone to study the use of seaweed, had actually made him *more* cautious about incorporating outside influences into his cooking.

"I don't have any fusion food on the menu. No ceviche, no *tataki*, no wakame. Because wakame is not from here." I noticed Jiménez had a single tattoo on his right bicep. It was an image of a *faro*—Spanish for lighthouse—with the words "Just a calm evolution" inked beneath it.

"For me, the level of salt is key to cooking," Jiménez said. "If you add soy sauce or other Asian ingredients to a cut of tuna belly, all you taste is soy sauce. With a few drops of *garum*, it's a different experience." Jiménez believed *garum* was the Roman way of salting food; few surviving recipes mention salt at all, while the majority stipulate some form of *garum*. "It opens your mouth to other flavors. My idea is to make people eat *garum* without *knowing* they are eating *garum*."

Over the next two hours, I was treated to a spectacular tasting menu, every course of which contained Flor de Garum as its *kakushi-aji*. It began with a single dollop of ice cream covered with shavings of black truffle, resting in a pool of extra-virgin olive oil; Jiménez invited me to try the ice cream first—it was blended with a few drops of *garum*, and just barely sweetened—and then mix it with the oil. It was followed by an upturned sea urchin, spines nestled in a bed of coarse salt, whose apricot-hued roe was surrounded by a prawn tartare made with *garum*, from which protruded three delicate spikes of sea asparagus. Jiménez came to the table to prepare one of his grandfather's signature dishes, marinated sea bass with oysters. Instead of "cooking" the raw fish in lemon, like a ceviche, he let it soak for a minute or two on the table in a bowl of *oxygarum*.

"The vinegar in the *oxygarum* changes the color," he said, showing me how the acidic marinade had whitened the sea bass loins, which he then laid atop a tartare of oyster flesh.

Even the *pan con chocolate y aceite*, a traditional Andalucían dessert made with dry bread and olive oil, incorporated *garum*; Jiménez had made the chocolate ganache, which he topped with dewfish roe, using a special *garum* made from bluefin tuna. Rather than overpowering the sweet and savory flavors, the fish sauce intensified and united them. *Garum* seemed to subject each dish to the culinary equivalent of italicization.

When I mentioned to Jiménez that the team at Copenhagen's Noma had recently published a recipe for a *garum* made out of fermented crickets, he shuddered, scandalized by Nordic enormities. "You know, chefs today think they are very smart," he said. "But we are not even 10 percent as smart as the Romans were two thousand years ago! We can use Google to look up recipes for kimchi foam and—cricket sauce. But here in Cádiz, we've always had the fish, the salt, the sun, the *garum*. It's just that not enough people today have the personality to say, 'I will stop here, and use the ingredients that we have here.'"

HOW DIFFERENT ALL THIS WOULD LOOK, I thought to myself, had Hannibal pushed on and succeeded in riding his elephants into Rome.

I was walking along an ancient Roman road, at the site of the ancient city called Baelo Claudia, an hour's drive southeast of Cádiz. Beyond the listing columns of the ruins of its forum, I could see the sands of Bolonia beach, whose sheltered coves, isolated behind coastal mountains, make it a favored spot for nude sunbathing. Just over the horizon lay the Moroccan city of Tangier, which, when it was known as Tingis, had provided the bricks for the Roman outpost's bathhouse. Some of the building materials are still scattered around the wrecks of cargo ships, whose silhouettes are visible as dark patches on the seabed just offshore.

Had classical antiquity been dominated by the Phoenicians rather than the Romans, the temples here might have been raised not to Jupiter and Minerva but to Our Lady of Byblos. Whoever lived here, though, the commercial heart of Baelo Claudia would likely have been the same: a complex of concrete vats near the shore, built for the express purpose of salting down tuna and mackerel hauled from the Strait of Gibraltar.

Why was salted fish such an obsession for the ancients, so much so that an entire industry was marshaled to produce and transport a pungent fish sauce? After all, the Romans were not people of the sea. The great cities of the Greek world—Athens, Sparta, Corinth, Syracuse, Rhodes—had gathered on the shores of the Mediterranean, as Plato put it, "like frogs around a pond." Rome, in contrast, was founded by Iron Age farmers, inheritors of Villanovan and Etruscan cultures, who settled on the hills overlooking the Tiber River, a long day's march from the sea. They thought of themselves as growers of grain, cultivators of grapevines, and pressers of olives, and saw nomadic pastoralists as slothful and barbaric. (My paternal-side origins in what's now Ukraine would have made me a contemptible Scythian: a drinker of milk and eater of raw flesh, and a herder of goat, sheep, or cattle.) Fisherpeople were generally regarded as abject maritime foragers, useful only for the food they hauled from the sea.

The story of Rome's founding, traditionally dated to 753 BCE, reveals much about the Romans' self-image as unspoiled agriculturalists. According to legend, Romulus and Remus were abandoned by their mother, a virgin priestess who had been impregnated by the disembodied phallus of Mars, the god of war, which rose from a sacred fire. After being suckled by a she-wolf, the twins were raised by a kindly shepherd, who taught them to herd animals and hunt. But then Romulus became a farmer, choosing for his domus—his settled homestead—the Palatine Hill, where he marked out his plot by plowing a boundary. This was the pomerium, the boundary, consecrated by augury, that would later surround every Roman settlement. When Remus contemptuously leapt over this paltry barrier, Romulus felled him with a powerful blow, declaring, "So perish anyone else who shall leap over my walls!"

"Wolf's milk, exile, and fratricide were an unusual ancestry," historian Robin Lane Fox has noted. (As is divine rape by fiery penis.) The real point of Romulus and Remus, anthropologically speaking, is that the Roman origin story involved drawing a boundary around an agricultural safe zone, beyond which lay savagery. Romulus divided the new state into two-acre parcels, which his followers could cultivate for themselves, and the subsequent history of the empire involved the relentless expansion of the pomerium of "civilization" into the *agrios*, the savage wilds, the realm of the meat-and-milk-consuming barbarians: Huns, Gauls, Goths, and my ancestors, the no-good Scythians. Forests and steppes won from barbarous nomads were turned into farmland and handed over to army veterans as a reward for their service. At the height of the empire, the pomerium stretched from Syria to the British Isles. Eventually, Rome itself became a machine powered by institutionalized slavery for bringing grain from Egypt, Sicily, and Sardinia, olive oil from Spain, and wine from Gaul back to the domus.

While Romans styled themselves honest eaters of the products of the land, their elite gastronomic culture was inherited from the seafood-loving Greeks. The first reference to a fermented fish sauce comes from the fifth century BCE, when Sophocles mentions a preserved fish *garos* in a satyr play; in a comic fragment, Plato jokes, "They are going to choke me to death by dipping me in rotten *garos*." The sauce, Latinized as *garum*, was probably first introduced to the gourmands of Rome by Greek chefs in the second century BCE.

"Captive Greece took captive her fierce captor," the satirist Horace would ironize a century later, "and brought culture to the rustic Latin lands." Appreciation of fish and seafood became a marker of wealth and culture among the Hellenized elite, who valued live fish for their freshness. In the villas of Baiae, near modern-day Naples, carnivorous morays were cultivated in fishponds; the livers of eels fed on human flesh were said to be particularly prized. In Petronius's *Satyricon*, nouveau riche Trimalchio awes his guests by setting his table with statues from which streams of peppered *garum* pour over living fish. By the time of the Emperor Vespasian, in the first century CE, Pliny the Elder reports that a pint of the highest-quality *garum* from Spain was worth eighty sesterces, as much as the most expensive perfume.

Garum's popularity among the elite made it a target for moralists. For the Stoic philosopher Seneca, *garum* was an "expensive bloody mass of decayed fish [that] consumes the stomach with its salty rottenness." Romans, by extension, ate a simple land-based diet of bread, stews made with lentils and fava beans, root vegetables, and small amounts of meat, or subsisted on the gladiators' fattening gruel of barley and beans. Medieval scribes in Christian monasteries—happy to preserve texts that condemned pagan decadence—probably contributed to the perception of *garum* as putrid and corrupting.

The archaeology, though, shows that *garum* was much more than the fetish food of the Roman elite. In the absence of refrigeration, fish spoiled quickly, so most people had to make do with preserved fish, which was packed whole or cut into chunks between layers of salt in terracotta transport vessels. In display cases at Baelo Claudia's museum, I'd seen several barnacle-covered amphorae that had been salvaged intact from the seafloor. Marine archaeologists have discovered dozens of wrecks laden with terracotta *garum* containers on the seafloor; one of the largest, a hundred-foot-long merchant ship found off Alicante, was carrying 2,500 fish-sauce amphorae when it sank. In the Cádiz area, eight- to ten-gallon double-handled vessels dominate; they tend to have wide mouths, straight long necks, ovoid bellies, and spikes on their bottoms, which were pushed into sand in the holds of cargo ships to keep them stable. While the fish fermented in the amphorae, their bones settled into the hollow spike, with the wide mouth allowing the liquid that rose to the top—particles of muscle tissue that formed a fishy paste known as *allec*—to be scooped out. The bulbous belly contained bones and flesh that continued to ferment into sauce.

Over one hundred fish-salting factories, or *cetariae*, like the one at Baelo Claudia, have been excavated in Spain alone. The industry was conducted by private traders, free of government control, and supported by a privately managed merchant fleet. Sprat and herring were processed as far north as Ploumanac'h, on the Atlantic coast of France; there are records of soldiers posted at Hadrian's Wall in the province of Britannia requesting fish sauce in their rations.

The evidence from Pompeii, a relatively small city in the Italian provinces, reveals that people at all levels of society enjoyed fish sauce. Cooks and servants arrived at the Bottega del Garum carrying small one-handled ceramic vessels that were filled from the shop's oversized dolia, in which locally caught fish were left to ferment into *garum*. Most of the vessels in Pompeii are inscribed with the name of Aulus Umbricius Scaurus. Formerly enslaved, Scaurus used profits from the fish-sauce trade to build an impressive villa whose mosaic floors are tiled with images of *garum* amphorae labeled *Liqua Flos*.

Some of Scaurus's finest was almost certainly manufactured in Baelo Claudia. Leaning on a railing, I peered into a complex of ten sunken concrete vats, some square, some circular. Atlantic bluefin tuna, which can reach lengths of 16 feet and weights of 1,300 pounds, pass through the Straits of Gibraltar on the way to their summer spawning grounds near Mallorca. Off the shores of Baelo Claudia, they were caught using a Phoenician technique known as the *almadraba*, in which migrating schools were forced to swim through an elaborate maze of nets before being speared in the final "death chamber." After being hauled ashore, they were cleaned and butchered on the patio of the *cetaria*, then thrown into the vats with salt and herbs. (There is evidence the largest of these complexes, which held over 300,000 gallons, were used to salt down entire whales.) Baelo Claudia—which covered thirty acres, was fed by three aqueducts, and was large enough to support a still-intact amphitheater—was a one-industry town, devoted to the manufacture of *garum*.

By 390 CE, though, Baelo Claudia had been abandoned. What caused its downfall? Multiple earthquakes, whose impacts are recorded in the crooked paving stones of the road alongside the *cetaria*, may have initiated a decline that was further hastened by a recession that gripped the empire. But another phenomenon, all too familiar to us today, may have been at work: the collapse of the fisheries. Baelo Claudia was famous for producing two of the costliest forms of fish sauce: *garum sociorum* ("*garum* for friends"), made from mackerel, and *haimation*, made from the blood and viscera of bluefin tuna. Zooarchaeologists have found the size of the vertebrae and fish scales recovered at Baelo Claudia steadily decreased over the course of decades. By the third century, organic evidence shows most fish sauce was once again being made from anchovies, sardines, and other small fish. In their quest for powerful sensations, the epicures of Rome had driven the apex marine species of the Mediterranean to the brink.

Today, though the International Union for Conservation of Nature has declared Atlantic bluefin endangered, a small population continues to spawn in the Mediterranean. Southern Europeans have built something of a culinary cult around bluefin, similar to the one sworn to *o-toro* in the sushi bars of Tokyo. Bricks of salt-cured, sun-dried bluefin tuna loin are sliced thinly and fanned out on plates on the counters of Cádiz, to be drizzled with olive oil. *Mojama*, as it's known, was probably first prepared in a Phoenician fish-salting factory, like the one I'd visited beneath the cobblestones of Cádiz.

Just beyond the orange-lichen-spotted stones of the *garum* factory was a beachfront restaurant, shuttered for the winter. Next to it I could see some vats beneath a tarpaulin. This was where Victor Palacios and a team of Italian archaeologists were trying to re-create *haimation* following a recipe from *Geoponica*, a Byzantine-Greek agricultural manual, using conditions identical to those in Baelo Claudia two thousand years earlier. They'd allowed the blood and viscera of a fresh-caught bluefin tuna to ferment outdoors, at ambient temperatures, in concrete vats.

Things weren't going well, Palacios had told me. The Italian team was unable to perfect the formula for *opus signinum*, the ceramic mortar invented by the Romans. Worse, though, the autolysis was incomplete. After more than six months, the salted bluefin hadn't fermented into anything close to a palatable sauce.

I wasn't displeased that they'd failed to figure out the secret of making *haimation*. The beauty of *garum*, I figured, was the way it concentrated the Mediterranean down to its sensual and nutritional essence. The ancients had achieved this by harvesting tiny schooling fish, the renewable foundation of the marine ecosystem. Today, giant purse seiners are subjecting anchovy and sardine populations to intense pressure. For the most part, they're being caught not to feed humans but livestock. Catching these flavorful fish for direct human consumption is a far better use of the sea's resources.

On the other hand, slaughtering a thousand-plus-pound bluefin tuna to render it into sauce—no matter how tasty—struck me as being not just wrong. At the risk of sounding like a Stoical scold, it was downright decadent.

WHEN I LEFT CÁDIZ, my suitcase packed with carefully wrapped bottles of Flor de Garum, I was pretty sure I'd come as close as anyone alive today to tasting the secret sauce of ancient Rome.

I was wrong. What I had in Cádiz wasn't *garum*, but an entirely different substance known as *liquamen*.

The day before my flight, I met Darío Bernal-Casasola, a classical archaeologist at the University of Cádiz who'd overseen both the excavations at Baelo Claudia and the recovery of the organic remains from Pompeii. Bernal-Casasola, who also consulted on the development of Flor de Garum, urged me to keep the modern re-creation in context.

"You have to think of *garum* like wine," he told me. "If you ask me, do Spanish people today drink wine? The answer is ¡Sí!—almost all of us. But we don't all drink the same wine. *Garum* was the same for the Romans. The emperor ate *garum*. The legionaries ate *garum*. The slaves ate *garum*. There was a huge diversity of varieties." Bernal-Casasola said the modern version, made from sardines and anchovies, would have corresponded to a medium-quality, household variety of fish sauce.

"This is the first time in modern history," he continued, "that a scientific reconstruction of *garum* has been attempted. But Flor de Garum isn't the *garum* of Cádiz. It's the *garum* they were making at the Bottega del Garum in Pompeii on August the twenty-fourth, 79 CE, the day Vesuvius erupted. Or, I should say, the closest we can approach to it. Because we can't be sure which herbs they were using, the proportions, or *exactly* which recipe they were following."

The biomolecular archaeologists who analyzed the remains from Pompeii, he pointed out, had only been able to identify some of the fish and plant species found in the dolia. "On American crime shows, they take a sample, they put them in a gas chromatograph, and they say, 'This is paint, this is blood.' That can't be done with ancient samples. The product had degraded over two thousand years. There are many opportunities for contamination."

But back home, as I began to cook with fish sauce in my own kitchen, this seemed like so much—you'll pardon the pun—carping. My sons, who made it clear they did not appreciate the odor of Flor de Garum heating in the pan, were puzzled by their father's latest obsession. But when I made two versions of one of Desmond's favorite winter meals, French onion soup, he asked for a second helping of the broth simmered with the *garum*. I added a tablespoon to a head of salted napa cabbage and Korean red chile flakes, and the result, after ten days of fermentation, was a spectacular Silk Road kimchi, a perfect union of Ancient Rome and the Far East. Flor de Garum made my sauces even better, imparting a herbal, umami intensity to my puttanesca. Though I didn't always tell my wife and kids I was using it, Flor de Garum became the reliable *kakushi-aji* in what they agreed were some of my tastiest meals.

Still, I couldn't shake the feeling that Flor de Garum wasn't as authentic as I'd thought. For one thing, it seemed very salty, so much so that a few drops too many could ruin a dish. I decided to share my concerns with Sally Grainger, a British researcher who had published several authoritative articles on the complex terminology of fish sauces. My timing, it turned out, was excellent: she was working on the final copy edit of *The Story of Garum*, a 300-page book on the archaeology, epigraphy, and ceramics of fish sauce.

"The team in Cádiz think fish sauce is Roman," Grainger told me, over a video call from her home in East Hampshire. "It's *not*. It's Greek. It was the Greeks who taught the Romans how to use it. Then the Romans took fish sauce and enthusiastically ran with it. They made an expensive sauce from fermented mackerel and tuna, which became known as *garum*. But that is not the *essential substance*."

Grainger worked as head pastry chef at London's Athenaeum Hotel before getting a degree in classical archaeology, and she now demonstrates Roman cooking techniques on YouTube from a kitchen she's set up in her garden. I'd come to think of her as the Julia Child of ancient gastronomy: she was genially pedantic, charmingly scattered, and genuinely authoritative.

Too many modern researchers, Grainger told me, subscribe to the "single-sauce hypothesis." She believes that what we call *garum* was actually two different sauces. The one described in the elite literature was a nearly opaque sauce made from blood and viscera, like the one manufactured in Baelo Claudia. This "black-and-bloody" sauce, as Grainger calls it, was served as a condiment for cooked foods, much like ketchup or sriracha is today. (This was the *garum* that would have poured freely from the statues on Trimalchio's table in *Satyricon*.) Behind kitchen doors, though, enslaved chefs cooked with a less costly sauce—one that many elite writers might not even have known existed—made from small fish. This was the "essential substance," the one the Greeks had originally called *garos*. To distinguish it from the black-and-bloody sauce, merchants renamed it *liquamen*, the trade name inscribed on many amphorae.

"What the team in Cádiz made is actually the essential substance, *liquamen*," Grainger told me. "They chose a recipe which was designed for making small batches in home kitchens, and which uses too much salt, as much as three parts for one part of fish. Other recipes, for bulk production, call for much less: seven buckets of fish for one bucket of salt." She was of the opinion that the Cádiz team rushed the fermentation, which, according to most ancient recipes, took three months, rather than twenty days, at ambient temperatures of about 90 degrees Fahrenheit. She praised Flor de Garum as a worthwhile experiment, but hardly the last word in modern recreations. She recommended the work of Garum Lusitano, a team that was trying to re-create the sauce from remains found at Tróia, a site in southwest Portugal.*

Grainger had tried her hand at making both *garum* and *liquamen* with fresh-caught fish. After talking her way onto the boats of amateur fishermen in Portsmouth, she'd filled glass aquariums in her backyard greenhouse with chopped mackerel and salt, letting them ferment during the warmest months of summer. "I could only get a tablespoon or so of blood from the mackerel, and the result was weird—it was highly nutritious, but it tasted of iron. One of my sauces went bad, and the smell was abysmal. Gagging! But the *liquamen* I made with sardines worked out. Scientists told me not to eat them, because of the risk of botulism. I ate it anyway, and I served it to people. It was a great success!"

Inspired by her experiments, and with my own supply of Flor de Garum running low, I decided to make my own. I bought some

---

* The Garum Lusitano team eventually succeeded in producing a *haimation* sauce from bluefin tuna, which Grainger told me was excellent; they even named a version made from sardines "Special Edition Sally Grainger" in her honor.

frozen whole fish from a Portuguese supermarket; Grainger had advised me to look for sardines under four inches in length, sometimes called sprats. I weighed out an amount of sea salt—from one of Cádiz's original Roman salterns—corresponding to 20 percent of the weight of the fish. It was important, Grainger told me, to make two or three cuts into the fish, to expose their guts, which would allow the bacteria within to break down the muscle tissue as quickly as possible.

But a serious challenge faced me: a Canadian winter was coming on, which meant our apartment would never get hot enough for fermentation to occur. I decided to try a hack I'd found on a German website. By using a yogurt machine, I could keep a sealed container at relatively high temperatures for long periods of time. Gratifyingly, the sardines completely digested themselves: within three days, all that was left was a brownish-gray slurry atop a layer of bones and scales. When I sent Grainger a photo, though, she told me to chuck it. The yogurt machine's default setting, 110 degrees Fahrenheit, while perfect for thickening milk, was far too high for fish sauce.

"You've cooked it," she told me. "The autolysis of the proteins will never be complete. You have to remember that *garum* is slow food."

I started another batch. This time, I invested in a plant propagator—basically an electrified rubber mat with a thermostat, the kind used to encourage seedlings or keep a pet iguana comfortable—which I placed in the insulated plastic cooler our family takes on camping trips. I put the sealed mason jar of salted sardines atop the mat, closed the cooler's lid, and set the thermostat for 90 degrees—a respectable Mediterranean summer temperature—vowing to myself that, apart from a daily shake to keep the fish and salt mixed, I wouldn't touch it for three months.

While I waited, I continued to investigate the role fish sauce played in ancient gastronomy. Much of what we know about Roman cuisine comes from the collection of recipes called *De re coquinaria*, or sometimes *Apicius*, after a wealthy first-century epicurean who famously hired a ship to take him to North Africa to confirm whether prawns there were better than those in his native Campania. (Apicius was probably a way of labeling someone a gourmet, as we call a lover a Romeo, or a miser a Scrooge.) The recipes, composed in Vulgar Latin, were almost certainly compiled by enslaved cooks between the first and fifth centuries. Almost two-thirds of the 465 recipes list *liquamen* as an ingredient. (*Garum* is mentioned on only two occasions, salt not at all.) In their brevity, they reminded me of Louis Saulnier's *Répertoire de la Cuisine*, a handbook for French Cordon Bleu chefs that manages to compress six thousand recipes into just over two hundred densely packed pages. To give you an idea, here's the complete text of Apicius's recipe for stuffed sea urchins:

> After boiling cleaned sea urchins, place them in a frying pan with leaves [what kind, we're not told], pepper, honey, *liquamen*, a little oil, and an egg, and then cook them again in a bain-marie, before serving them with a sprinkling of [more] pepper.

Not much, in other words, for the modern chef to go on. Fortunately, Grainger had published a translation of the compilation; using her *Cooking Apicius* as a handbook, I began to assemble an ancient Roman pantry, or the closest I could get in twenty-first-century Montreal. A bottle of Muscat from Greece would stand in for *passum*, or aged raisin wine; I improvised the syrup known as *defrutum* by slowly simmering red grape juice with dried figs. Mediterranean herbs were harder to come by; locally grown Scots lovage (*Ligusticum scoticum*) would have to stand in for lovage (*Levisticum officinale*). Rue, a bitter and mildly toxic herb with a pleasingly funky aroma, came from the garden of a woman in our neighborhood who grows it to keep the squirrels away from her tomatoes.

For several weeks, my family put up with late dinnertimes as I tried to wrangle obscure and unfamiliar ingredients into nutritious meals acceptable to two picky boys. A lentil and leek pottage (Apicius 5.2.3) made with mint, honey, coriander, rue, and a tablespoon of *defrutum* was judged interesting, if a little weird, by Desmond. I found it an unexpected but delicious mix of sweet, salty, herbal, and savory. (Victor took one look, pushed it away, and demanded more of the macaroni I'd cooked as a backup.) But the real family-pleasers were the *patinae*, omelet-like dishes made by combining beaten eggs with fish, mushrooms, spinach, nettles, and other ingredients; the one our boys most approved of (Apicius 5.3.4) was a combination of whole and mushy peas with a touch of coriander and lovage, oven-baked in a cast-iron pan like a frittata.

All of these dishes involved fish sauce. A splash of Flor de Garum turned every *patina* I made from blandly eggy to richly flavored. I decided to make an *oenogarum*, heating vinegar, red wine, honey, Flor de Garum, and caraway seeds, and thickening it with a cornstarch and butter roux. The result was a purple-hued sauce, which tasted like stewed plums; it was a hit with the kids on spelt-and-fava rissoles, and made a perfect sauce for baked sea bream or grilled branzino.

Grainger told me she saw *liquamen* as an umami unifier of flavors: "Roman food is highly spiced. It's sweet and sour; the sauces are very dense. But they can easily be acrid, bitter, and discordant. And what fish sauce does is bring it all to a balance, so nothing dominates, and all those subtle undertones of herbs and spices can come to the fore, in a harmonious whole."

One thing had been established beyond a doubt: there was nothing putrid, rotten, or inedible about Roman fish sauce. Used properly, it was delicious. As Grainger puts it in *The Story of Garum*, "Ancient fish sauce was a complex magical ingredient, that should no longer be a subject of jokes and innuendo but recognized for what it was; fundamental to an ancient Mediterranean cuisine, and used by virtually everyone in their daily lives."

I've come to suspect there was a reason for the obsession with fish sauce beyond its deliciousness—one that may explain why the ancients set up hundreds of *cetariae* on the shores of the Mediterranean. Fish sauce is rich in vitamin B12 and amino acids; it's been calculated that it provides up to 7.5 percent of the protein in contemporary Vietnamese diets. (Unfortunately, neither modern nor ancient fish sauces contain omega-3 fatty acids, which are destroyed in the fermentation process.) For the common people of the Roman Empire, whose diets were light in meat, it may have been the most reliable source of high-quality protein at their disposal.

The real attraction of *garum*, though, is the way it imbues foods with intensity, vivacity, even wildness—the exact qualities so often lost by the time agriculture manages to get food to our tables. The fact that urban elites in ancient Rome obsessed over this quintessence of the Mediterranean Sea makes perfect sense to me. Since Romulus plowed out his pomerium on the Palatine Hill, Romans had symbolically turned their backs on the wilds, opting instead for the world of the domus—the domesticated landscape centered on growing grain and grazing livestock. I suspect that many of them, safely ensconced in their villas, longed for the lost sensorial intensity available to the hunter-gatherers, the nomads, the fisherfolk—the people whose ways of life they were busy usurping. *Garum* may have been their way of reinjecting wildness into lives that had become distant from nature and divorced from the drama of the struggle for food, sex, and survival. Lives that had become, in a word, tame.

As a descendant of barbarous nomads long-since subjugated by the Romans—a citified Scythian whose own struggles with domesticity sometimes manifest in an atavistic longing to light out for the frontier—I thought I knew exactly how they felt.

FOR THE TIME BEING, I had a problem. My homemade *liquamen* was weeks from being ready, and my last bottle of Flor de Garum was nearly empty. With the exchange and shipping fees, importing a new stock from Cádiz could prove costly. I'd developed a fish sauce dependence; without it, my favorite dishes tasted flat and lifeless. This was one addiction, though, I wasn't inclined to kick. I needed to find a substitute, and fast.

I was cheered by the suggestion that *garum* had never actually disappeared. Many scholars have argued that it lives on, under different names, in a variety of preserved fish preparations. One candidate was *colatura di alici*, which has been made on the Amalfi Coast by Cistercian monks since the Middle Ages. I found a bottle in Montreal's Little Italy, and though it was promisingly amber and fragrant, on the tongue *colatura* proved to be an up-front assault of salt and fish, without much umami nuance. The problem, according to Grainger, is that *colatura*, though artisan-made in wooden barrels, uses anchovies that have been gutted, meaning that the flavor-building process of autolysis doesn't occur at all.

It turned out that I was looking on the wrong continent. I knew that Asians, longtime connoisseurs of umami, had their own traditions of making fish sauces. Although some scholars have speculated the Romans brought *garum* to East Asia overland via the Silk Road, Grainger points out there is absolutely no evidence for this. Instead, she subscribes to the "independent evolution" theory. "Salting fish can be seen as an intuitive practice," she has written, "which undoubtedly happened spontaneously on many a beach where early man fished with primitive equipment."

My own experiences with Asian fish sauces inclined me to agree. I'd tried *patis* from the Philippines, *nam pla* from Thailand, and *yu-lu* from China; most brands were industrially made, and because they were oversalted to cover the off-tastes of spoiling fish, they had to be corrected with sweeteners. To my surprise, Grainger offered a ringing endorsement of a brand of *nước mắm* from Vietnam, which she believed had an excellent claim to being an independently evolved Asian version of *garum*.

I contacted Red Boat's founder, Cuong Pham, a software engineer who came to California from Saigon as a child in the 1970s. He'd returned to Vietnam, where his mother's cousin once had a fish sauce factory, and discovered that Phú Quốc, an undeveloped island in the Gulf of Thailand, had a reputation for making the best.

"It all started because I just needed to get some fish sauce for my mom," he recalled, with a chuckle. "I realized Phú Quốc was the real deal." Cuong now owns two fish boats and produces 130,000 gallons of fish sauce for the world market a year. Fresh-caught anchovies are preserved in wooden barrels in sea salt and aged at ambient temperatures, which average 90 degrees Fahrenheit year-round. As Grainger points out, these are the same ingredients and conditions that would have produced high-quality Roman *liquamen*.

Cuong sent me samples of his fish sauce, which included two bottles of sauce aged in old bourbon barrels that had also been used to make maple syrup. This Phamily Reserve was rich and smoky, but what really impressed me was the premium sauce called 50°N (a reference to the nitrogen content; the more nitrogen, the more protein). As far as I could tell, it was identical to Flor de Garum—minus some of the herbal notes in the Spanish re-creation—and it brought the same intense umami quality to anything it was used in.

My hunt for the *kakushi-aji* was at an end. Until my own homemade *garum* was ready, Red Boat 50°N, made with a sustainable stock of anchovies from a well-managed artisanal fishery, would serve as my hidden umami ingredient.

It was a few weeks after I talked to Cuong Pham that Grainger—who is nothing if not thorough—reminded me that one mystery remained to be solved. Modern science had allowed us to analyze organic samples and re-create *liquamen*. But we still couldn't be sure what the "black-and-bloody" sauce—the one elite writers glorified as *haimation* or *garum sociorum*—tasted like.

Grainger left me with a lead. For at least three hundred years, a traditional sauce has been made in Japan's Ishikawa Prefecture from the fermented blood and viscera of squid. *Ishiri* is opaque, and the presence of blood imparts the same metallic taste Grainger detected in her attempts to make black-and-bloody sauce. *Ishiri* is not a cooking ingredient; like *garum sociorum*, it's meant to be used on finished dishes, as a condiment.

"After tasting it," Grainger reported, "I realized that it had many similarities with the black-and-bloody viscera sauce that is the true *garum*."

But when a friend's student shipped me some *ishiri* from Japan, I was disappointed. It arrived in soy-sauce-sized plastic bottles. The sauce was as black as squid ink, and the flavor was harsh and metallic. I've tried *ishiri* in many dishes and still haven't developed a taste for it. If *ishiri* is indeed *haimation*'s modern equivalent, it may be one Roman flavor that will always remain alien to me.

ONE DAY, as the buds were starting to appear on the maple branches outside our apartment, I decided I was ready to take my *liquamen* out of the camping cooler. The sardines had been reduced to a creamy brownish slurry, the color and consistency of gravy. Churning it up, I could see bones and scales floating in the chunky liquid. I took the mason jar out to our front balcony, to forestall further, and well-justified, recriminations from my family about nauseating odors. I poured the mess into a jelly strainer, a tripod with fine-meshed nylon suspended from it, and let the liquid *drip-drip-drip* into a bowl. As the bowl filled, I could see the liquid was a coruscating gold. Even after an hour of slow draining of the muck, it yielded only ten ounces of liquid. But that would be enough to last me for a couple of weeks.

And then, after taking a deep breath, I spooned up a few drops and let the liquid settle on my tongue. It was salty, beyond fishy-smelling, and—glorious. Richer than Flor de Garum, subtler than *nước mắm* or nam pla, fit for Trimalchio's table. My obsession had come to an end. Not only had I found the *kakushi-aji*, the hidden flavor of the ancients, now I knew how to make it myself.

5

YORKSHIRE DALES

Hard Cheese

I WATCHED AS THE PROCESSION OF CHEESES trundled past on the belt: a wedge of Coolea, a Gouda-style cheese from Ireland served with a hunk of clotted cream fudge, followed by a runny slice of Tunworth, then a carrot-hued triangle of Sparkenhoe Red Leicester. It took all my willpower to not lunge and grab them all, before anyone else could snatch them away.

I was sitting on a stool in London's Seven Dials Market, a cavernous brick building, once a Victorian-era warehouse for cucumbers and bananas, converted into a multistory venue where street-food vendors peddle their wares indoors year-round. Beneath glass domes, on plates color-coded from cream to red according to price, twenty varieties of British cheeses were borne at a stately pace along a 130-foot-long conveyor belt. It was as riveting, in its way, as gazing at an airport carousel in the hopes an errant piece of luggage would miraculously scroll by.

At regular intervals, a cheesemonger in a striped black-and-white smock would lower a cloche over a newly sliced wedge and add it to the parade. The belt looped back on itself, which gave you the opportunity, if you'd regretted not securing a morsel as it passed from right to left, to reach over and snag it on the return voyage. Provided, of course, one of your fellow turophiles (or cheese-lovers, as our breed is unfortunately known) seated around the counter hadn't beaten you to it.

I'd been prepared to dislike chef Mathew Carver's Pick & Cheese, which was modeled on the rotary sushi concept, popularized around the world by such chains as YO! Sushi and Moshi Moshi. Instead of salmon futomaki, each plate carried a different British cheese, paired with such well-chosen sides as apricot harissa, charred leeks, and shortbread. In my opinion, conveyor belts demean sushi—which, rather than being left to oxidize, ought to go straight from the master's hands to the guest's plate—but they seem well suited to cheese, which is best enjoyed at room temperature. Letting the cheese stand alone, perfectly portioned under a glass cloche, was an invitation to contemplate its essence.

Cheese is, after all, a miracle. From only three ingredients, an almost infinitely variegated range of flavors and odors can be manifested in solid and delicious form. Depending on how you manipulate them, salt, rennet, and the milk of a ruminant mammal can metamorphose into a dainty pyramid of spreadable young Valençay goat cheese, or a massive eighty-three-pound wheel of hard, savory Parmigiano-Reggiano. Like the finest of wines, a well-made cheese is a poem, in which formal constraints create the conditions for aesthetic transcendence.

I'd finally plucked three cheeses from the conveyor belt: a Sharpham Cremet from Devon, like the stanza of an amorous Shakespearean sonnet in double-creamy goat's milk; a Spenwood, a little haiku in sheep's milk, deceptively simple in its Pecorino-like melding of the salty and the sweet; and a truffled Baron Bigod, a Falstaffian limerick of a cheese made with the milk of Montbéliarde cows, which oozed, Brie-like, with peppery, mushroomy flavors. On the counter before me, this trio of verses-in-dairy, set next to a balloon of amber wine from Austria that caught the last failing rays of the evening sun, called to mind a still life from the Flemish Renaissance.

All right, I'm done. Forgive my lapse into vintage *Gourmet* magazine-era food porn—I'll try not to let it happen again—but I'm making a point about the way we talk about cheese in the English language. In Italy, Spain, Holland, and France, cheese is afforded a degree of gravitas. In English-speaking countries, people who take cheese seriously are suspected of fussiness, triviality, and—worst of all—sensuousness. In the United States, the land of spreadable Velveeta, rubbery Kraft Singles, and "cream cheese product," the subject is liable to conjure up images of Wisconsin's "cheeseheads," known for wearing foam-rubber triangles of Day-Glo orange Swiss cheese on their heads at Green Bay Packers' games.

In Britain, too, an aura of mirth surrounds the topic of cheese. The name Gloucester conjures the annual Cooper's Hill Cheese-Rolling and Wake in the village of Brockworth, where, every spring since 1826, thrill-seekers have tumbled after giant wheels of Double Gloucester rolled down a fifty-degree incline, often breaking bones in their pursuit. A wedge of mold-veined Stilton brings to mind G. D'Arcy "Stilton" Cheesewright, thick-necked nemesis to Bertie Wooster in P. G. Wodehouse's Jeeves stories, who has a penchant for blithering on about the cheese board at the Drones Club. And for many people, the names Red Leicester, Caerphilly, Lancashire, and Dorset Blue Vinny will trigger a recitation of Monty Python's Cheese Shop sketch, in which John Cleese unsuccessfully solicits forty-three cheeses from proprietor Henry Wensleydale, whose establishment's chief virtue is that it is uncontaminated by any actual cheese.

Which is why I found the approach taken by Pick & Cheese so refreshing. There was no cutesiness, no cheesy puns on the menu. To my surprise, though, there was also no sign of the cheese I'd crossed an ocean to find. Wensleydale, the oldest named cheese in England, has been made continuously in the Yorkshire Dales for over seven hundred years. It is senior to Cheddar, more venerable than Cheshire, and at least as old as Cantal, the oldest named cheese in France. Wensleydale has survived the dissolution of the monasteries under Henry VIII, the enclosures of the commons, the nineteenth-century industrialization of dairying, the rationing of the Second World War, and the buyouts of creameries by foreign multinationals. In his 1945 essay "In Defence of English Cooking," George Orwell, chafing under wartime austerity, recalled the glories of the nation's cuisine, among them dark plum cake, horseradish, Cox's Orange Pippin apples, and a select handful of British cheeses: "There are not many but I fancy Stilton is the best cheese of its kind in the world, with Wensleydale not far behind."

Its status as a national myth was forever cemented when, in a popular cartoon special, the cheese-loving inventor Wallace rode a Claymation rocket to the moon with his clever dog Gromit, and discovered that it tasted exactly like Wensleydale. Yet true farmhouse Wensleydale is all but unobtainable in Britain. The mini-truckles of crumbly, acidic, white Wensleydale retailed in supermarkets—often labeled with a likeness of a grinning Wallace and Gromit—bear virtually no resemblance to the full-flavored, unpasteurized, blue-veined cheese of yore.

The server at Pick & Cheese, who told me he had grown up eating cranberry-studded Wensleydale with Eccles cake at Christmas, said that, for the real thing, I should try the cheese shop around the corner. Coincidentally, it was named after Thomas Neal, the same man who had built the cucumber-and-banana warehouse now occupied by Pick & Cheese.

Which is how I found myself crossing a hidden courtyard in Covent Garden to Neal's Yard Dairy, the shop responsible for launching Britain's first modern artisanal cheese revival in the 1970s. On the counter sat two large cylinders of a cheese with mottled gray rinds, topped by precut wedges whose yellow paste showed through plastic cling wrap. At the eye-watering price of £51.90 per kilogram,

Stonebeck Wensleydale was by far the most expensive cheese in the shop. I inhaled deeply—taking in a lungful of that ineffable cheese-cellar odor of mold and curds—and asked the black-capped counterman to cut me three hundred grams.

Working out the conversion later, I realized it had set me back twenty bucks, the most I'd ever paid for a slice of cheese that thin in my life. I consoled myself that I had in my possession the rarest of curiosities: Britain's most ancient cheese, made from the milk of a now critically endangered breed of dairy cattle.

I was about to learn two important lessons. First, cheese is so changeable that, uniquely among foods, it may be impossible to re-create what it tasted like in the past. Second, I hadn't paid too much for Wensleydale at Neal's Yard. If anything, I'd actually been *undervaluing* the dairy I ate. As I was about to discover, we'd all be better off paying the true price for the animal protein we put on our plates.

WHOEVER YOU ARE, you should probably be eating more cheese, particularly of the farmhouse variety. Not only is it good for your body, it's also good for the planet. In fact, seeking out farmhouse cheese—which is simply cheese made on the same farm where the milk is collected—and making it a regular part of your diet is a readily attainable, very concrete step toward healing our broken agricultural systems.

Not convinced cheese will do you, and the world, good? Bear with me. Before the Neolithic agricultural revolution, our ancestors were unable to digest the lactose, a highly nutritious sugar, in milk after they'd reached adulthood. Babies thrive on breast milk because their stomachs produce an enzyme known as lactase, which snips lactose into its digestible components, glucose and galactose. After weaning, though, lactase production rapidly diminishes. To this day, only 35 percent of humans can digest lactose beyond the age of seven or eight; for the rest, consuming liquid milk is a surefire prescription for farts, diarrhea, and a burbly tummy.

About twelve thousand years ago, somewhere in the Fertile Crescent, a mutation occurred in the genes that code for lactase. A copying error in a single letter in the genome resulted in a gene variant, or allele, that allowed adults to continue producing lactase. Those with the allele were better able to enjoy the full nutritional benefit of liquid milk into adulthood. Lactase persistence, as it's known, emerged around the same time as such settlements as Çatalhöyük in Turkey, where people first gathered to domesticate wheat, barley, and other grains. This was not mere coincidence. The wild ancestors of goats, whose natural range is the Zagros Mountains of Iran, Iraq, and Turkey, were probably attracted to the grains being grown around human settlements—as, eventually, were the ancestors of cattle and sheep. Keeping these camp-followers close at hand by herding and penning them would have provided meat, as well as a backup supply of milk for infants. Human adults who happened to have the gene mutation for lactase persistence would have prospered by having access to an additional supply of nutrients when other food sources ran low, thus helping them to pass on their milk-tolerating mutant gene.

Now, here's the thing about cheese: because fermentation turns the nutritious sugars in liquid milk into digestible lactic acid, it contains only residual levels of lactose.* This means that everybody—except the most severely lactose intolerant—can digest such fermented dairy products as butter, kefir, yogurt, and cheese. (This explains why China, where lactase persistence is rare, has nonetheless become the world's largest growth market for cheese.) Liquid milk will coagulate into solid curds when you add rennet—the complex of enzymes found in the stomachs of young ruminants that allows them to digest their mothers' milk—or such acids as lemon juice and vinegar.

---

* Though sheep's and goat's milk are naturally lower in lactose, this doesn't necessarily mean sheep and goat *cheese* are the lowest in lactose. The key factor is how complete the fermentation process is. As a rule, soft young cheeses have more residual lactose; hard aged cheeses like Parmesan have almost none at all.

An oft-repeated origin story about cheese has it that one day, a nomadic herdsman filled his drinking gourd, which happened to be made from a calf's gut, with milk instead of water. After a hard day's ride, he found that his milk, transformed by the presence of rennet, had been magically churned into solid curds of delicious, and easily digestible, cheese. The problem with this story is that there would have been no reason for the apocryphal nomad to fill his gourd with liquid milk; prior to the emergence of lactase persistence, he wouldn't have been able to digest it.

Anthropologists now favor another creation myth: Neolithic herders discovered cheese when they cut open the stomachs of newly slaughtered suckling kids, lambs, and calves, and found them filled with coagulated milk—ready-made cheese curds. Another possibility is that, in the warm climate of the Fertile Crescent, ambient heat alone would have been enough to initiate coagulation. Either way, people would have been aware of the nutritional value, and deliciousness, of cheese before the lactase persistence gene was widespread.

About 8,500 years ago, when climate change was causing soil degradation, erosion, and deforestation in the Levant and what is now western Turkey, there was a marked increase in livestock grazing, as shown in the archaeological record. As crops failed and wild food became scarce, anybody who could digest the milk of domesticated ruminants was more likely to survive to pass on their genes. Just four millennia after it emerged, the mutant gene was widespread in human populations. If a Paleo dieter ever tells you human bodies are adapted to a pre-Neolithic, hunter-gatherer lifestyle, just point to the lactase persistence gene. It's one of the best examples, along with the way bodies in the Himalayas and Andes have adapted to survive at high altitudes, and how West Africans developed immunity to malaria, of how rapidly the human genome can evolve under the influence of environment and culture.

The earliest archaeological evidence of cheese-making dates to a 7,400-year-old site on the banks of the Vistula River, in central Poland.

In the 1970s, fragments of red clay, which looked as if they had been baked after being pierced with pieces of straw, were identified as some kind of sieve. It wasn't until 2011 that a team at the University of Bristol found the signature of dairy fats on the potsherds, evidence the pottery was used to strain liquid whey from curds.

The earliest fully intact cheese—as opposed to traces of milk fat on pottery—comes from Egypt. It was discovered wrapped with canvas and packed in a ceramic jar in the tomb of Ptahmes, mayor of Memphis in the thirteenth century BCE. Intended for enjoyment in the afterlife, it turned out to be a blend of sheep's, cow's, and goat's milk but also contained the deadly bacterium that causes brucellosis, which would have meted out swift justice to hungry tomb raiders.

The practice of dairying, and with it the lactase persistence gene, continued to spread north by way of the Balkans. The livestock-keeping, milk-drinking agriculturalists from the Middle East, packing the mutant gene in their genomes, came to outcompete and outnumber the indigenous hunter-gatherers of Europe. (Lactase persistence is a useful enough trait that it arose independently, by way of mutations in entirely different genes, among shepherds in West Africa and South Asia.) By one estimate, people with the gene variant may have produced up to 19 percent more fertile offspring than those who lacked it. Ninety percent of Scandinavians and 72 percent of English and Scottish people have the gene; in Greece, the number is 40 percent, and in Tuscany, just 8.9 percent. I attribute my own tolerance for dairy to my Ukrainian heritage and genes that may go back to the nomadic, livestock-keeping Scythians, whose ability to drink liquid milk so shocked the Romans.

Milk, which supplies everything young mammals need to grow and thrive, is a spectacularly nutritious food. Its protein, which comes mostly in the form of casein, is bundled into microscopic spheres called micelles, held together in a matrix of calcium, a mineral essential for healthy bones and teeth. Fat is contained in large globules that carry eye-popping levels of vitamins A and D. (Milk is also an outstanding source of B12, an essential vitamin scarce in vegetarian diets.) Cheese concentrates all the nutritional virtues of milk into a compact, transportable food that can be eaten months—or in the case of a Gouda or Parmesan, years—after the original milk would have soured. Many farmhouse cheeses have the further advantage of being made with raw milk, fresh from the udder, which teems with living white blood cells, probiotic bacteria, and active enzymes. Finally, whether it's raw or pasteurized, farmhouse cheese comes from animals that have been allowed to feed on grasses and wildflowers in pastures, meaning that it's unusually high in omega-3 fatty acids and healthy unsaturated fats.

The Neolithic farming package, which included dairying with goats, sheep, and cattle, took a while to make it from the Fertile Crescent to the British Isles, finally crossing the Channel—with the gene for lactase persistence along for the ride—about six thousand years ago. Writing in the first century, the Greco-Roman geographer Strabo observed of the ancient Britons, "Their habits are in part like the Celti [of Gaul, or modern France], but in part more simple and barbaric—so much so that, on account of their inexperience, some of them, although well supplied with milk, make no cheese."

The Romans, who occupied Britain in 43 CE, may have scorned liquid milk, but they were keen turophiles and left plenty of evidence of their love of curds in the archaeological record. Legionaries received a daily one-ounce ration, probably of a hard, easily transportable sheep's-milk cheese resembling modern Italian Pecorino or Spanish Manchego. Supplying the 45,000 members of the standing Roman army in Britain with rations would have required quite an industry. Cheese factories, and the distinctive round clay molds for making rennet-curdled sheep's cheeses, have been found in excavations of villas and encampments from Londinium to Hadrian's Wall.

After the Romans left England—or were thrown out, depending on who you ask—in 410, the history of cheese-making in the British Isles goes all hazy. For a while, a Romano-British elite, nostalgic for the good life, may have continued to consume cheeses made the old way, until Saxon invaders drove them into Wales and Brittany. Cheese makes sporadic appearances in the legal documents, laws, and charters of Welsh and Saxon kings, and in the records of Irish monasteries.

The truth is, we have no idea what kind of cheese people were eating in early medieval Britain. This is not the case in France, where Benedictines and other monastic orders devoted to self-sufficiency perfected labor-intensive cheeses such as Munster, Maroilles, and Brie de Meaux, which King Charlemagne praised by name after sampling it at Jouarre Abbey in 774. We do know that cheese in some form was made and eaten by medieval Britons, and they were probably healthier, less prone to starvation, and happier because it existed. The modern history of cheese-making in Britain really begins, like so many other things, with the coming of the French in 1066.

For better, and sometimes for worse, cheese-making, and the complex of practices that went along with it—herding, pasturing, dairying—is deeply entwined with the story of our species. If cheese has been reduced to the unhealthiest of foods—a bland pizza topping—it's the fault of industrial food makers, who have deployed considerable ingenuity to strip it of flavor, texture, and nutritional complexity.

Cheese has brought humans joy since Neolithic times. If there's a villain here, it is those who, in the name of affordability, safety, and uniformity, have made cheese into a caricature of its true self.

IN EUROPE, CHEESE IS NEVER JUST CHEESE. It is a symbol of place, of soil, of terroir. In France, even the most rubbery, pasteurized, processed supermarket brand of Camembert trades on its ties to the Norman countryside and the enduring *gloire* of peasant traditions. In the culture wars surrounding Brexit, Conservatives and Leavers held up "territorial" cheeses as examples of the sturdy, traditional products of a mythical Great Britain that, once purged of Continental influence and competition, would once again flourish. Some environmentalists, meanwhile, vilify cheese—along with liquid milk, factory farms, and veal-fattening pens—as a symbol of a Dairy-Industrial Complex responsible for animal cruelty, climate change, and the monocultures hastening the loss of biodiversity.

Guardian journalist George Monbiot, the main proponent of the latter view, believes that raising livestock for food is an abomination. In his documentary *Apocalypse Cow*, the vegan activist argued that the British Isles should be "rewilded," and wildlife allowed to roam free through forests, marshes, and grasslands as they reemerged from fields and pastures liberated of farms. The human population, cleared from the land into cities, could subsist on almond milk and artificial protein. To make his case, Monbiot flew to Helsinki to sample a gray pancake synthesized in a lab from oats and bacteria. "That is lovely," he declared for the camera, adding, none too convincingly, "I would eat that every morning."

Left out of the picture, or at best reduced to caricatures in condescending media profiles, are Britain's cheesefarmers (the term of art for makers of farmhouse cheese), who, being human, are confoundingly complex in their backgrounds and political outlooks. Charles Martell, responsible for reviving Gloucester cheese in the 1970s, declared himself an ardent supporter of Brexit, much to the delight of the European press, who noted that his wife was Ukrainian and his territorial cheese was made with the labor of Polish and Romanian farmhands. Meanwhile, the only maker of authentic raw-milk Stilton in Britain, which is retailed as Stichelton—the Old English name for the eponymous Sherwood Forest village—is a transplant from upstate New York named Joe Schneider.

My next stop was the warehouse of Neal's Yard Dairy in Bermondsey, where chief buyer Bronwen Percival greeted me with a wide-open Californian smile. She grew up in San Diego County, where her family kept goats on a small acreage in the Cuyamaca Mountains. Percival's book *Reinventing the Wheel*, which she co-authored with her husband, Francis, is the best account I've read of why seeking out and enjoying farmhouse cheese is a form of resistance to the uniformity brought by industrial agriculture.

Percival showed me around the offices and storage areas of Neal's Yard Dairy's warehouse, located in a viaduct beneath the tracks of the London and Greenwich Railway, one of the world's first passenger railways. "It's nice to have brick arches," she said, "because they're fairly well insulated and keep the cheese cool in the summer." After we'd put on smocks and hairnets, she took me on a tour of a turophile's paradise. In four of the railway arches, wooden shelves were stacked to the ceiling with big cylindrical truckles of Westcombe, Hafod, Cheshire, and Wensleydale. I told her the abundance of cheeses in Neal's Yard Dairy was the exact opposite of Monty Python's Cheese Shop sketch.

"Well, that was a pretty accurate depiction of a land bereft of cheese," said Percival, with a laugh. When the original Covent Garden shop opened in 1979, owners Nick Saunders and Randolph Hodgson first focused on making their own dairy products,* but they soon struck out from London to establish contacts with farmhouse cheese-makers. The problem was, Percival pointed out, there were very few left. "The extinction had already taken place. There were a few vestigial producers who were making a handful of Cheddars, Cheshires, and Lancashires, but people had stopped making farmhouse cheeses in favor of selling liquid milk, which they could get a guaranteed price for."

In their book, the Percivals document how the industrialization of dairying wiped out diversity on every level, from the microbes in milk to the grasses and wildflowers in pastures to the livestock breeds in farms and finally to the richness of human communities in rural areas. Before the nineteenth century, a fantastic variety of

---

* One of their first clients was John Cleese, who, arriving on a day when all they had in stock was their homemade yogurt, was given the opportunity to use the line "It's not much of a cheese shop, is it?"

cheeses, of varying quality, were made on small farms. All of them were coagulated with rennet, usually obtained from the stomach of a cow, goat, or sheep, and fermented with the microbes naturally present in the whey from earlier batches, in the raw milk itself, or even in the cracks and crannies of pails, wooden shelves, and old stone walls. The coming of the first railways—like the ones conveying the trains rumbling over our heads at Neal's Yard—in the 1830s allowed liquid milk to be brought to cities. Together with canals and turnpikes, railways helped fashion a distinctive British cheese: low in moisture, high in acidity, and, above all, hard—qualities that made cheeses easy to transport, especially when shipped as large truckles, like the barrel-shaped Stiltons, Cheshires, and Cheddars stacked on the warehouse shelves around us.

Cheese-making was first industrialized on the other side of the Atlantic. Jesse Williams, a farmer with sixty-five cows who wanted to process the milk from his son's farm, opened the first true cheese factory in Rome, New York, in 1851; within thirteen years, there were over two hundred such cheese factories in New York State alone. Factory Cheddar from the New World, wrapped in cloth for transport, began to arrive at the port of Bristol to be shipped by rail to London, where it retailed for half the price of authentic British Cheddar.

Two scientific breakthroughs contributed to the gradual extinction of farmhouse cheese-making. Chemist Louis Pasteur's process for killing pathogens in wine through rapid heating was applied to liquid milk in the 1880s, as an attempt to end the scourge of tuberculosis. The Danes used pasteurization to kill the spoilage bacteria in cream, which they then fermented and exported to Britain in the form of a cheap, stable, mild-flavored butter. When the same process was applied to raw milk, it wiped out pathogens but also killed the beneficial bacteria necessary to ferment the milk into cheese. A Danish chemist named Christian Hansen, who had already developed a purified extract to replace rennet, founded the company that offered a solution: to the blank slate of heat-purified milk, cheese-makers could add a few chemically isolated strains of lactic acid bacteria. Prepackaged sachets of starter culture did for the world of cheese what Fleischmann's powdered yeast did to sourdough bread: it eliminated a fantastic range of diverse flavors. (Another maker of starter cultures, DuPont, boasts that every third cheese currently made in the world uses its Danisco range.) According to the Percivals, the combined impact of pasteurization, starter cultures, and obsessive hygiene has led to what they call a "holocaust" of raw-milk microbes.

"This is not a term that we use lightly," they wrote in *Reinventing the Wheel*. "The quest for control has caused the catastrophic destruction of the microbial communities on which cheesemakers rely to make their raw-milk cheeses distinctive." Bronwen Percival believes this lost diversity extends to our gut. Before pasteurization, the bacterium *Helicobacter pylori,* whose presence may have a beneficial impact on the immune response, was found in just about everybody's gut; now it's present in the stomachs of fewer than 6 percent of young Americans, and its absence has been linked to a rise in allergies and asthma. "The jury's still out, but I think it's a plausible hypothesis that by putting a diversity of microbes into our digestive tract, we're stimulating our immune systems in ways that have all kinds of notable health effects."

In Britain, the near-disappearance of farmhouse cheeses is only partly explained by the rise of factories, pasteurization, and starter cultures. In 1933, the Milk Marketing Board was set up to stabilize the price of liquid milk. During the Second World War, all farmers were forced to sell their milk to the board, and factories were limited to making Cheddar and a few other varieties of strictly rationed cheese. Before the war, there were one thousand registered producers of farmhouse cheese, a third of them making Cheddar; by the time rationing ended, in 1954, just 140 farmhouse cheese-makers remained. France also experienced prewar industrialization—by the 1890s, Camembert was already a mass-produced, mass-marketed product, designed for rail shipments from Normandy to Paris—but the French didn't nationalize their milk supply during the war. Today, there are just 350 artisanal cheese-makers in the United Kingdom, only a few dozen of them true farmhouse producers, compared to 4,500 in France.

The truth is that farmhouse production accounts for a vanishingly small percentage of the cheese consumed around the world. Since 1997, forty-pound blocks of Cheddar have been traded, along with wood pulp and pork bellies, as commodities on the floor of the Chicago Mercantile Exchange. In the past, the standard family farm had a dozen or so cows, with breeds adapted to the climate and landscape; today the largest factory farms in California have single-breed herds of nineteen thousand animals. And, of course, while the milk we get comes from lactating cows, goats, and sheep, most of their offspring are slaughtered and eaten. As cheesemonger Ned Palmer, a former employee of Neal's Yard Dairy, wrote, "The hard fact is that if you consume dairy products you are to some extent involved in the death of animals. Calves, lambs and kids are, to put it bluntly, surplus to requirements in a dairy herd unless they are needed to replace a milking animal that has retired."

Percival knew all this, yet still passionately stood by the idea that good cheese is worth not only fighting for but also paying for. "The charge of elitism comes up all the time. But I believe that's because there's been a debasement of this very precious food." In the nineteenth century, she pointed out, people paid a high price for Cheddar and other cheeses relative to what they earned. "I'm not saying we should go back to that, but we should recognize that the dairy industry has become hugely extractive, and inflicts a lot of hidden costs on the environment. As a society, we should be eating a lot less animal protein, whether it's cheese or meat. What we do eat has to be sustainably produced. And yes, that's going to be more expensive."

Farmhouse cheese is about as sustainable and ethical as farming gets. It's also, in my opinion, one of the most life-enriching foods you can eat. In this way, raw-milk cheese is like dark chocolate, vintage wine, or homemade sourdough bread: you don't need a lot to feel deeply, lastingly satisfied.

I asked Percival what she thought of George Monbiot's idea that agriculture itself was the culprit, and allowing farmland to revert to nature was the best way to heal the planet.

"So we'll all survive on yeast extract or something?" she scoffed. "He believes the only truly valuable biodiversity is completely natural. And biodiversity that's man-made, or partly man-made, has no value whatsoever." The best response to that, she said, was to pay a visit to a farmer who was making territorial cheeses in a nonindustrial, traditional way. "You'll see seminatural landscapes, meadows, and pastures that are incredibly biodiverse. Along with cows, they support wildflowers, insects, animals, all kinds of ground-nesting birds that wouldn't survive in a forest."

But I was way ahead of her. My next destination was the original home of the legendary cheese of Wensleydale. My train was leaving in an hour.

WALKING THE YORKSHIRE DALES, a series of five river valleys that crisscross the Pennines, the chain of low hills that runs up the spine of northern England to Hadrian's Wall, is heaven. Driving them—especially if you happen to be a jet-lagged North American not used to shifting with your left hand while working the clutch of a right-hand drive car—is hell. I'd picked up a rental car outside York's train station and quickly regretted it. Every time I dared turn my head to take in the vista of a meandering emerald dale flecked white with sheep, an oncoming lorry seemed to be barreling toward me on a shoulderless two-lane road constricted between drystone walls. By the time I'd reached the parking lot outside Jervaulx Abbey, I was a jittery, white-knuckled wreck.

Yet it took just half an hour of wandering through the vine-draped ruins of the twelfth-century abbey to calm my nerves. The Dales are the cultural domain of the Brontë sisters and James Herriot, the vet who authored *All Creatures Great and Small*, and a visit to the monasterial complex, nestled in rolling meadows, was a gentle introduction to a storied, seemingly timeless landscape. A century after the Norman Conquest of 1066, a group of Cistercian monks from Savigny, France, in rebellion against the perceived excesses of the Benedictine order, settled in the wilds of northern England to follow the rule of Saint Bernard, devoting themselves to lives of seclusion, self-sufficiency, and manual labor. After abandoning an earlier site, the abbot led his community to Wensleydale, which, though infested with wolves, had the advantage of being surrounded by the fertile lands bordering the nearby River Ure. After a few difficult years, a small community of monks set up a grange, run by the lay brothers, who, unlike the choir monks, were permitted to leave the grounds of the abbey. Granges were Britain's first large-scale agricultural institutions since the Roman occupation, and the brothers excelled at the hard but rewarding work of making bread, beer, butter, and cheese.

I wandered beneath arches hung with creepers and vines, occasionally clambering over what remained of lichen-covered limestone walls while staying mindful of a sign, put up by Jervaulx's private owners, that read "You are entering a ruined Abbey and not a playground." The destruction meted out after Henry VIII dissolved the monasteries was impressive. After the last Abbot of Jervaulx was hanged in 1537, the lead was stripped from the buildings' roofs and sold by weight. The church at the center of the complex, originally the length of an American football field, had been reduced to its floorplan, though one intact wall was still topped by the frames of ten soaring lancet windows. Deprived of its roof, the abbey's ceiling was now the heavens.

I walked through the "meat kitchen," which contained the remains of three circular ovens. Beyond that was a rectangle of turf that a map at the entrance identified as the abbot's lodging. It was in the cellar below his rooms that the kitchener, responsible for food storage, and his staff of lay brothers washed the rinds and turned the rounds of the cheese that would come to be known as Wensleydale. The earliest record of Cistercian cheese-making in Yorkshire dates to an inventory written in 1150.

What exactly did this proto-Wensleydale taste like? That's harder to say than you might imagine. The flavor, consistency, and even color of a cheese depends on the time of year it's made, the pasturage or feed the animals have access to, and the microbes and molds in the environment. While archaeologists have a good shot at reconstructing many other ancient foods, cheese is one case where we might really need to wait for the invention of a time machine.

The Wensleydale that people eat today is a hard white cow's milk cheese, similar to Lancashire, another British cheese known for its acidity and crumbliness. The Wensleydale made by the monks of Jervaulx would have been soft, open-textured, and channeled with veins of tangy blue mold. That sounds like a description of a creamy white-and-blue Roquefort—which makes sense, as the Cistercians' roots were in France. Conditions in the Dales are also pretty similar to those in the Causses plateau, home to the famous caves of Roquefort, where a wet and windy climate and the presence of limestone encourage the growth of mold.

The biggest distinction between modern Wensleydale and its medieval namesake, though, is the source of the milk. I walked back to the parking lot under the wary gaze of a dozen or so black-footed, white-faced Cheviot sheep, a breed recognized for its hardiness since at least 1372. The Cistercians were the first order to introduce large-scale sheep farming to England, eventually selling the wool on an industrial scale to Flanders. For this, they deserve both praise and damnation.

Praise, certainly, for what they *did* with the milk. And damnation for the damage their sheep, more than any other kind of livestock, have inflicted on the land.

I MET ANDREW HATTAN in the village of Pateley Bridge. He'd insisted on driving me the last three miles to his farm, which, he explained, would be on a road more treacherous than anything I'd driven so far. In the passenger seat of his four-by-four, a forest-green Škoda, I was grateful I'd taken him up on his offer. The rough stone track, corrugated by rainfall and punctuated with mud puddles, would have left my little Citroën folded and spindled. Though we were at just over a thousand feet above sea level, something about the cold clear light, and the lack of trees and man-made structures—apart from those ever-present drystone walls—reminded me of the roof-of-the-world feeling of crossing the Bolivian Andes.

The remoteness of Low Riggs, whose tenancy Andrew and his wife, Sally, took over in 2007, is one of the distinguishing features of farms in the Yorkshire uplands. The 460-acre property, officially classified as "severely disadvantaged" meadow, pasture, and moorland, once belonged to Byland Abbey, another Cistercian house. After the dissolution of the monasteries, the land was passed on to Richard Yorke, the mayor of York, whose family used it to raise sheep, like the monks before them, until the nineteenth century. Andrew showed me a stone over the door of the farmhouse, which was built with tawny-red bricks of local millstone, carved with the date 1655. Much of the interior dates from 1858, when it was completely rebuilt; judging from some charred oak lintels Andrew had found, he guessed the two-story interior had been gutted by fire. The family who'd occupied it before them had owned the farm since 1962.

"The building wasn't damp-proofed when we moved in," Andrew said. "It had electricity and a phone—just. For heat, there were electric heaters and open fires. The family before us basically lived in the back kitchen. It was a sort of wipe-your-wellies when you went out, rather than when you went in, kind of place."

After making sure to wipe my own shoes, I was greeted by Andrew's wife, Sally, who works part-time as a dental officer for the

National Health Service, and Rachael, their daughter, in the kitchen, which remained the warm heart of the home. (Their son, Sam, would make a brief appearance at dinner, before politely retreating to his room to attend to preadolescent pursuits.) Filling my glass with brown ale, Andrew explained that neither he nor Sally had a tradition of farming in their families. Sally had grown up in the suburbs of Leeds, in West Yorkshire. Andrew, the son of teachers, was born in Nigeria, but the family moved to rural Yorkshire when he was a boy.

"By the age of twelve, I had the farming bug really badly," said Andrew. He worked on a sheep farm as a teenager and then went to agriculture college in Edinburgh. For his postgraduate work, he studied the high-yielding breeds that were arriving from the Americas, managing a herd of four hundred Holsteins at the University of Reading. Originally from Holland, the big, black-and-white, spindly-legged Holsteins have become freakishly efficient machines for turning brought-in feed—corn, alfalfa, soy, and other products of industrial monocultures—into milk; known as "white-water factories," they can produce over thirteen gallons of milk per day. (One champion Holstein with the cuddly name Selz-Pralle Aftershock 3918 averaged fifty gallons a day in 2017.) In the United States, 95 percent of all cows are Holsteins, the majority confined to factory farms where milking robots are laser-guided to their udders.* Andrew was tasked with putting the university's Holsteins in respiration chambers to measure how they turned different kinds of feed into methane, feces, urine, kilojoules of heat, and eventually gallons of milk.

"It was pure reductionism. It really made me think. Sixty percent of what we put into them went up the chimney as heat. But they were

---

* Holsteins were first imported to the United States in 1852, but after an outbreak of foot-and-mouth disease, they were crossed with another Dutch breed, the Friesian, which had arrived in Canada thirty years later. The nine million dairy cows alive in the United States today are descended from just two bulls, and not that many more females, meaning the genetic diversity of the entire population is equivalent to fifty individuals—putting the milk supply at huge risk should medication-resistant pathogens arise.

still producing fifty liters of milk a day." Holstein milk, which is low in fat and protein, doesn't make particularly good cheese. "I had to milk them three times a day. I'd come home to Sally, and my clothes stank so much, I'd have to take them off outside. It was full-on."

By the time the Hattans were given the opportunity to take over Low Riggs, Andrew swore he'd never milk another cow. Since the time of the Cistercians, the barren landscape of the Yorkshire uplands has been formed by sheep. The Hattans took on a flock of Swaledales, a horned sheep bred not for its wool but for providing fat hardy lambs that thrive in the lowlands. After buying some tups—as rams are called in Yorkshire—from Scotland, they had success breeding high-performing hybrids. Eventually they had a thriving flock of 450 ewes, but there were two problems. The first was the impact they were having on the land.

"Sheep are environmentally disastrous, especially in the quantities we have in the United Kingdom," said Andrew. "They're foragers, browsers, with noses that are designed to pick out just the nice bits and then move on."

Wherever sheep graze, plant diversity plummets. There are currently thirty million sheep in the United Kingdom, and as comforting as the sight of fluffy flocks on rolling hills might be to a certain kind of Briton, their presence usually indicates that at some point commoners—in the most literal sense of the word—were driven from their ancestral lands so aristocratic property-holders could make a profit. This they did by using the former commons to raise sheep to supply the wool industry. What is left, after centuries of overgrazing, is a green-and-pleasant barrens, devoid of shrubs, trees, and even wildflowers. Sheep, like goats, are best suited for marginal and rocky lands—like, for example, the sunbaked hills of Sardinia, the birthplace of hard, salty Pecorino cheese. In most of the British Isles, though, sheep are a poor fit. They are also shockingly profligate consumers of water, requiring 6,400 gallons to produce a pound of meat, compared to about 5,400 for cattle and just 750 gallons for pigs.

"Up here," said Andrew, "we have peaty soils, and the sheep were grazing them so hard the grass wasn't growing back."

The second problem, pointed out Sally, as she served plates of beef-and-mushroom stew with new potatoes alongside homemade bread, was that the sheep business doesn't pay all that well. The Hattans decided to take advantage of a European Union scheme that would provide a subsidy if they kept cattle native to the region. They started with twenty Galloways, a hardy slow-growing breed known for producing high-quality beef. But the breed's outdoors-loving ways meant their hooves quickly churned the wet winter soils into what Andrew called "pudding." Sally said, "They were *too* self-contained. Hardy, but also wild and woolly." With a grimace, Andrew added, "And *quite* maternal. Separating the mother and calf could be ... dangerous."

Andrew remembered his mother telling him about some unusual cows on a farm where she used to vacation as a child. Before the war, many farms on the Dales had kept Northern Dairy Shorthorns, a dual-purpose breed, valued for both milk and beef. With the coming of high-yielding Holsteins, their numbers had dwindled to thirty living females, and by the 1980s Northern Dairies were registered as critically endangered by the Rare Breeds Survival Trust.

"We decided that, if we were going to keep cattle," said Andrew, "they should be keeping *us*." Aware their EU subsidy was set to diminish (thanks to Brexit, it would soon completely vanish), the Hattans decided they had better find a way to derive maximum benefit from their acreage with a high-quality, high-value product: farmhouse cheese.

For Andrew, that meant a return to milking cows, something he'd sworn never to do again. They contacted a local vet who had made it his hobby, with the help of farming families in Cumbria and Cornwall, to keep the Northern Dairy Shorthorn breed alive. The Rare Breeds Survival Trust, a fifty-year-old conservation charity that has prevented many farm animal breeds native to Britain from going extinct, had collected the semen from seven Northern Dairy bulls. Starting small, the Hattans brought in a small number of cows, turning a disused 1850s outbuilding into a milking parlor, which they connected with pipes to a brand-new "make room," the building where the milk is coagulated and pressed into cheese. The first wheels of Stonebeck Wensleydale were made from milk collected between mid-April and the end of September. Bronwen Percival was among the first to sample them, and her delight in the flavor, and obvious desire to showcase Stonebeck at Neal's Yard Dairy in London, convinced the Hattans they were on the right path.

By then, the plates had been cleared, and it was time for the cheese course. I'd brought some cheeses the owner of La Fromagerie, a cheese shop in London's Marylebone, had picked out for me, including a Stichelton, the raw-milk version of Stilton, and a Corra Linn, an aged Scottish sheep's cheese reminiscent of a Spanish Manchego, and Sally set out some walnuts and pearl onions pickled in malt vinegar.

At the center of the plate was a slice of the cheese I'd crossed an ocean to try—Stonebeck Wensleydale. The rind, textured with a fine grid after a couple of months wrapped in calico, was as mottled as desert-boot camouflage, in hues of wet and dry sand. The rich-yellow paste was supple, yet crumbly. And the odor and taste—the two are, of course, indissociable—conjured up fresh-cut grass and summer pastures sprinkled with wildflowers. This wasn't dry, bland, industrial Wensleydale to be scarfed down with Christmas cakes, nor was it anything like the Roquefort-style sheep's cheese I imagined the Cistercian brothers had made. The Hattans had made something that, while a pure product of the Yorkshire Dales, was also purely their own.

Like the best cheeses I've had, almost all of which have been made from unpasteurized milk, Stonebeck Wensleydale drilled down into a deep part of my mammalian brain—something certainly connected to infancy, suckling, and contentment—and left me calm, happy, and a little bit sleepy. Which was all for the best, because, by then, it was time for bed. It had been a long day, and the following morning, I had a date with a very special herd of cows.

A CHILL AND WINDY MORNING IT WAS, too, for this was October in northern England, but the sky, when the fast-moving clouds got out of the way, was as blue as an alpine lake. Andrew was waiting for me, in shorts and a zip-up jumper, but before taking me to see the cows, he invited me to look more closely at the grass below our boots.

"Since the 1960s, the fields here were farmed the conventional way, with inorganic fertilizer, and treated with herbicides to spray out the weeds. When we got here, all the biodiversity was gone. It normally takes twenty years for a field to recover." Two of their fields had been left fallow for the last fourteen years. "They'll hopefully be officially registered as species-rich next year." On the borders of the fields, the Hattans have been slowly restoring the native woodlands, planting pioneer species like alder, wild cherry, birch, mountain ash, blackthorn, and holly. The network of roots is helping to stabilize the steep slopes along a gill, or stream, while reducing runoff and preventing landslides. The trees and shrubs provide habitat for otters and dippers, little diving birds that use their wings like fins, propelling themselves underwater in search of prey. The emerging woodlands also support grouse, which in turn attract human hunters, a species Andrew tolerates, if with gritted teeth.

"Since we've reduced our sheep, we've had an explosion of floral diversity in our meadow havens. Trees are springing up everywhere." Cows are more gentle grazers than sheep, feeding on the whole plant rather than just the tasty bits, and also keep unwanted species in check.

I asked Andrew what he thought of Monbiot's crusade against traditional agriculture. "I'd quite happily have George on the farm," he said, with a chuckle. "He doesn't worry me at all." Andrew believed that restoring the northern hay meadow, a fantastically diverse—yet human-managed—environment, was better than rewilding the Dales and abandoning them to a "state of nature." "If there were no grazing, you'd get a monoculture of rushes along the stream, and then the thistle and bracken would take over." He pointed to a tangle of prehistoric-looking orange ferns. "Bracken is an ancient plant, very successful and competitive, that, unchecked, takes over everything."

By early summer, the meadows here are crazy-quilted with meadow vetchlings, buttercups, common lady's-mantles, and wild white clover—up to 45 distinct plant species in a couple of square yards, 150 of them in a field. This rich flora provides habitat for pollinating insects and ground-nesting birds, as well as underground communities of microbes, fungi, and invertebrates. A well-tended Dales meadow stores twice as much carbon as natural grasslands.

On one point, though, Andrew agreed with Monbiot. "If rewilding meant we had wolves here, then good, they'd eat all the sheep, and we need fewer sheep in the UK." Grass-fed cows, he reckoned, were doing the landscape a service. By spreading their manure as they grazed, they were reinvigorating the land with nitrogen, phosphorus, and potassium, naturally boosting the fertility of the soil.

We trudged up the sloping pasture behind one of the stone barns, weaving our way through flattened pats of soil-enriching manure. A dozen cows eyed us watchfully, neither advancing nor retreating. Some were creamy white, some mottled red and white, and others were roan, their auburn coats lightened with a sprinkling of white hairs. "Some of these have some introgression of Holstein blood into them," said Andrew, "but the fact is they were all originally from Northern Dairy families." They were also surprisingly small. In the millennia since wild aurochs were tamed, selective breeding has turned *Bos taurus*, domesticated cattle, into monsters like Italian Chianina, which tip scales at 3,300 pounds, and the Miniature Zebu, which weighs a tenth of that. Northern Dairy Shorthorns tend to weigh in on the small side. "A modern Holstein will be fifteen hundred pounds; ours weigh a thousand." They also yield about half as much milk as their hulking cousins. They make up for the low volume with nutrition: their milk is up to 4 percent fat and 3.6 percent protein—ideal numbers for cheese-making.

Northern Dairies are beautifully adapted to the uplands. Woolly coats keep them warm when the weather is foul; their small stature means they can shelter from the wind behind drystone walls; and their low weight means the ground isn't churned to mud under their hooves. They are also, Andrew made it clear as he patted the flanks of a roan with a creamy white tail, endearing beasts. "People tend to say they're docile. I don't know if they're any more docile than other breeds; we've got a mixed bag. But they are agile, very good at running downhill. In the summer, at milking time, five in the morning, they'll *run* down to the milking parlor. I've never seen that, with any cows."

The cheese-making season had ended three weeks earlier—the only reason the Hattans had the leisure to welcome a guest—but Andrew agreed to walk me through a typical summer day's work. On Mondays, Wednesdays, and Fridays, starting at quarter to four in the morning, chilled milk, piped from the milking parlors the previous day, is added to the morning's fresh milk. Andrew then adds rennet and starter culture—a prepackaged brand, though the Hattans aspire to make their own soon—before driving his kids to school. By the time he returns, around eleven, the milk has coagulated, and it's time to cut the curd. The curds are then hung in bags, where solids form as liquid whey begins its long *drip-drip-drip* into the vat below. Around 3:30 in the afternoon, Andrew returns to crumble and salt the drained curd, and put it into cloth-lined molds, where it's left overnight.

The following morning, the semisolid wheel is placed into a cast-iron cheese press, where it's compressed beneath a stone suspended between side posts with shoulder-straining turns of a screw. ("Absolute man-eater it is," muttered Andrew, glaring at the Victorian monster with grudging respect. "Weighs a ton.") After pressing, the wheel is moved to an aging room, where it's left to mature, with over four hundred of its peers, on wooden shelves. Andrew showed me the youngest cheeses, made at the beginning of October, whose thin rinds were brilliant white; those made in August had already developed character, their rinds thickening and mottling. The Hattans get £62.70 for a seven-pound, three-ounce wheel, which means that when the shelves are full, there's over £28,000 of inventory in the aging room. If Andrew were to sell the milk in liquid form, he would get a mere £1.10 a gallon. Transforming it into cheese increases its value almost sevenfold.

"It's expensive," he admitted. "But it has to be. The geography, our isolation, dictate that we have to export something from the farm that is concentrated value. We can't bring in great loads of feed. We need to be as self-sufficient as possible." The Hattans are aware that, in reviving raw-milk farmhouse Wensleydale, they've achieved something special, even if Andrew expresses it with a typical Yorkshireman's understatement. "The fact that we have *the* breed, *the* farm in the Yorkshire Dales, *the* hay meadows, and *the* old cheese recipe, and we're actually making cheese similar to what was made eighty years ago—well, that's quite nice."

I told him that the consensus in London was that he made a wonderful cheese: when the subject of Stonebeck Wensleydale came up, cheesemongers gushed.

"I would say that's not *because* of me. It's in *spite* of me." He cast an uphill glance at a trio of Northern Dairies, contentedly munching on grass. "But really, it's not about me at all. It's the cows."

IT'S TRUE THAT STONEBECK WENSLEYDALE, as well as the crumbly white pasteurized version sold in supermarkets, is not the same cheese the Cistercians recorded making in 1150 CE. What I found incredible, though, is that there is a nine-hundred-year-long tradition of making raw-milk cheeses in the Yorkshire Dales. Wensleydale should have gone the way of so many other farmhouse cheeses, killed by industrialization and wartime rationing, making it another course in humanity's lost supper. Instead, it's still being enjoyed, thanks to the efforts of the Hattans.

The secret of Wensleydale, of course, is that it has never been just one cheese. After the monasteries were wrecked and the lay brothers scattered, knowledge of cheese-making was passed to the peasantry; farmers' wives in turn transmitted their know-how to their daughters, who created similar cheeses under the names Swaledale, Teesdale, Nidderdale, and Coverdale, after the valleys in which they lived. (There's evidence that even in the monastic period, much of the labor was done by female cheese-makers known as *deyes*, from which the word *dairy* is derived.) A series of disease outbreaks in sheep, which began as early as 1270, meant that by the seventeenth century, sheep's milk had been almost completely replaced by cow's in the cheeses of the Dales.

In descriptions predating the Second World War, a distinction is made between young white Wensleydale—which probably resembled today's crumbly supermarket product—and an aged and "pickled" Wensleydale, which was held in greater esteem. "Ripened Wensleydale," wrote one turophile in 1937, is "soft and flaky, will spread like butter, and has the delicate blue veining well distributed throughout the curd. The flavour is rich, sweet and creamy—not acid or bitter."

The Hattans had shown me prewar manuals, with notes penciled in the margins, that described the making of two kinds of Wensleydale. The blue version had to be "pickled," cured in a bath of brine before maturing. Andrew admitted that he was obsessed with re-creating blue Wensleydale. In his first years of cheese-making, a few wheels had naturally developed blue veins. As a test, he'd inoculated some batches with *Penicillium roqueforti*, the strain of bacteria that goes into Roquefort, which would likely have been naturally present in the Cistercians' cheese. It worked well, but Bronwen Percival strongly discouraged him from continuing the experiment. She argued that any "bluing" should arise from bacteria naturally occurring in the environment. Andrew said that he understood her concerns but said he wasn't quite ready to dispense with the consistent results allowed by ready-made starter cultures.

If I wanted to get the story about what became of the prewar blue Wensleydale, Andrew recommended I pay a visit to Andy Swinscoe, who had set up a kind of museum of Dales cheeses. Though it was only twenty miles west of Low Riggs, thanks to twisting mountain roads—and a never-ending succession of slow-moving tractors—it took me an hour and a half to reach the Courtyard Dairy. Swinscoe and his wife had converted an eighteenth-century stone barn into a shop dedicated to championing the cheeses of northern England. They lived upstairs, and let local cheesefarmers use the surrounding fields to graze their sheep and cows. In a shed near the parking lot, Swinscoe showed me a brilliant contraption: a cheese-vending machine, which, should one be struck with a sudden midnight craving, allowed for the purchase of a Baron Bigod or a sheep's milk halloumi after the dairy had closed.

Andrew had warned me that Swinscoe, a lanky fellow in a white smock and cap, was a "cheeky chappie," and I got an idea of his wit when I watched him at work behind the glass cases, where thirty kinds of northern cheeses, most of them farmhouse, were arrayed.

"Now," he announced, with studied gravity, "it's very important that you're rude to most customers, especially Trevor." Trevor, clearly a regular, had just walked in. "We need to give him the same level of service everybody gets—disdain."

Taking her cue, the woman working next to him looked poor Trevor up and down and shouted, "Now get out!"

Taking off his apron, and some of his cheekiness with it, Swinscoe led me to the little museum in an adjacent building. I told him I was curious about how Wensleydale had changed from its original blue monkish incarnation to its current white industrial form.

"We know that Wensleydale became a cow's milk cheese between two and three hundred years ago," he said. "Today, sheep here are used for lamb, for their meat. They are sheared, but the wool is of no value anymore." Swinscoe dates the beginning of the decline in farmhouse cheese to the 1890s, when cheese merchant Edward Chapman, tired of the variable quality of farmers' cheeses, set up his own centralized cheese-making operation in an old woolen mill in the town of Hawes. Competitors imitated him, and around the same time, new roads allowed trucks to reach the farms, which in turn allowed even remote farmers to sell their excess milk in liquid form rather than as cheese. T. C. "Kit" Calvert, who would become the first historian of Wensleydale, bought the Hawes Creamery in the 1930s, and when the war broke out, he worked hard to make sure Wensleydale—along with Cheddar, Cheshire, Lancashire, and a few others—was one of the cheeses included in the ration books. As of 1941, most people were allowed two to three ounces a week— enough to cover a few crackers—though vegetarians and outdoor workers were given as much as a pound.

"Austerity Wensleydale," as it was known, was not the rich, spreadable, blue-veined form of the cheese but the more quickly made white and crumbly form. By the time the war ended, there were only nine farmhouse producers of Wensleydale left; the last farmhouse maker gave up in 1957.

"The ration book was the final nail in the coffin," said Swinscoe. "And after rationing, white Wensleydale became *the* Wensleydale." Under current legislation, the old pickled blue version, because of its high moisture content, wouldn't qualify as a real Wensleydale. Nor, Swinscoe suspects, does the Hattans' Stonebeck. And that, he believes, is just wrong.

"The simple fact of the matter is that the Hattans are making the cheese that reflects this region most, as it was one hundred years ago. Because they're using Northern Dairy Shorthorns, because of what they feed them, because of the way they make their cheese. With factory Wensleydale, it's sold after two weeks! The Wensleydale of the Hattans we're selling at the moment is aged about four months."

Swinscoe believes that what the Hattans and other cheesefarmers do has a deeper meaning. "The traditional Yorkshire Dales hay meadows their cattle graze on are an important part of Britain's history. But most meadows are under a stewardship scheme." The government pays landowners, in other words, *not* to farm the meadows, in an effort to restore biodiversity—a form of rewilding. "My argument is, all they're doing is turning them into a museum piece. What the Hattans have found is an economic reason to keep that breed alive, and the meadows alive. In order to make the cheese taste better. And it does!"

That's exactly the point: the entire farming system behind Stone-beck, from grass to milk, is legible on your tongue and in your nose when you put a slice in your mouth. This is something that's true of any great cheese.

"Look, I agree, we should all be eating less dairy and meat," said Swinscoe. "But an old-fashioned dairy farm, with small fields, diverse pasture, traditional breeds, is a *good* thing. It's good for wildlife, for biodiversity, and for soil health, which is going to be one of the next problems the UK and the world is facing."

There's another, very human reason that the Hattans' story is important. Around the world, farmers are in crisis; from Saskatche-wan to Rajasthan, rural areas are experiencing a quiet pandemic of depression and suicide. In England, as in most of North America, the average age of farmers is now fifty-nine. To make a profit growing a single crop, farmers need more acreage, and ever bigger and more sophisticated equipment, which puts them deeper in debt. Many of them are miserable, and their children, seeing their misery, have no desire to take on the farming life. In most places, large corporations are the ones who really profit. One-third of the world's milk supply is under the control of twenty multinationals.

In Yorkshire, Swinscoe had watched things going the other way. When Courtyard opened a decade earlier, there wasn't a single farmer within fifty miles making raw-milk cheese; now, because out-lets like his exist, there are five. "You speak to the farmers who have gone back to less intensive farming, and they like what they're doing. They're there with their animals. It's nice. It feels right.

"The most important thing, though, is *taste*. If it doesn't taste good, we haven't got a business. It's that simple. And it's got to taste better than anybody else, because if it doesn't, why would people come and buy Andrew and Sally's cheese, which is more expensive and harder to find? The only way we can get them interested in the first place is to let them taste. And once they've tasted, that's when we can start telling them the *real* story."

He didn't need to convince me. In the hope of tasting real Wensleydale, I'd crossed the Atlantic and risked my life on the backroads of the Yorkshire Dales. It had been worth it. I might have come for a unique flavor, but I was leaving with a wonderful story.

6

PUGLIA

The Death of the Immortals

IT HAD BEEN A LONG WINTER—another long winter—of snowstorms and lockdowns and travel restrictions. When things got really dreary, I'd take a swig of olive oil, the stuff the Greeks in my neighborhood shipped over by the container-load from Crete, and make a meal of tzatziki, dolmades, and Kalamata olives. The yielding flesh of the brine-cured olives, combined with the peppery bite of the oil at the back of my throat, always lifted my spirits.

"The entire Mediterranean seems to rise out of the sour, pungent taste of black olives between the teeth," novelist Lawrence Durrell wrote in *Prospero's Cell*. "A taste older than meat or wine, a taste as old as cold water. Only the sea itself seems as ancient a part of the region as the olive and its oil, that like no other products of nature, have shaped civilizations from remotest antiquity to the present."

Durrell wrote those words on his beloved island of Corfu, which is where I'd first read them, serenaded by the electric buzz of cicadas in the treetops. When I pictured a happy place, I imagined myself on the Costa Brava, the shores of Corsica, the beaches of Croatia, or just about anywhere on the Mediterranean, watching the olive leaves shimmying under the gusts of a *xaloc*, *mistral*, *tramontana*, or some other mischievous southern wind.

"The first olive tree on the way south marks the beginning of the Mediterranean region," wrote Fernand Braudel. For the French historian, Mediterranean civilization was defined by the "eternal trinity" of wheat, vines, and olives. But wheat has long been a global commodity, and grapes, which were first domesticated in Georgia on the Black Sea, are now cultivated from the Yarra to the Okanagan Valley. *Olea europaea*, in contrast, can only really thrive in a narrow band between 30 and 45 degrees latitude, a zone that, north of the equator, neatly encompasses the Mediterranean. While olive trees have been successfully transplanted to California, Chile, and Australia, their true homeland remains the shores of Homer's wine-dark sea. The best definition of the Mediterranean, as Braudel saw it, was as the place where the olive tree grows.

So, from the window seat of a high-speed train from Rome to Bari, I watched eagerly for the silvery-green canopies that would signal my arrival in the Med. But just my luck: it was an unusually cold March, the lower slopes of the Apennine Mountains were blanketed with white, and the only splashes of color under a lowering gray sky came from the violet blossoms of almond trees. As the tracks crossed into Puglia and began to run parallel to the Adriatic coastline, I could just make out the blur of green treetops bent under a driving rain. It was only after arriving in the hilltop town of Ostuni that I realized I was well and truly in the olive zone. The street outside my hotel was lined with undersized urban olive trees; gouts of wet snow fell between their unmistakable lanceolate leaves.

The following day, though, the sun broke through the clouds, and all thoughts of winter were banished. A naturalist named Filomena Tanzarella had agreed to show me around the Piana degli Ulivi Monumentali, one of the world's great concentrations of ancient olive trees. Flo, as her friends call her, drove me up to the edge of the Murgia, the plateau that dominates the center of Puglia. From a panoramic lookout point, we gazed down over a broad plain that extended toward the coast. Perpendicular to the coast were furrows of greenery known as *lame*, remnants of fossil streams, their courses marked by rich alluvial soil, that still channel rainwater underground from the Murgia to the Adriatic when the rains come.

In this part of Italy, Tanzarella explained, there are no major rivers, and sometimes not a drop of water falls from June to September. For millennia, sun-drenched, water-poor Puglia has been an ideal environment for the harvest of a hardy drought-tolerant cash crop. Sixty million olive trees now grow from the Grotta del Soffio in the south to the town of Foggia in the north—240 trees for each person in Puglia. With its shallow extensive roots, an olive tree can survive in dry rocky soil on fewer than eight inches of precipitation a year. Below us was a carpet of green, a quarter of a million *monumentali*— massive olive trees, many of them thought to be over two thousand years old. Tanzarella pointed to a die-straight road that cut through the orchards.

"The first huge engineering project of the Romans was the Via Appia," she said, "which they built in the third century BCE, to allow soldiers to go south and conquer new lands. Then they built the Via Traiana, which comes down to the Adriatic coast. They planted olive trees all along it."

After driving down a series of switchbacks to the coastal plain, we followed a two-lane road lined by waist-high walls. These were the celebrated drystone walls of Puglia, which have been declared an "intangible heritage of humanity" by UNESCO. (They reminded me of the more sinuous stone walls that stitched together the crazy quilt of the Yorkshire Dales.) To build them, limestone was gathered from local fields, and pounded into place with hammers. The absence of cement lets rainwater flow freely through the stones, preventing it from pooling in the fields, and the moisture that remains in the cracks allows pollinating insects to survive through the dry summer months. At regular intervals, the extravagant fronds of prickly pear cactus, an import from Mesoamerica known to Italians as *fichi d'India*—their fruit is prized as a sweet after-dinner palate-cleanser—bristled from the stones. The walls, which mark the property limits of centuries-old rural estates, enclosed rank upon rank of massive olive trees. In some places, the stones dipped or curved from the true to accommodate living branches.

By then, I couldn't stand it any longer: I needed to get close to an olive tree. I begged Tanzarella to pull over. Drawn as if by a magnetic force, I hopped over a wall. Clay-rich red earth, still wet from yesterday's rain, caked the soles of my shoes. A scourge of olive-eating starlings swept over the treetops, thousands of black birds moving as one, like a storm-loosened banner tormented by a whirlwind. From time to time, the hollow boom of a hunter's rifle echoed over the plain.

But it was the *monumentali* that set the tone, marking this landscape as one of the world's enchanted places. Compared to some of Greece's trees, which tower so high that pickers on long ladders are unable to reach the upper branches, these weren't especially tall. Trees in Puglia undergo pollarding, a technique that involves pruning away the upper branches, which over decades results in a broader crown, shorter trunks, and fatter easier-to-reach olives. The contortions of their trunks made me think of gnarled hands and lacquered guts, or the agonies of Michelangelo's *Slaves* emerging from blocks of marble. Some branches had grown horizontally and had to be propped up by Jenga towers of cinder blocks, so the trees resembled dowagers bent over crutches. Unlike solitary oaks lording over meadows, the *monumentali* conveyed no aloofness, yet each was an individual, and an eccentric one at that. These were *charismatic* trees.

"They always twist clockwise," observed Tanzarella. "Nobody knows exactly why. Some people say they follow the sun; other people think it is connected to the polar axis." She pointed out a tree that had corkscrewed on itself through two full revolutions. "It takes a really long time for the trees to twist. When you see one like that, you know it's really old."

A metal tag stamped with a seven-digit number was nailed to each trunk. Tanzarella explained that in the 1990s rich northerners paid farmers to dig up the shallow roots of some of the largest trees. "The destiny of most of them was to die, because they couldn't survive the humidity and the cold. So now they are all geolocated with tags, and we know if they're being removed."

I approached a tree with a large cavity in its trunk. Farmers carve away the interior of some trees, a process meant to encourage new growth and bigger olive yields. The gnarled brown wood around me oozed timeworn antiquity, while the canopy above exploded with vital dark-green leaves. It was like encountering the lustrous mane of a teenager atop the head of a haggard crone. I understood why some Pugliese compared the *monumentali* to witches, and believed that, when they turned their backs on them, the trees magically shifted shape.

The contrast between ancientness and youthful vigor is part of what makes the olive tree such a potent symbol. The olive tree, Athena's gift to the people of Athens, provided the wood that made Heracles's club. Odysseus carved Penelope's marriage bed from a living olive tree. Its leaves and branches stand for peace, forgiveness, and hope—think of the dove returning with an olive branch in its beak to Noah's ark after the flood—which is why uprooting an olive tree, as the Spartans did when they put Attica under siege, or as Israeli settlers do today in Palestinian groves, is considered an unspeakable act of aggression. The oil pressed from its fruit kept the menorah in the Temple of Jerusalem burning for eight miraculous days, anointed the beard and shawl of the Prophet Mohammed, and to this day confers beauty, luster, and health on those who consume it or anoint their bodies with it. For the people of the Mediterranean, land planted with olive trees is no longer wild but has been tamed—brought into the domus—and made useful to humans.

The base of the hollow tree, I noticed, was scattered with windfall olives. I picked up a handful: they were purplish-black, oval, and no bigger than the nail of my index finger. Tanzarella recognized them as Ogliarola salentina, the cultivar favored by the Romans for making oil. She said the same kind grew on her own property. She and her husband made a bit of money by pressing the olives from their 150 trees and bottling the extra-virgin under the name Columella, in tribute to the Roman agronomist.

Such small holdings were typical of southern Italy, where over generations properties have been subdivided into parcels, most smaller than two acres. It's believed that, until recently, a quarter of a million Pugliese were still pressing oil from their own trees. This is in contrast to Spain, the world's largest producer, where a handful of cultivars—especially the oil-rich Picual—are grown in super-high-intensity groves on estates of thousands of acres. Though Italy is thought to possess five hundred of the nine hundred named cultivars in the Mediterranean, just two—Ogliarola salentina and Cellina di Nardò—account for 85 percent of all olives grown in the southern provinces. Despite the antiquity of its olive-growing traditions, Puglia is close to being a monoculture. And like all monocultures, it's vulnerable to pathogens.

A decade ago, the olive trees of Puglia began succumbing to a mysterious ailment known as olive quick decline syndrome. I'd been following the progress of the disease, which by some reports was advancing northward at the rate of 1.2 miles a month. Before arriving, I'd read that the Piana remained unaffected, which is why I was surprised when Tanzarella pulled over to the side of the road for a second time and pointed out a tree that looked shriveled and sick. I grabbed a leaf, which cracked beneath my fingers. It was rust-colored and inward-curled, like a stick of dried cinnamon, and the canopy drooped.

Coming across a sick tree in the Piana was very bad news. It meant the bacteria that causes the disease, *Xylella fastidiosa*, might already be reproducing in the vascular tissues of some of the world's most ancient trees. This would condemn them to a certain death, for

Xylella has no known cure. Tanzarella's property was less than ten miles away, and she was worried that the bacteria could infect her trees.

A new hope had emerged, though, which was one of the reasons I'd decided to visit Puglia. Reports were coming in about ways of preventing *Xylella*, rooted in the region's natural diversity. If a time-hallowed monoculture has lately proven to be Puglia's curse, its lucky charm may well lie in genes that were hiding in plain sight in the fields around us, or being borne aloft in the beaks of starlings.

DONATO BOSCIA REMEMBERED exactly where he was when he realized something was wrong with the olive trees of Puglia. "It was the tenth of August, 2013, at seven thirty in the morning," he told me. "My in-laws have a beach house near Gallipoli. The night before, my brother-in-law asked if I could come take a look at a small piece of land he owns, where he has about seventy olive trees, most of them centuries old. He told me they looked a little strange. We went the next morning, and I saw something I hadn't seen in thirty years of studying plant diseases. Big branches that were brown and dry. Desiccated olives on the affected branches. I started to explore nearby towns, a few kilometers away, and saw fully collapsed olive trees. From that moment, my vacation was over."

Boscia is a soft-spoken man with a patient manner, tired eyes, and a kind smile. He'd invited me to meet him at the Institute for Sustainable Plant Protection, a cramped warren of labs, offices, and greenhouses on the campus of the University of Bari. Trained as a plant pathologist, he has become the lead researcher on *Xylella fastidiosa* for Italy's National Research Council. Ten years earlier, though, he had no idea what was sickening Puglia's olive trees. Nor did he have any inkling of the chaos that the discovery of the disease would unleash.

"The regional plant protection service had a meeting and concluded the problem was due to a severe attack of the leopard moth. I talked to an old farmer, over ninety years old, who told me the moth had always been around, digging galleries in trees, but he had never known it to cause whole trees to collapse."

The lab began the painstaking process of sampling infected trees to exclude known pathogens. Boscia's mentor, the virologist Giovanni Martelli, mentioned that it reminded him of a disease he'd encountered while studying at the University of California, Davis. Pierce's disease, which was spread by flying insects, had a similar effect on grapes—its devastation of vineyards in the 1890s led it to be called Anaheim disease—but there was no indication the pathogen could affect olives. Nonetheless, Martelli, who died in 2020, suggested Boscia's colleague Maria Saponari run a routine check for the Pierce's disease pathogen. It had been dubbed *Xylella fastidiosa*, an allusion to the difficulties it caused scientists who tried to propagate it in the lab.

"I got an email from Maria at five o'clock one morning. She'd just got the DNA sequence from a company in Korea, and it came back one hundred percent positive for *Xylella*. I said, 'Houston, we have a problem.'" Boscia was a virologist, and *Xylella* was a bacterium, but his team quickly pivoted to face the emerging threat.

"The climatic conditions in Gallipoli are almost a photocopy of the ones in the Los Angeles area at the time Pierce's disease started. And in the south of Puglia, we had an abundant population of a very efficient vector, as well as the sensitive plant species: a continuous forest—almost a carpet—of olive trees."

He started by informing the regional and European authorities that the southernmost part of Puglia, the Salento peninsula—the stiletto heel attached to the Italian boot—was facing an outbreak of a novel pathogen. By the end of 2013, surveys revealed that twenty thousand acres of olive trees were already showing symptoms of *Xylella*. The European Commission mapped out an infected zone, drawing a line from east to west north of Gallipoli. South of this line, Puglia's plant protection service began a program of eradication, uprooting sick olives and destroying almond trees and other susceptible plants within a 110-yard radius of infected trees. A twelve-mile-wide containment zone was established to the north, where inspections were stepped up and sick trees removed. Beyond that was a six-mile-wide buffer zone, where trees were still considered healthy but would be closely monitored. The limit of the infected zone now extends seventy-one miles north of the site of the original outbreak, to the town of Fasano, on the edge of the Piana. In a decade, the zone has expanded a hundredfold to cover three thousand square miles. Boscia estimates that ten million trees, though possibly many more, have already died.

Identifying the insect vector that transmitted the disease was easy. The *sputacchina*, or meadow spittlebug, an amphibious-looking insect about the length of a large mosquito, is known for the bubbly white nests it leaves on plants; in late summer, when it lays its eggs, it looks like a salivating giant has wandered the fields, gobbing on the greenery. Also known as the froghopper, the *sputacchina* has wings and strong legs that allow it to leap high into the tree canopies, where it shelters from the summer heat. When a spittlebug carrying *Xylella* makes a meal of an olive leaf, the bacteria spread through the plant's xylem, or vascular tissue, to the roots, where they begin to reproduce. The pathogens create a kind of gel that clogs the xylem, preventing water and nutrients from reaching the crown, whose leaves quickly wither and die. The Salento peninsula, where Boscia detected the first case, was an especially rich breeding ground for spittlebugs.

"In Fasano," said Boscia, "it might take three people a whole day to collect thirty *sputacchine*." This was not the case in the Salento. "Near Gallipoli, it takes two people only a couple of hours to collect four hundred. In the north, it's like the groves are under sniper fire; from time to time, the spittlebugs might take out one tree. In the south, it's more like they are under constant machine-gun fire: *tak-tak-tak!*"

As more trees died, panic gripped Puglia. Farmers chained themselves to sick trees, picketed public buildings, and blocked trains. Some environmentalists suggested sinister links with the Trans Adriatic Pipeline, a natural gas conduit intended to reduce European dependence on Russian energy, whose construction involved the relocation of several thousand olive trees. Anticipating the reaction to the coronavirus pandemic, denialists and conspiracy theorists spread rumors about the disease's origins on social media. Monsanto, some claimed, had engineered the bacteria so they could replace Puglia's trees with their own patented genetically modified olive cultivars. Others maintained the Mafia was using *Xylella* to clear agricultural land to build luxury resorts. Politicians embraced the accusations: Beppe Grillo, leader of the populist Five Star Movement, called *Xylella* a *gigantesca bufala*, "a gigantic hoax," and made a show of insouciance by ornamenting his office with an infected tree.

Meanwhile, the team at the University of Bari struggled to limit *Xylella*'s relentless northward march, even as it raced to discover the disease's origins. Saponari coauthored a paper pinpointing the bacterium: it was *Xylella fastidiosa* subspecies *pauca*, genotype ST53, identical to a strain common in South America. An analysis of mutations in the gene linked the disease's source to an ornamental coffee plant imported from Costa Rica in 2008, which corresponds to the first time farmers remembered seeing sick trees in Italy.

It was obvious to Boscia and his team that controlling spittlebugs would limit the spread of *Xylella*. This could be done with insecticide, and spraying was already used by many farmers to control olive fly infestations. Getting word out was key, but, incredibly, some politicians in Puglia actively hampered the effort. In 2015, government prosecutors, apparently under orders from the region's newly elected governor, accused Boscia and ten other scientists of orchestrating the epidemic to further their careers. After four years of investigations, all charges were dropped. Boscia was commended by the international John Maddox Prize committee—in the same year they recognized Anthony Fauci—for his courage promoting evidence-based science "despite facing lawsuits and a smear campaign that he started the outbreak." But the damage had been done: while the conspiracy theorists were sowing confusion, *Xylella* had continued its spread. Boscia worries the neighboring region of Calabria and the islands of Sardinia and Sicily will be next in the line of fire.

The official reaction—or lack of reaction—had a certain twisted logic. Puglia is one of the poorest parts of Italy, and olive trees are key to not only its identity but also its economy. Since the beginning of the epidemic, the region's olive industry has shed 33,000 jobs. News of the killer bacteria has stained the reputation of Pugliese extra-virgin abroad, with some buyers expressing concerns about increased pesticide use affecting the purity of the oil. (The oil-makers I met insisted they treated the trees in the spring, long before the harvest starts in late October, and that only natural citrus-based insecticides are used.) Tourists who come from afar, the thinking goes, would rather luxuriate beneath a timeless green canopy than in a petrified forest of dead trees.

"Can you imagine?" marveled plant pathologist Pierfederico La Notte. "The Puglia region made the first public information video about *Xylella* in 2021. It took them eight years!" Boscia had walked me down a corridor to his younger colleague's sunlit office. I'd already seen the infomercial, which showed a father and son pushing a rototiller between ancient trees. Tilling the soil this way kills 95 percent of spittlebugs by cutting up the grass and weeds where the larvae live in the spring. I told La Notte that at Brindisi's international airport, the only poster I could find alerting visitors to the epidemic was discreetly hidden beside restrooms next to a luggage carousel. He groaned. "All because they are afraid to have a bad influence on tourism, on the image of Puglia!

"*Xylella* changed my life completely," continued La Notte. "I feel responsible not only for my territory, my land, and my son's future, but also because Puglia is on the front line for protecting the Mediterranean." La Notte's wife presses organic extra-virgin olive oil from their own trees. Their property lies north of the infected zone, near the regional capital of Bari, but La Notte believes it's only a matter of time before their trees are infected. Spittlebugs are extremely mobile: they can travel hundreds of miles in a day by clinging to trucks and car bumpers, which explains why so many infected trees are found along roadsides. In the Salento peninsula, many properties have been abandoned, and untended grass and weeds give the insects plenty of habitat for egg-laying. La Notte believes that tilling needs to happen north of the infected zone, to anticipate the advancing *Xylella* wave.

"We take all the necessary measures on our farm. But if our neighbors don't do the same, it's a disaster." From the start, La Notte realized lab and fieldwork wouldn't be enough. To fight rumors, he helps moderate an authoritative, evidence-based Facebook page called "Info Xylella," which provides crowdsourced updates on the disease's progress.

What maddens La Notte is that the European authorities seem to have learned nothing from *Xylella*. "Ornamental plants are still not regulated. We continue to import fungi; we continue to import viruses. In Italy alone, there are at least thirty points where imported plants can enter. Chile, with three thousand miles of coast, has just two. Australia, more or less the same. But in Europe, the nursery lobby is very strong, and farmers are too numerous and divided to act as an effective lobby."

Both La Notte and Boscia find the way the bacteria have homed in on the region's most iconic trees especially heartbreaking. "The older the tree is," Boscia told me, "the more sensitive it is to *Xylella*." Three-quarters of a million of Puglia's olive trees are *secolari*, more than a century old, and 320,000 of those are classed as *monumentali*, meaning they are not only ancient but also massive.

One by one, the Pugliese have watched their beloved giants, which often have names in dialect, blacken and die. First to go was the Salento's largest tree, La Ulia te la Chiesa; then Lu Matusalemme ("The Methuselah") at Borgagne, at 3,000 years thought to be Italy's most ancient tree; followed by Lu Gigante di Alliste, thought to be 1,500 years old. Many of the dried-out trees end up burning to the ground, victims of summer wildfires or arson, reportedly by farmers who have decided to clear their land the easy way.

"Some areas look like the day after a nuclear catastrophe," Boscia told me. "You will see. It's like whole fields have been through an aerial war."

From time to time, though, the scientists had heard reports from farmers that, in the midst of parched groves, a few trees still had green canopies and remained in relatively good health. It was a simple observation that presaged a remarkable breakthrough. Identifying the cultivars that had resisted the disease could be the key not only to saving an age-old olive oil industry but also, as it turned out, Puglia's oldest and grandest trees.

IS ANY TREE MORE ENTWINED with the story of humanity than the olive? It's been our constant companion since the earliest days, making its first appearance in the Mediterranean half a million years ago, around the same time our species diverged from *Homo erectus* on the African savannah.

Olea europaea subspecies *europaea* is believed to have arisen from a cross between two African trees, ironwood and Laperrine's olive, a near-extinct native of the Saharan mountains. The fact that it has twenty-three chromosomes, exactly the same number as our species, is a coincidence, albeit a suggestive one. An olive is a drupe, like a cherry, mango, or peach, but it's inedible when ripe, thanks to the presence of oleuropein, a bitter phenolic compound that repels insects. There's a reason an apple—or maybe it was a pomegranate—features so prominently in the Garden of Eden story: it could be plucked, ready to eat, from the branches of the Tree of the Knowledge of Good and Evil. An olive must be repeatedly soaked in water, and preferably treated with lye from wood ash, to be made edible. (I've tried brining fresh olives at home. It's time-consuming work, and the results I got were pretty lackluster.) Cultivating an olive tree calls for forethought; to enjoy its fruit requires culture.

When the glaciers in Europe retreated after the Last Glacial Maximum, the olive trees that had survived the Ice Age were concentrated in distinct refugia on the shores of the Aegean Sea, around Gibraltar, and in the Near East. Abundant evidence of humans gathering the fruit of wild olive trees, known as oleasters, in these areas dates to about twelve thousand years ago. According to a genome profiling of 1,846 trees from over a hundred locations, we first started cultivating the tree 8,000 years ago, somewhere on the border between Turkey and Syria, in the historic homeland of the Kurdish people.

The first solid archaeological evidence of domestication comes from Tel Tsaf, a site in the central Jordan Valley of Israel, in the form of charred olive wood dated to seven thousand years ago. The date of this find roughly coincides with a dramatic spike in olive pollen in the southern Levant. From there, cultivated olives spread west, through Cyprus, Greece, and Italy to the Iberian Peninsula. Our friends the Phoenicians—the presumed inventors of *garum*—may have helped spread the olive tree to Tunisia, Algeria, and Morocco through their North African stronghold of Carthage. Phoenician shipwrecks are full of distinctive amphorae for transporting olive oil.

The combination of two technologies made olive oil into the fuel—*and* the food, *and* the cosmetic, *and* the medicine—that ran the economies of early Mediterranean civilizations. Grafting allowed farmers to cut shoots from favored trees and insert them into the rootstock of a wild or domesticated olive tree. As it grew, the grafted shoot, or scion, hijacked the entire operation, making the tree produce the desired tasty or oil-rich crop. Milling allowed farmers to use heavy circular stones of granite or basalt to crush olives to extract every drop of oil. From Gibraltar to the Holy Land, remains of oil mills are even more common than *garum* factories. *Gethsemane* is the Aramaic word for "olive press," and the eight contorted trees that today overlook the garden on Jerusalem's Mount of Olives may well grow from roots that nourished the same olive varieties crushed in the original mill.

In the Roman Empire, captives, centurions, and senators alike were nourished by olive oil, which was, in the words of author Tom

Mueller, "the ancient world's answer to sweet light crude." The quantities consumed were astonishing. I once spent a morning walking around Monte Testaccio, a hill with a half-mile circumference in a working-class district of Rome. As tall as a ten-story building, it could be mistaken for one of the seven historic hills of Rome; at its summit, roosters crowed and green parrots flitted among palm trees. Where the grass and shrubbery had been worn away, I could see strata of shards of red terracotta. The entire hill, in fact, is one vast midden of smashed olive oil amphorae, which, according to inscriptions, were mostly shipped from the extensive plantations in Andalucía and North Africa. By one estimate, there are 25 million amphorae in Monte Testaccio, representing 460 million gallons of olive oil. Olive oil was distributed free of charge in Rome, part of the grain dole known as the *Cura Annonae*; each citizen is estimated to have consumed over two quarts *per month*. Skeletal analysis shows that at the time of the eruption of Vesuvius in 79 CE, olive oil made up almost one-quarter of the calories in the diet of the people of Herculaneum.

The largest surviving cache of ancient extra-virgin, incidentally, also comes from Herculaneum, in the form of an oil dispenser one researcher described as containing "white-yellowish, brownish and blackish glomeruli with a waxy consistency." What it tastes like is anyone's guess. Not surprisingly, no researcher has yet dared to drizzle a dash of two-thousand-year-old glomeruli on a plate of arugula.

ABOUT HALF A MILE from the route of the Via Traiana, the road built by the Emperor Trajan to connect the port of Brindisi to Rome, I drove through the gates of the Masseria Brancati. *Masseria* is the term for the main buildings of historic feudal agriculture estates, which in Puglia now often do double duty as luxurious hotels or rural homestays.

Corrado Rodio, a member of the seventh generation of his family to grow olives here, met me at the front door. In a hallway, he paused to show me a framed photo of his great-grandfather, who modernized the mill in the 1880s. Rodio, though he was dressed in a beret and a duffle coat rather than a Homburg and a waistcoat, could have passed for his ancestor's twin: both had olive-shaped eyes, salt-and-pepper moustaches and beards, and jet-black brows. Rodio pulled on a pair of rubber boots and invited me to follow him down a twisting flight of polished stone steps into the cellar beneath the farmhouse. Nimble as a billy goat, he punctuated every new marvel with an emphatic *"Guarda!"* ("Look!") or a full-throated *"Incredibile!"*

We began in the *frantoio ipogeo*, the underground mill over which the *masseria* was built. This part of Puglia is rich in karst, a water-soluble limestone that is often riddled with caves. Rodio held out a handful of flintstones he'd found while digging in the cellar. The previous day I'd visited a cave in the Murgia plateau, less than three miles away by crow's flight, which contained the remains of the Woman of Ostuni, who had been carefully buried with a headdress of shells painted in red ocher, and was eight months pregnant when she died. The flintstones on this property, ideal for hunting prehistoric megafauna, were identical to the ones discovered next to the Paleolithic woman, whose bones have been dated to 29,000 years ago. The way Rodio saw it, the story of his *masseria* encompassed the entire human history—and prehistory—of Puglia.

"Guarda!" he said, leaping across a coffin-sized depression cut into the limestone floor. "This is the oldest part of the mill. In Neolithic times, people may have put their olives here." Puglia was once part of Magna Graecia—Greater Greece—a loose collection of settlements in southern Italy founded by colonists from the eastern shore of the Adriatic. They shared the territory with the indigenous Messapians, a tribe who lived in walled settlements until the Romans completed their conquest of the Salento peninsula in 267 BCE. Next to the depression was a circular groove, about the size of a manhole cover. "This was the base of the press. And here is a little tank, a half meter in height. It's really primitive. I think the oil and the water pressed from the olives would have been stored here." Caves like

these remain cool year-round but rarely dip below 57 degrees Fahrenheit; any colder than that, and crushed olive paste becomes difficult to process. Rodio believed the remains of the first olive mill on this site were Messapian, though perhaps even older. *"Incredibile, no?"*

The Romans were the next people to use the cellar. Rodio led me to a circular basin in the middle of the floor, in the center of which a massive round stone had been placed. *"Guarda!* This is a Roman-style olive press."* The Romans used the *trapetum*, a rotary crusher consisting of two convex stone half-circles mounted on a cylindrical central post, which was turned by donkeys, horses, or a pair of perspiring humans. The stones were raised one Roman inch (0.97 inches) above the basin, and as they rolled, they crushed the ripe olives into a paste, which was then placed into woven sacks or onto mats. These were compressed with a lever, and no doubt a lot of grunting, to extract the oil.

"Some mills in Puglia were working the same way, with the same tools the Romans used, up until the Second World War." Rodio led me outside and pointed to a walkway beneath the observation tower that had been built over the mill. "The first documents we've found for this *masseria* come from the Brancati family, five hundred and fifty years ago." Rodio pointed out horizontal slits in the wall, which allowed arrows and shotguns to be aimed at raiders. "The *masserie* were built on the model of Roman agricultural towns. When pirates and robbers came from the sea, everybody would hide inside the walls. They could survive for months; they were completely self-sufficient." Rodio takes his olives to a nearby cooperative, where they are milled using a stainless-steel centrifuge, which allows several hundred pounds of olives to be pressed at their ripest, within hours of harvest.

"The Romans were capable of producing an oil of absolute excellence. But with ancient systems, you can only make excellent oil if the olives are healthy, fresh, harvested the same day, and if the millstones are clean. If they are dirty, or the olives are left too long before they are pressed, it is impossible to achieve excellence." The best Roman oil, the kind the emperors and a few lucky farmers had access to, may have been superior to anything that comes out of a modern centrifugal press. (Grindstones leave the pits and skins intact, releasing less sharp-tasting chlorophyll and producing oil with a mild, buttery flavor.) But the oil everybody else ate, from nobles to hoi polloi, was more likely than not fusty, grubby, and, by the time it got to Rome, on its way to being rancid.

Inside the farmhouse kitchen, Rodio poured out samples from five bottles of oil pressed from his olives. Holding the plastic cup in my palm, which heated the oil to release the aromatics, I performed the *strippaggio*, the sharp intake of breath through gritted teeth that coats the taste buds and draws an oil's volatile substances, via the retronasal route, toward the brain's smell receptor cells. I find the whole slurpy-slurpy rigmarole of a formal olive-oil tasting a bit embarrassing, and my palate certainly isn't trained enough to pick out all the notes of almonds, lemon, and green tomatoes that professional olive oil sommeliers claim to detect. But the Masseria Brancati's *fruttato medio* struck me as being extraordinarily good. Rodio explained it was made from olives milled that December, making it less than three months old. The bottle I was sampling was made with the variety the Romans favored, Ogliarola salentina olives. Unlike modern cultivars, selected to arrive at maturity at the same time, Ogliarola olives on the same tree matured in stages, allowing slow-moving mechanical mills to process them over weeks and months.

As Rodio told it, I was eating oil from trees that had been producing olives since the time of Julius Caesar. Ancient as the trees may have been, their oil tasted fresh, grassy, and vibrant, and produced the telltale back-of-the-throat tingle that indicates it is charged with polyphenols.

Outside, Rodio's olive trees were standing up to another dump of springtime sleet with admirable stoicism. He drove me through the grove in a pickup truck, introducing me to some of the grandest of his trees. La Capanna ("The Cabana") was a squat, centripetal whorl of trunk with a thirty-three-foot circumference from which a trio of stems protruded.

"Two adults and two children can sleep comfortably inside the trunk of La Capanna. Once we fit nine people and a dog inside! *Incredibile!*" A little farther down a dirt road, we stopped next to the oldest tree on the estate, which had taken an abrupt turn to the horizontal, so that its trunk grew parallel to the ground. "It's called the Grande Vecchio"—the "Great Old One"—"but my children called it L'Elefante." Over the centuries, its trunk had twisted on itself through three complete revolutions, so that it now bulged like an overwound rubber band on a toy airplane. A weather-worn stack of masonry blocks, which Rodio said had already been in place when his family took ownership of the *masseria* in the nineteenth century, prevented the trunk from touching the ground. "The Grande Vecchio could be three thousand years old, maybe older."

Rodio admitted it was impossible to know the exact age of his trees. Unlike Douglas-firs or ponderosa pines, which record changes in climate in annual growth rings, ancient olive trees have heartwood which decomposes or is deliberately cut away. Olive trees in Israel, Crete, and Portugal are said to be several millennia old,* but these claims are based on the none-too-exact method of measuring the diameter of the trunk and dividing it by an average rate of annual growth. The real problem comes down to the definition of *tree*. The actual wood of a monumental olive tree may not be particularly venerable, but its roots can be very ancient indeed. Like the walls of some Japanese temples, which are torn down and rebuilt from their foundations every few generations, a new structure can arise from the roots even after a tree appears to have been killed by wildfire or frost. I'd come to think of *Olea europaea* less as a fixed solid than as a process for embodying Mediterranean soil and sunlight—a Zen master of the arboreal world.

---

* This may be true: an as-yet-unpublished study out of France combining radio-carbon dating, CT-scan tomography, and a variety of other techniques has found that a famous stand of olive trees on Mount Lebanon may indeed be seven thousand years old.

Which meant that when Rodio told me I was tasting oil from trees that were over two thousand years old, I was willing to take him at his word. The oldest known work of Latin prose, Cato the Elder's *On Agriculture*, written in 160 BCE, refers to the distinctive olive variety cultivated in the Puglia region as *Salentina*. Most of the trees in the Piana are planted in rows at a spacing corresponding to sixty Roman feet. This is the exact distance recommended by the first-century Cádiz-born writer Columella, in situations where vegetable crops are planted between olive trees, which is the tradition in this part of Puglia. Rodio suspected that trees outside the grid—such as the Grande Vecchio—were not planted by the Romans but had started as oleasters, wild olives, onto which Ogliarola salentina shoots had been grafted.

"When an old tree is sick," said Rodio, "I graft a shoot from a healthy tree on it. My father did the same, and my great-grandfather. The Romans did it, and probably the Messapians before them. The stem that grows from the roots might be only fifty years old, but it lives on ancient roots. That is the true immortality of the olive tree.

"You ask me what the olive tree represents to me. It is everything. When I was a boy, olive oil brought riches to my family. Before they started to cultivate the trees industrially in Spain and Tunisia, olive oil was precious." He fell silent for a moment, reflecting. "It is like *I* am an olive tree. They really feel like part of me."

I brought up the fact that *Xylella fastidiosa* had already been detected in this part of the Piana. Rodio told me he had taken all the recommended precautions, treating his trees with an organic pesticide and tilling the soil in the spring.

"My neighbor has *Xylella*. Five of his *monumentali* trees, and six young ones, are infected. And I am so afraid. For us in Puglia, olive groves represent landscape, beauty, tourists, riches. But they are also a treasure trove of biodiversity. In one old tree, you'll find hundreds, if not thousands, of living beings. Insects, spiders, mice, snakes, the starlings that make their nest in the branches, the foxes, and sometimes the dogs and cats that shelter in the trunks. When their roots die and rot, they add water to the soil. When you think of the fungi, the bacteria we don't see . . . *incredibile!* When these trees die, all that life will disappear."

I sensed that something in Rodio might die too. He had recently planted eight hundred trees in the hopes they would prove resistant to the bacteria. But he was most worried about what would become of the *monumentali*. The potential solution was a radical one: the trees would have to be pollarded down to the trunk, their green crowns removed—a virtual decapitation—and then grafted with healthy shoots.

"I don't know if I'm capable of cutting them. All these trees, I have them in my heart. If it was a sure thing that it would save them . . ." From beneath darkly furrowed brows, Rodio gazed at the Grande Vecchio. "I have to think about it."

BEFORE LEAVING THE MASSERIA BRANCATI, I asked Rodio a question. Did he ever, I wondered, eat butter?

"*Mai!*" he'd replied, without hesitation. "Never!"

I'd suspected as much. By now, the health-conferring benefits of the Mediterranean diet will be familiar to most people. The diet features large amounts of fruits, vegetables, unrefined cereals, lentils and beans, dairy in the form of cheese and yogurt, generous splashes of flavonoid-rich red wine, and more seafood than meat. Most of all, though, it calls for oceans of olive oil.

Some of the longest-lived populations in the world inhabit the Italian islands of Sicily and Sardinia and such Greek islands as Crete and Ikaria,* where olive oil is the fat of choice. Genetic factors, as well as strong family and community connections, are thought to play a role in their inhabitants' longevity, but the fact that olive oil is

---

* The oldest of these islanders, it is true, also lead singularly active lives. Many are shepherds, who spend their days outdoors, following their goats and sheep at a leisurely but steady pace up and down hills. Some report drinking upward of a quart of red wine a day, and remaining sexually active into their nineties.

so popular in these Mediterranean Blue Zones, as the regions with the healthiest centenarians have been dubbed, is pretty suggestive. As is the fact that PREDIMED, a Spanish study of 7,500 adults at high risk of heart disease and stroke, found that those who consumed four tablespoons or more of extra-virgin olive oil—that's a quarter cup a day—showed 30 percent fewer cardiovascular events compared to those who consumed a low-fat diet.

If studying the archaeology of food has taught me one thing, it's this: we are what we eat. Fossilized bones, teeth, and tissues bear the signatures of meals eaten thousands of years ago. The fact that more attention isn't paid to the fats we put into our bodies perplexes me. High-quality extra-virgin olive oil, historically available only to well-placed peasants and the discerning rich, is cheaper and more available than it has ever been. Yet around the world, people eat six times more butter and margarine. If extra-virgin olive oil isn't already your main source of fat, you would almost certainly benefit from a complete oil change. Bear with me for a couple of paragraphs, and I'll explain why.

In the twentieth century, fat—especially the saturated fat that comes from animals—was demonized as an artery-clogging short-cut to heart attacks, cancers, and strokes. (When I was growing up, this inspired people to switch to hydrogenated margarine, which turned out to be charged with verifiably lethal trans fats.) Actually, fat is fantastically energy-rich, packing nine calories per gram, twice the amount of either sugar or protein; for most of human existence, it's been one of the rarest and most precious of nutrients. Current dietary wisdom recommends eating reasonable amounts of full-fat dairy and cheese and butter, preferably from grass-fed animals. While coconut, walnut, and avocado oil can make good cooking oils, they tend to be more expensive than olive oil.

What most of the world consumes is soybean, corn, cottonseed, and rapeseed oil, also known as canola. ("Vegetable oil" could be any of the above; the term allows manufacturers to slop whatever com-modity oil they have on hand into the bottle.) None of these were significant parts of the human diet before 1900. Soybean oil, the most consumed of the refined cooking oils, is particularly detrimental to both the environment and human health. Much has been made of the overproduction of corn in the United States, but an equal amount of land—85 million acres—is devoted to growing soybeans, which are planted in alternate years to fix nitrogen in the soil. Soybean oil use has increased 320 percent in the last sixty years, neatly tracking the rise in diet-related diseases. Now the world's seventh most consumed foodstuff, it is near ubiquitous on supermarket ingredient lists. Industrial soybean cultures, along with palm oil plantations, are also responsible for deforestation in the Amazon and displacement of Indigenous Peoples, particularly in Brazil, the main supplier of soybean oil to China and India.

While soybean oil and chemically extracted seed oils aren't exactly toxic, they aren't good for your health, especially in the long term. Michael Pollan, Paul Greenberg, and other authors have shown how, in the course of a few generations, healthful omega-3 fatty acids have been displaced by omega-6 fatty acids, which are thought to contribute to the chronic inflammation responsible for cancer, diabetes, cardiovascular illness, and many of the other "diseases of civilization." The ratio of omega-6s to omega-3s in soybean oil is twelve to one; in corn oil, it's sixty-six to one. A good olive oil is closer to two to one. In fact, the proportion of linoleic acid (an omega-6) to linolenic acid (an omega-3) in extra-virgin is identical to the ratio found in human breast milk.

Olive oil also contains 230 minor components, the most interesting of which are the polyphenols, responsible for a freshly pressed oil's bitterness and that sting at the back of the throat. Formerly referred to, imprecisely, as antioxidants, these are the compounds that plants produce to protect themselves from sunlight or insect attack. Nicotine, coumarin, caffeine, and the tannins in teas are polyphenols, as are the pigments in leafy greens and blood oranges; the latest research shows these micronutrients interact with the gut microbiome to stimulate the immune system. Consuming them produces a powerful anti-inflammatory response and is thought to be an effective way to head off disease.

For me, the choice between oil pressed from hours-old olives in a mill and oil extracted from soy or seeds using a neurotoxic solvent is an easy one to make. I pick extra-virgin every time. I keep two bottles in my kitchen: a well-priced twenty-five-ounce bottle for everyday sautéing, and a more expensive sixteen-ounce bottle of flavorful Italian, Spanish, or Greek oil for dressing salads and finishing dishes. I always check the bottle for the production date—polyphenols degrade quickly, so I try to buy oils from olives harvested no more than eight months earlier—and favor brands that name the cultivar used. Coratina, Picual, and Koroneiki olives are especially high in polyphenols. Our family sometimes goes through two full-sized bottles a month, which is as much as the ancient Roman ration. I'd be surprised if Desmond's and Victor's stamina and high energy levels—perhaps even their lustrous hair—didn't have a lot to do with all the olive oil their parents work into their diet.

Olive trees alone clearly won't resolve the world's unhealthy fat crisis. To begin with, some people, odd as this seems to me, don't like the flavor of olive oil. Second, olive trees will never supply the world's edible oil needs. Though olive oil has a relatively low carbon footprint—one study from Tunisia showed that a quart of well-produced olive oil helps sequester twenty-two pounds of carbon dioxide—and olive trees are tolerant of drought conditions, radically scaling up production would almost certainly lead to a reduction in biodiversity.

It turns out that the species-rich olive groves such as Puglia's Piana are an anomaly. The norm is now the super-high-intensity plantations in North Africa, California, and Spain, where trees are grown to fit under the cabs of towering olive harvesters that drive along closely planted rows, stripping olives from branches as fast as a person can walk. Even with such highly industrialized monocultures, Mediterranean nations often fail to supply their own needs. Bad crop years can cause price spikes, and as author Tom Mueller revealed in his exposé *Extra Virginity*, these can fuel a lucrative black market in adulterated and counterfeit olive oil. When it comes to supplying the world with extra-virgin, there may not be enough Mediterranean to go around.

Given *Xylella fastidiosa*'s advance through Puglia, though, all this might prove irrelevant. If the bacterium breaches the containment zone and reaches other Mediterranean territories, eating olive oil will stop being a healthy option and once again become a near-unattainable luxury.

THE FIRST DEAD TREES APPEARED just south of Squinzano. I was driving the ss16, a state highway that parallels the Adriatic coast, and every now and then, a tree with browned leaves and bare limbs would flash by, its clawlike branches suggesting arthritic fingers frozen in a death clutch. Within a few miles, the living trees were outnumbered by the dead. By the time I reached the outskirts of Lecce, I was driving through a forest of skeletons.

As the motorway plunged toward the tip of the Salento peninsula, the extent of the *Xylella* disaster became clear. The fields on either side of the motorway were bare. Property owners had cut down their stricken groves, or allowed them to burn. Puglia, like much of Italy, has lately been facing severe summer droughts. Olive groves provide cooling shade; their network of roots prevent the soil from eroding; and when their canopies are healthy and green, they serve as a natural fire retardant, crucial at a time when increasing summer temperatures are making wildfires more severe. With the disappearance of the forest that structured its ecosystem for centuries, the Salento was now rushing toward desertification. With its thickets of prickly pear cactus, it looked more like northern Mexico than southern Italy.

About a dozen miles from land's end, I pulled into the parking lot of Forestaforte, an olive mill near the town of Gagliano del Capo. Beyond a hangar-like room, dominated by an array of stainless-steel malaxers, extractors, and a centrifuge, a secretary showed me into Giovanni Melcarne's office. For the last five hundred years, Melcarne's family has made a living pressing oil from the olives of Salento. On this afternoon, he seemed preoccupied and tightly wound. A decade of living through a plague had clearly taken its toll.

"I have a farm, I have this mill, I'm an agronomist, and I'm the president of the DOP of Terra d'Otranto," said Melcarne, as he fidgeted with an e-cigarette between sips of ginseng tea. Locally produced olive oil, he explained, benefited from a "protected designation of origin," a label that added value to each bottle. By law, Terra d'Otranto had to be made with the Salento's most ancient cultivars, Ogliarola salentina and Cellina di Nardò, exclusively from olives gathered in the province of Lecce. This is no longer possible, as *Xylella* has killed virtually all the trees. "Medium-sized farms like mine, which invested everything in quality, in innovation, are the ones that have suffered the most." Melcarne has been forced to sell some of his state-of-the-art olive milling equipment at a discount to foreign firms.

"I'm a very pragmatic person. The way I see it, problems aren't solved by crying over spilled milk," said Melcarne. While farmers, campaigners, and politicians were pointing fingers and spreading conspiracy theories, he looked for a solution. Three years after the first outbreak, he contacted the plant pathologists at the University of Bari. Donato Boscia and Pierfederico La Notte agreed to come look at a tree in another olive farmer's grove. In a landscape of dried-out brown leaves, a single branch on this tree was still green. The farmer explained to Melcarne and the scientists that he'd grafted a shoot from another variety onto the Ogliarola trunk; astonishingly, the scion seemed to be keeping the entire tree alive.

The miracle cultivar turned out to be Leccino, a cold-resistant olive known for producing a mild, almond-flavored oil. Leccino had first been planted in Puglia in the nineteenth century, when some farmers were already worrying about the south's overreliance on a couple of ancient varieties. La Notte put out the word to gene banks around the world, including the Worldwide Olive Germplasm Bank, which keeps hundreds of Mediterranean varieties alive in its green-houses and orchards in Córdoba, Spain. Over 270 cultivars were grafted onto the trees in Melcarne's fields, but in the end, only one other variety, an Italian cultivar with the clinical-sounding name FS-17, proved resistant. Melcarne used his life savings to graft thirty-five acres of his own trees. The resistant shoots brought new life to the trees, and in 2019, he celebrated by pressing the first batch of what he dubbed Courage Oil. He has since obtained a derogation that allows for Terra d'Otranto DOP extra-virgin to be made with the resistant cultivars. So far, about five thousand acres have been replanted with FS-17 and Leccino.

"That's very little," pointed out Melcarne. "At the current rate of planting, we'll need fifty years to recover. As soon as I realized the bacteria was in the region, I knew the big challenge would be saving the *monumentali*. My father slept under those trees. He cared for the soil. He harvested the olives one by one." Grafting offers a chance to save the *monumentali*, but only if it's done before they're attacked by the bacteria. "That's something many farmers still haven't under-stood." It took Melcarne and the scientists several years to realize that crown grafts—chopping off branches and inserting the grafts into the severed extremity—worked the best. But as Corrado Rodio had made clear while contemplating the Grande Vecchio, to mutilate a giant tree, especially when it was still healthy, was a wrenchingly hard decision to make.

Convincing farmers to switch to new cultivars has also proved to be a barrier. The origins of Leccino lie not in Puglia but in medieval Tuscany. FS-17, a patented cross between the Frantoio and Ascolana tenera cultivars, was developed by scientists in the 1980s. I've tried oil made with both cultivars, and they make excellent extra-virgin. But some farmers fear that the conspiracy theories will come to fruition, and post-*Xylella* Puglia will turn out be a vast monoculture domi-nated by a couple of resistant varieties. Sustainability advocates have argued the *Xylella* outbreak provides an opportunity for a deeper change. Replacing olive groves with vineyards, vegetables, and fruit trees would help diversify agriculture in Puglia, while providing the shade and root networks that could help reverse desertification.

Melcarne was sympathetic to these arguments, but he was committed to restoring the traditional olive tree landscape. If he could find native-born varieties that stood up to *Xylella*, he figured more of his neighbors might be willing to plant them. "If you go around the Salento, you see it's full of wild olive trees, many of which aren't affected by the bacteria." Starlings and other birds swallow olives whole—a strategy for getting around the bitter taste of oleuropein— and carry the pits to new locations, depositing a few drops of feces, which helps fertilize the plant as it grows. While the trees cultivated in groves are clones, propagated by grafts, every olive pit is a genetically distinct plant—which could potentially be a new cultivar. Melcarne put out a call on Facebook, and farmers responded by bringing him healthy plants they found on their properties. These weren't oleasters, the shrub-like precursors of the olive tree, but feral plants, the wild offspring of domesticated trees. "Some of the wild plants actually produce pretty big olives. So far we've found four exemplary plants, and now we're in the final phase of testing. If all goes well, we'll be able to certify them as resistant by the end of the year."

Scooping up his vape, Melcarne led me through the parking lot to a greenhouse. Hundreds of plants, ranging in size from shoots to large saplings, were lined up in planters. This was the project closest to his heart: Melcarne hoped to preserve the historic cultivars of Puglia by crossing them with resistant varieties. "Many of these are crosses with Ogliarola and Cellina di Nardò. I inoculate them with *Xylella* to see which ones will resist. At the end of this year, I'll have between ten and twelve kinds in production, of which seventy percent will be resistant. They're small right now, but we already have six hundred plants in production.

"To compete in the market, we need to give consumers—the most cultured consumers, anyway—different kinds of oils, with different flavors. And the more varieties we have, the more chances we have to protect ourselves from plant diseases."

In the end, it wasn't a gene bank that was providing the best hope for saving southern Italy's crucial olive oil industry. In Puglia, home to one of history's longest-running monocultures, it was the natural diversity preserved in traditionally managed fields and orchards—and transmitted by little black birds—that was coming to the rescue.

DONATO BOSCIA SUGGESTED that before leaving Puglia, I visit a farm that had some success saving ancient trees with grafts. The Petruzzi family lived near Fasano, at the northern limits of the containment zone, where *Xylella* had yet to arrive. As I parked next to their farmhouse, a trio of shepherds, accompanied by hard-working sheepdogs, were herding a flock of sheep through a gap in the drystone walls. While *Xylella* had been detected in the vicinity, most of the orchards in this part of the Piana were still green and lush. This was a classic Mediterranean landscape, one that hadn't changed much in two thousand years. I was glad my last impression of Puglia wouldn't be of spectral forests and barren fields.

I walked through the estate with Donato Petruzzi and his wife and daughter, following a *lama*, an underground stream, whose course was marked by lush growths of almond, lemon, and fig trees. Petruzzi owned 250 monumental olive trees, and he was determined to keep every one of them alive. He showed me where workers had performed crown grafts on the trees. This was the operation that Corrado Rodio had dreaded, and the results weren't particularly pretty: the biggest limbs of the grand old trees had been severed, and shoots from resistant FS-17 and Leccino trees inserted into the wood. Tourniquets of fiberglass had been wrapped below the cuts, to protect the fragile scions from being attacked by insects. A small tree could be grafted for €40; a big tree might cost €140. The real challenge, Petruzzi's daughter Stefania pointed out, was finding the skilled workers capable of practicing this ancient art.

Petruzzi, who was now retired, had worked as the regional representative for the Italian Farmers' Confederation in Bari, and brought an insider's view to the epidemic. As painful as the preventive measures were, he was willing to take them. "The problem is many people around here still haven't realized *Xylella* is coming. If they went south to Lecce, they would see how bad things are. The bacterium is going to arrive here, sooner or later." The first grafts had been done five years earlier. Some trees were now producing healthy crops of olives. "I remember seeing this one planted," he said, pointing to one of the smaller trees. "It was sixty years ago. Last year it produced a quintal"—220 pounds—"of Leccino. And the oil was good." But he admitted he preferred the oil from the olives the tree had been producing since he was a young man. If a cure for *Xylella* was ever found, he thought it would be possible to make this tree bear Ogliarola salentina olives again.

As I left, Petruzzi said he had something to show me. Reaching into a treetop, he plucked an elongated fruit from a branch. It was a caviar lime, he said, a citrus fruit that chefs in Italy paid top prices for. I broke it open and took a suck on the tightly packed pulp sacs within; it was bracingly tangy, with a pleasing hint of marmalade-like bitterness. I took one long last look at the scene around me, the violet flowers of almond trees in bloom, the *fioroni* figs, the still-green lemons dangling from branches. All this diversity beneath the shimmering crowns of the olives struck me as quintessentially Mediterranean, and exactly what the sustainability advocates hoped the *Xylella*-devastated parts of the Salento peninsula would become. It was about as close to a vision of paradise as a place could get.

The fruit I'd sucked on, *Citrus australasica*, also known as the Australian finger lime, wasn't native to Puglia. It had been introduced to this landscape by humans, part of our age-old pursuit of flavor, nutrition, and delight. Of course, exactly the same thing was true of *Olea europaea*, the olive tree, which was deliberately spread through the

Mediterranean from the Fertile Crescent and has created one of the most appealing and fruitful of all the landscapes created by humanity.

Our species, whose origin stories lie in lost Arcadias, has always sought to re-create paradise on Earth. In places like Puglia, we actually succeeded. But many of us have forgotten that these Edens didn't just happen: they are the product of millennia of care and toil. If we really value them, the responsibility to preserve them falls on us.

7

CAPPADOCIA
Lost and Found

ACCORDING TO THE STANDARD NARRATIVE, humanity's long fall from grace has occurred at the expense of the other species with whom we share the planet. The human-caused extinctions began with the phenomenon known as prehistoric overkill. Shortly after *Homo sapiens* washed up on shore, Australia's megafauna—which included hippopotamus-sized wombats, marsupial lions, and six-foot-tall thunderbirds—was wiped out. In North America, the arrival of humans was followed by the disappearance of ninety genera of mammals, among them the saber-toothed *Smilodon*, the two-thousand-pound camel, and the giant beaver. More recently, the same happened to the giant lemurs and pygmy hippos of Madagascar, flightless moas of New Zealand, Steller's sea cows of the Bering Sea, and passenger pigeons of the Great Lakes.

Where humans went, other species vanished. Now that there are more than eight billion of us, a sixth of all birds, a fifth of reptiles, a quarter of mammals, and a third of reef-building corals are heading for extinction. Before our species came along, the normal background extinction rate saw one species of mammal disappearing every seven hundred or so years. (At the same time, the natural process of speciation meant new species were constantly arising.) Under our watch, the loss rate has accelerated to one mammal species every four years. The spread of humanity, from this perspective, is one long story of erasure.

Occasionally this narrative gets turned on its head, as a species considered extinct rises from the grave. Some of the most spectacular resurrections have involved prehistoric fossil taxa, including the Majorcan midwife toad, the Wollemi pine, and the coelacanth, a massive lobe-finned fish thought to have disappeared 66 million years ago, before it was discovered browsing on cuttlefish off the shores of South Africa in 1938. Others, declared extinct "beyond a reasonable doubt" in recent times, have been rediscovered in the wild, among them the minuscule mouse-deer, which a night-vision camera caught picking its way through a Vietnamese forest in 2019. A plant or animal that pulls off this neat trick is known as a Lazarus taxon, after the man Jesus was said to have brought back to life after four days in the tomb.

The first case of species extinction in history involves an edible plant. (Earlier examples of prehistoric overkill, while they certainly occurred, predate written records.) For a little over seven centuries, one of the most sought-after products in the classical world was a golden-flowered plant with vaguely valentine-shaped fruits. For Greek physicians, silphion was a cure-all, prized for everything from abdominal pain relief to wart removal. For Roman chefs, who knew it as silphium or laser, the plant's root was a pantry staple, crucial for spicing up an everyday pot of lentils or adding the finishing touch to an extravagant dish of sterile sow's womb or scalded flamingo. Julius Caesar was said to have removed 1,100 pounds of silphion resin from the imperial treasuries in Rome, where it was stockpiled alongside gold and silver.

Then, just as suddenly as the silphion plant bloomed—according to one chronicler, it appeared for the first time in 638 BCE, after a "pitchy" black rain descended near the coast of what's now Libya—it disappeared. The last stalk, according to Pliny the Elder, who died in the eruption of Vesuvius in 79 CE, was shipped from Africa to Nero as a curiosity, and may have ended up in the ample belly of the gluttonous emperor. For many, the disappearance of silphion is a cautionary tale. Long before we shot the last passenger pigeon and fished Atlantic cod to collapse, human appetite was capable of extirpating a species from the wild.

I'd long been aware of the legend of silphion. Since the Middle Ages, botanical explorers have sought the plant on three continents, always in vain. In 1629, the physician Prospero Alpini made the unlikely claim that he'd located silphion growing in the medical garden of Padua. (The plant's leaves and resin bore no resemblance to the original, and Alpini sowed lasting confusion by naming this garden-variety species *Laserpitium*.) From the early nineteenth century, a succession of Italian travelers excitedly claimed to have rediscovered silphion growing in Libya. In 1817, a Genoese doctor identified *Thapsia garganica*, a plant with heart-shaped fruits and a resin used by indigenous Libyans, as a likely candidate. It turned out to be deadly for camels and not much better for humans; its resin provoked vomiting and diarrhea. In 1996, the Italian scientist Antonio Manunta made a splash with *Cachrys ferulacea*, which has heart-shaped fruits and produces an agreeably scented resin. The plant's leaves, however, don't correspond to the ancient descriptions, and it's commonly found in Italy and Greece, places the ancients made clear that silphion couldn't grow.

The most plausible candidate was proposed by French medical historian Suzanne Amigues. She argued that a tall fennel-like plant with celery-like leaves and a resin that whitened on contact with air matched the ancient descriptions. "These facts," she wrote, "permit us to affirm that *Margotia gummifera* is the contemporary species closest to silphium, though not that it *is* silphium."

I didn't really buy it. *Margotia gummifera* grows all over the Iberian Peninsula, and several studies have concluded it has little value as a medicinal plant. If silphion had survived—and that was a big if—it wouldn't be as a plant with no known culinary or medical applications that has long grown like a weed all over Spain and Portugal.

So when I found an article entitled "Next Chapter in the Legend of Silphion," in which yet another obscure species was hailed as the long-lost spice of antiquity, I was intrigued but wary.

"Recently," I read in the abstract, "a rare and endemic *Ferula* species that produces a pleasant-smelling gum resin was found in three locations near formerly Greek villages in Anatolia. Morphologic features of the species closely resemble silphion, as it appears in the numismatic figures of antique Cyrenaic coins . . . Initial chemical and pharmacological investigations of this species have confirmed the medicinal and spice-like quality of its gum resin."

If the legendary silphion had indeed survived into the twenty-first century, it would be the most spectacular case of a Lazarus taxon in the history of gastronomy. The paper had been published in the peer-reviewed journal *Plants*, and the research came from the venerable Faculty of Pharmacy at the University of Istanbul. After a few video calls with the author, I began to plan a voyage to the interior of Turkey.

BEFORE LEAVING, I decided to go see Philippe and Ethné de Vienne, a couple famous in Quebec as "spice hunters." I'd long been a fan of their shop Épices de Cru, an Ali Baba's cavern of intoxicating odors and sensations tucked away in one of the inner corridors of Marché Jean-Talon, the largest outdoor food market north of the Rio Grande. On a winter day, browsing shelves filled with jars of comet's tail pepper from Java and grains of paradise from West Africa, or such proprietary spice mixes as their Apicius blend (celery seeds, long pepper, and fennel), feels like a short but restorative tropical vacation.

I rode my bike to their offices and warehouse in the east end of Montreal. Ethné, originally from Trinidad, is slender and gracile, and her youthful career as a fashion model in Holland still manifests in her close-cropped hair, horn-rim glasses, bold jewelry, and photogenic smile. Philippe, the descendant of a noble French family from the Dordogne Valley, is a reformed gourmand, trying to eat more healthily after decades of work as a chef and caterer, and a midlife diagnosis of multiple sclerosis. One of the couple's first collaborations involved orchestrating an Indonesian rijsttafel, with Philippe as chef and Ethné translating from an old Dutch cookbook. Every summer, they'd return from vacations with their children with suitcases filled with obscure herbs and spices, a habit that became the foundation of their business. I wanted to get their take on the ethics of seeking out the legendary silphion in Turkey.

"We are food consumers," Ethné told me, as we sipped cups of tea in a boardroom that doubled as a library of obscure cookbooks and culinary treatises. "We have always wanted the best that the world has to offer." As a child, Philippe lived in the suites at Boston's Copley Plaza Hotel, which his mother managed, growing up on room service caviar and beef Wellington. "We were fortunate to grow up in the one percent," said Philippe. "And we rejected it." The couple have made a career writing cookbooks, appearing on French-language television, and scouring the world in search of such obscure spices as andaliman, a Szechuan-style pepper they tracked down in a hill village of Sumatran cannibals, and blue fenugreek, the cornerstone of the cuisine of Georgia.

I asked them if they'd ever heard of a modern herb or spice being driven to extinction by human consumption. "There are certain things we refuse to sell, especially wild plants, because they're being overharvested," said Philippe. Early on, they'd sold the flour of a Turkish orchid used to make salep, a hot beverage famous in the Ottoman Empire. Because it takes thousands of bulbs to make a pound of the flour, *Orchis mascula* has been driven to near extinction. Épices de Cru no longer carries salep, but they do retail the voatsiperifery pepper, the fruit of a woody vine that hangs from trees in Madagascar. A decade ago, chefs in France fell in love with its uniquely floral, camphor-like flavor, and the high prices they were willing to pay led people in Madagascar to tear down vines, or even chop down entire trees, to supply the market. But since then the lianas have been replanted and raised in gardens, and Ethné and Philippe were confident the voatsiperifery pepper they sold was sustainably harvested.

Such cases were pretty rare, they pointed out. Most herbs and spices were cultivated, rather than wild-harvested. "My main ethical concern with spices," added Philippe, "is the way the big corporations that control the trade do contract farming." The biggest player in the industry is the American giant McCormick & Company, which, like Coca-Cola in the beverage trade, has bought up such proprietary blends as Old Bay seafood seasoning and Cholula Hot Sauce, as well as such national wholesalers as France's Ducros. Spice growers, who are often Indigenous, are bound in exclusive contracts to the big corporations, to whom they become indebted. When artisanal merchants like Philippe and Ethné show up and ask people to name their price, it's often the first time spice growers make a real profit from what they produce.

They took me to the back of the offices, where, with childlike enthusiasm, they pulled out plastic bins to show me seasonings they'd gathered from their travels. There was fermented Svanetian salt from Tbilisi, Georgia; scaly grains of long pepper, beloved by the ancient Romans, from India's Malabar Coast; grains of paradise from Ethné's birthplace of Trinidad; fluorescent-orange rose petals from Iran; Syrian seven spice from the souk in Aleppo. Every spice came with a story of adventures had, connections made, friendships established.

"We're not trying to convince anyone to like something," Ethné said. "We just want people to know we're not crazy! I tell them, Can you believe that I almost passed out from pleasure when I tried this pepper on the plantation? Try it, and you'll see I'm not crazy!"

We spent so much time trading stories that I forgot to ask them directly whether they endorsed my plan to go to Turkey in search of the long-lost silphion. But judging by their attitude, I got the feeling that not only did they approve but that they were hoping I'd be crazy enough to try some—and, at the very least, let them know what it tasted like.

"WELCOME TO SILPHION LAND," said Mahmut Miski. The professor chuckled nervously at the audacity of his pronouncement, but given the setting, it seemed apt. We were standing in an orchard surrounded by fieldstone walls in the boulder-strewn foothills of Mount Hasan, a still-active volcano in western Cappadocia. Miski had led us to a thicket of grooved buff-colored stalks shaded by oak trees. He stooped to pull a gnarled root ball from the rocky soil. This was the chemical factory of the plant, and it perfumed the air with a pleasant, slightly medicinal odor, halfway between eucalyptus and pine sap. "To me, the smell is stimulating, as well as relaxing. You can see why everybody who encounters this plant becomes attached to it."

I'd met Miski the previous day, outside the train station on the Asian side of Istanbul. On the Konya-bound high-speed train, Miski explained that he'd first stumbled upon the plant while doing postdoctoral research forty years earlier. He'd received a grant to collect specimens of *Ferula*, a genus of flowering plants in the Apiaceae family, which includes carrots, fennel, and parsley. Turkey, which has the greatest diversity of flora in the temperate zone, is home to half of the two hundred or so known *Ferula* species, many of which have yielded novel disease-fighting compounds.

Miski explained that he'd been collecting another plant near the village of Dikmen when two boys asked him if he'd like to see a giant *chakshir*, the local name for *Ferula*-type plants. They led him along a precipitous dirt road to an isolated property where their family eked out a living growing barley and chickpeas. Behind waist-high fieldstone walls, the brothers showed Miski several unusually tall *Ferula* plants, whose thick stems oozed an acrid-tasting resin. They told him that sheep and goats loved to graze on its leaves, and Miski observed that flies and other insects that were attracted by its pearl-colored sap began to mate.

Miski subsequently learned the plant had first been collected in 1909 by a German businessman living in Turkey, and was identified as a new species by Evgenii Korovin, the renowned Russian botanist, who named it *Ferula drudeana* in a 1947 monograph. Since then, the plant had disappeared from the literature. Miski's hunch that *Ferula drudeana* would prove to be a chemical gold mine turned out to be correct: in his lab, stereoscopic and chromatographic analyses of the root extract identified thirty secondary metabolites (substances that, while they don't contribute to the primary business of helping a plant grow or reproduce, confer some kind of selective advantage). Miski told me the plant would likely yield dozens of yet-to-be-identified compounds of medical interest.

"You find the same chemicals in rosemary, sweet flag, artichoke, sage, and galbanum, another *Ferula* plant," marveled Miski. "It's like you combined half a dozen important medicinal species in a single plant."

It was only after a return visit to the site in 2012 that Miski made the connection with silphion. In his paper in *Plants*, Miski enumerated *Ferula drudeana*'s similarities to silphion as it had been depicted on ancient coins: thick branching roots, similar to ginseng; frond-like basal leaves; a grooved stalk rising toward extravagant circular clusters of flowers; celery-like leaves; and papery fruits, or mericarps, depicted in a shape resembling an inverted heart.

The similarities in appearance weren't the only compelling link. The original silphion was said to have appeared suddenly, after a great downpour. Miski observed that when rains came to Cappadocia in April, *Ferula drudeana* would spring from the ground, growing up to six feet in just over a month. Because the ancient silphion resisted cultivation, it had to be harvested in the wild, a task entrusted to desert nomads; the pioneering physician Hippocrates reported that two attempts to transplant it to mainland Greece failed. Among contemporary botanists, *Ferula* plants have a reputation for being unable to reliably germinate outside of their native habitats. Miski told me that his first attempts to transplant *Ferula drudeana* also failed; it was only by using cold stratification, a technique in which seeds are tricked into germinating by exposing them to cold, wet conditions, that his team was able to propagate seedlings in a greenhouse setting.

After our train arrived in Konya, we picked up a rental SUV at the station and drove to the city of Aksaray, once a relay point for caravans crossing Anatolia, now a rest stop for long-distance buses. In the parking lot outside a tea shop, we stopped to pick up Mehmet Ata, who, as a boy, had led Miski to his family's property. Now a grandfather, Ata shared stories of scaling Mount Hasan, which rises dramatically, to over ten thousand feet, out of the Konya Plain. We followed a serpentine road up one of the mountain's western flanks to the village of Dikmen. Ata showed us his childhood home, now abandoned, which consisted of a warren of dark rooms carved directly into volcanic rock. His family had taken possession of the home sometime after 1923; before then, the village had been inhabited by Greeks, who were known to have carved labyrinthine "troglodyte" dwellings into rock all over Cappadocia, often to avoid Ottoman tax collectors. In the aftermath of the Greco-Turkish war following the partitioning of the Ottoman Empire, over 1.5 million Greeks were expelled from western Turkey. The area we were exploring had been an enclave of Greek culture for well over two thousand years.

Miski maneuvered the SUV at a walking pace, weaving between boulders along the same dirt road he'd hiked decades earlier. The terraced hillsides reminded me of arid sunbaked environments I'd seen on some Aegean Islands. The property was in a kind of basin; on one side, closely spaced stone walls climbed like rows of seats in an amphitheater; on the other, the basin opened to a plunging view of the outskirts of Aksaray. Ata told us that most of the walls had been built before his family had taken over. He believed that the grapevines that still clung to the slopes had been planted by their wine-drinking Greek predecessors.

We left the SUV outside a wooden barrier that had been erected to protect the orchard from goats, sheep, and other livestock. Ata told us his father, a farmer, used to harvest wheat with a sickle, and showed us the oval-shaped clearing where the grain had been threshed.

I followed Miski as he scrambled over lichen-covered boulders to the spot where he'd first found the plants. With some difficulty, he managed to locate a trio of intact *Ferula drudeana* plants; their dried-out stems, one of them about five feet long, protruded from between rocks. The ground was strewn with broken stalks; picking one of them up, I noticed it was grooved and as light as balsa wood. Miski checked on some seedlings that had been germinated in a green-house in Istanbul, then replanted in the orchard by Ata. These were in good condition, but still a little small, and wouldn't be ready to flower for several years.

Miski was apologetic; this was October, and there wasn't much to see. The time to come, he reminded me, was when *Ferula drudeana* burst into flower after the spring rains. I'd seen photos taken in mid-May, and the orchard was gilded with sprays of yellow flowers atop the stalks. Miski reckoned there were about 150 plants here. An equal number grew 150 miles to the east. This was where *Ferula drudeana* had been first collected, in a tectonic valley with a Mediterranean microclimate, near Farasha, a town that also had a long history of Greek inhabitation. The two populations turned out to be genetically identical, a fact Miski finds significant. "Other *Ferula* species show evidence of being spread in the wild, by birds or the wind. These *drudeana* populations have preserved their identity and chemical profile, signaling they weren't spread by wild propagation but were brought here at some point by humans."

Miski passed me the root ball, which had been partially unearthed, probably by an animal. Covered with a dark-brown coat, as hard as bark, it suggested the cross section of an elephant's trunk. Several thick branches protruded downward, like a ginseng root. If this really was silphion, I was holding the chemically productive part of the plant that ancient cooks would have grated into food. I took a deep whiff; the plant might have been dormant, but the odor was ambrosial. I asked Miski what Ata could tell us about the plant.

"He says that they used to pound the root into a powder, and eat it like a cream, or boil it into a tea. He has a close friend whose first wife divorced him because he was infertile. He gave him some of this *chakshir* to eat, he says, and now he has two children." Animals, Ata added, loved to browse on its leaves, and it was rumored that goats and sheep that passed through areas where *Ferula drudeana* grew bore twins or triplets.

Before wrapping the root ball in paper and carefully putting it in my backpack, I broke off a piece from the interior and, to Miski's evident surprise, popped it into my mouth and gave it a meditative chew. It was fibrous and slightly bitter on my tongue, but not unpleasant. Chemically, something interesting was definitely going on. I pointed out to Miski that if he were right about this plant, I might be one of the first people in the last fifteen hundred or so years to actually eat silphion.

"Well," he said, after thinking it over for a moment, "certainly the first *Westerner*."

THERE WAS AN OBVIOUS PROBLEM with Miski's contention that *Ferula drudeana* was the long-lost silphion. The foothills of Mount Hasan are eight hundred miles northeast of the shores of Libya. How, then, had a plant so notoriously resistant to transplanting hopscotched the Mediterranean and ended up blooming in the interior of Turkey?

Though the ancients occasionally contradicted each other in describing the plant, on one point everyone, from the Greek medical writer Theophrastus to the moralizing Pliny the Elder, was unanimous: the best silphion came exclusively from a narrow zone around the city of Cyrene, a site now occupied by the modern Libyan settlement of Shahat, about 110 miles east of the port of Benghazi. The geographer Strabo, writing in the first century BCE, was explicit: "The country which produces silphion is narrow, long and somewhat arid, extending in length about 1000 stadia [115 miles] towards the east, and in breadth about 300 stadia [34 miles]."

Cyrenaica, as the region became known under the Romans, was founded by Greek settlers who were driven from the island of Santorini by drought. Seeking a place with a climate suitable for farming, they established the city of Cyrene, seven miles inland from the coast, in 631 BCE. "Libya is like a leopard's skin," observed Strabo, "for it is spotted with inhabited places that are surrounded by waterless and desert land." While Cyrene was sited on one of the leopard's spots—an oasis, essentially, with a climate similar to mainland Greece—the land where silphion grew was located to the south, on the stony steppe that gradually slopes into the sands of the Sahara. To the west, on the other side of the Gulf of Sidra, lay Carthage, the city founded by Phoenicians that would become Rome's trading and military rival.

The settlers from Santorini, led by King Battus, founder of the Battiad dynasty, established friendly relations with indigenous Libyans. The well-watered plateau was indeed fertile, with three harvest seasons, and the land produced barley, rice, saffron, onions, and garlic. Cyrenaica became one of the granaries of the ancient world, shipping 28,000 tons of grain to Athens during a famine in 330 BCE. Trade in silphion was a royal monopoly, but since it couldn't be cultivated, the Battiads apparently relied on nomads to gather the plant from the desert. Strabo described a clandestine trade with Carthage, in which silphion, perhaps pilfered from the royal warehouses, was swapped for wine. The resin harvested from the living plant was shaken with flour, meal, or bran, creating a stable product for shipment across the Mediterranean. Possessing the "silphion of Battus" became synonymous with having "all the gold in the world."

Coins struck under the Battiad dynasty, between the sixth and second centuries BCE, give us the best sense of both silphion's importance in the Cyrenaic economy and what the plant actually looked like. Some of the coins depict the plant in remarkable detail. A thick, grooved stem rises from two or three levels of frond-like leaves arranged on opposite sides of the stalk, and topped by a circle of what looks like beads. This corresponds to a typical feature of *Ferula* species: the umbel, a cluster of flowers protruding, like the ribs of an umbrella, from a central point. On other coins, a gazelle stands on its hind legs, stretching to nibble on the upper leaves. Others show a seated female figure, generally interpreted as the nymph Cyrene—both the namesake and the symbol of the city—stretching a hand toward a stalk of silphion. The obverse of many of the coins depicts what Miski believes is one of the most distinctive features of *Ferula drudeana*: a pair of mericarps, the fruit of the plant, whose broad papery sheaths allow the seeds to be wind-wafted to distant patches of soil. The overlapping mericarps look like a pair of buttocks pressed against glass. Turn the image upside down, though, and it's a dead ringer for the heart on a Valentine's Day card.

The resemblance has led to the widespread misconception that silphion was some kind of ancient contraceptive, or even an aphrodisiac, and that the coins were meant as a salacious advertisement for Cyrenaic luxuries throughout the Roman Empire. The notion was first spread by North Carolina State University historian John M. Riddle, who wrote in *Eve's Herbs*, a book published around the time Viagra hit the market, "Anecdotal and medical evidence from classical antiquity tells us that the drug of choice for contraception was silphium." Exhibit A, wrote Riddle, is the image of the nymph Cyrene on the coin: "One hand touches the plant and the other points to her reproductive area." That is a stretch. The most that can be said, in fact, is that the nymph's hand is in her lap. As for Valentine-shaped hearts, they weren't used as symbols of romantic love until Victorian times. And the last coin depicting silphion was minted in 308 BCE, almost three centuries before Augustus's reign marked the beginning of the empire, which means it could hardly have been an advertisement for Cyrenaica in imperial Rome.

Riddle speculated silphion's contraceptive properties were one of the reasons for a mysterious population decline that struck Rome at the height of its prosperity. In the classical medical literature, silphion was a remedy for baldness and dental pain, for pleurisy and epilepsy, and a balm, according to one lyrical translation, for both the "dog-bitten" and the "scorpion-smitten." It was everything, in fact, *but* a contraceptive. There are also absolutely no references in the ancient texts to silphion being used as an aphrodisiac. (The confusion seems to have arisen through wishful thinking about an allusion to "silphion-bearing Cyrene" in one of Catullus's love poems.) The idea that it might have been a contraceptive comes from an ambiguous mention in Dioscorides—a Greek physician who lived in what is now Turkey, and one of the few authorities who seems to have actually seen the living plant—that when consumed with pepper and myrrh, silphion "moves the menstruation." The furthest Pliny—who admits he never saw the plant—will go is to say that after a miscarriage, the leaves could be used to clean a woman's womb and expel the fetus.

Erica Rowan, an archaeobotanist at the University of London who specializes in ancient Roman foodways, doubts silphion was ever widely used as a contraceptive, abortifacient, or aphrodisiac. "When laser or silphion is mentioned in ancient medical texts," she told me, "it's always with ten other things, like ox's urine and black pepper." Women certainly employed herbs for birth control, but Rowan believes hard-to-find silphion wouldn't have been one of them. "There are other more common herbs that could cause abortions. Most people would probably have used something cheaper—and more local."

If the sexual practices of the Roman elite weren't responsible for silphion's disappearance, what was? Strabo, writing after Cyrenaica was annexed by Rome in 96 BCE, wrote the "silphion plant was near to extinction when the barbarians, because of some grudge with the local people, invaded the country and destroyed the roots of the plant." The "barbarians" the geographer referred to were probably indigenous Libyan nomads on the steppes south of Cyrene.

"It is not easy to find," wrote Pliny, whose *Natural History* was published in 77 CE, "because the tax-collectors, who are in charge of the pasture-land, thinking of a bigger profit, devastated it to use as forage for their livestock." Another writer noted that the flesh of sheep fattened on silphion stalks is "wonderfully delicious."

According to one hypothesis, the ex-magistrates who governed Cyrenaica after it was made a senatorial province tried to profit as much as they could from the land's riches during their one-year tenures in office. Since silphion was the province's cash cow, they may have overharvested the plants to line their pockets as quickly as possible, or even marketed silphion-fed sheep as a kind of ancient version of well-marbled Kobe beef.

Analyses of tree rings and pollen records tell another story. Silphion's disappearance may have been caused by one of the earliest documented examples of human-induced climate change. During the early years of Greek settlement, Cyrenaica's climate was much lusher than it would be later; following Strabo's analogy, the leopard spots where people lived and cultivated crops were much larger. Studies of a rare tree known as the Saharan cypress show its growth rings were wider between 500 and 250 BCE. According to these dendrochronological analyses, there were high levels of moisture at the time the area was most renowned for silphion production, with the process of desertification accelerating dramatically around 500 CE.*
Pollen samples, dated by the appearance of nonnative olive trees introduced by the Greeks, show signs of the presence of sheep and other livestock. Today, Libya is 95 percent desert—almost all sand, in other words, and no spots.

Combining the evidence from ancient texts and modern archaeology, a plausible account of a local extinction event can be pieced

---

* An intriguing reference to silphion growing is found in letters written three centuries after Nero was supposed to have received the last stalk. In 406 CE, Synesius, the Greek-speaking Bishop of Cyrene, congratulated his brother for raising silphion in his garden, and regretted to inform a friend in Constantinople—modern-day Istanbul—that a shipment of ostriches, olive oil, saffron, and "a great deal of silphium juice" would be delayed.

together. The Greeks planted wheat and barley, but under the Romans cultivation of grain intensified: large landowners rented their estates to tenant farmers, and these highly taxed sharecroppers were under pressure to increase crop yields and raise more livestock. Just as the Amazon rainforest is now felled to pasture cows, Libya was deforested to provide more pastureland for Roman sheep, increasing soil erosion, reducing rainfall, and kick-starting the process of desertification. As the population of Cyrenaica peaked at 135,000, farming estates expanded south of Cyrene, into the narrow band where silphion grew. Since Greek times, cutting the plant's root, rather than harvesting it, had been forbidden, but by allowing their sheep to get fat—and delicious—on silphion, the farmers found a way to get around the law.

The warming and drying of Libya's climate, then, was initiated when sharecroppers started to cut down trees and expand their farms to supply the populations of Athens and Rome with grain. As Miski had explained to me, *Ferula drudeana* and similar species won't germinate until they've gone through up to two months of cold, moist, winter-like conditions. Faced with warmer winter temperatures, the destruction of its habitat, and foraging sheep, silphion didn't stand a chance in Cyrenaica.

"Silphium not only represents the first recorded instance of species extinction at the hands of humankind," one recent study has concluded, "but also the first instance of such extinction induced primarily by climate change of any cause or scale."

What happened in Cyrenaica, it's important to note, fits into the larger story of declining soil fertility, hastened by a thousand years of extractive Roman agricultural techniques. Some scholars believe this was an underlying cause of the fall of the empire—and something we in the modern world ignore at our peril. The earliest farmers in the area around Rome had planted multistory canopies of olives, grapes, cereals, and fodder crops to feed their livestock, but after Romulus, they turned to iron plows. "Using an ox and plow saved labor but required twice as much land to feed a family," wrote geomorphologist David R. Montgomery in *Dirt*. "As plowing became standard practice, the demand for land increased faster than population." By 75 BCE, the hinterland around Rome could no longer feed the metropolis, and a failed harvest in Gaul caused famine. The empire set about turning North Africa into its granary, planting the coast with dense olive groves. "With hungry rioters in Rome," wrote Montgomery, "it is likely that the Senate annexed Cyrenaica for its ability to produce grain." Plowing the Roman way gradually, but inevitably, exhausted the soil faster than it was replenished by natural processes.

By the third century, the theologian Tertullian, a native of Carthage in North Africa, was lamenting humanity's impact on the environment, in terms that sound strikingly modern: "Cultivated fields have overcome woods; flocks and herds have driven out wild beasts ... thick population meets the eye everywhere. We overcrowd the world. The elements can hardly support us. Our wants increase and our demands are keener, while Nature cannot bear us."

A millennium-long process of soil degradation was reaching its climax. "Rome did not so much collapse as consume itself," wrote Montgomery. "While it would be simplistic to blame the fall of Rome on soil erosion alone, the stress of feeding a growing population from deteriorating lands helped unravel the empire." From this perspective, the extinction of silphion in Cyrenaica was a minor localized tragedy in a much larger story of empire-wide environmental decline.

Conditions in Turkey's interior today, interestingly enough, may be more like those in ancient Cyrenaica than anything in modern desert-ridden Libya. Winters in the village of Dikmen, at an elevation of about 4,900 feet, are cold and rainy enough to allow *Ferula drudeana* to germinate. Those fieldstone walls, some of them centuries old, offer protection from grazing animals. Miski speculates that two thousand or so years ago, a Greek trader or farmer might have tried planting silphion seeds that had been sent to him, or that he'd brought, from North Africa.

"Because it takes at least ten years to mature, they might have planted it, then forgotten all about it," mused Miski. "But the plant kept on growing in the wild, and ended up populating this small area. The descendants of the original farmers wouldn't have known what the heck it was." Both locations where the plant grows in Turkey had Greek populations stretching back to the time of Alexander the Great; to this day, the five-thousand-strong Romeyka community on the Black Sea, though now Muslim, speaks a form of Pontic Greek dating to the seventh century BCE.

"The ancients were very good at transporting things," points out Erica Rowan. "There's no reason why people from Cyrenaica couldn't have brought the seeds to Cappadocia and planted them. They're similar enough, with a Mediterranean climate. And this *Ferula* species does look like what's shown on the coins."

Shahina Ghazanfar, a research associate who specializes in the taxonomy of Middle Eastern plants at the Royal Botanic Gardens at Kew, London, agrees. "Morphologically, *Ferula drudeana* seems to be the most likely candidate. The opposite leaves, which aren't found in the other species, are particularly convincing. The striated stems, fruits, the root—all seem to point to the idea that this *Ferula* species could possibly be a remnant cultivated plant in Anatolia that was known as silphion."

In the absence of a well-labeled herbarium being unearthed in Herculaneum or Pompeii, there was one promising—if not surefire—way of confirming that *Ferula drudeana* was the silphion of the ancients. Somebody was going to have to eat it.

"Everything depends on whether or not you can make dishes with it," Rowan told me. "There are a lot of plants that we could eat, in theory, but they don't add flavor. Silphion's medical properties were important to the ancients, but its defining characteristic was that it was a seasoning."

Which got me to thinking about the root ball I'd tucked into my backpack. After driving Ata back to Aksaray and dropping off our car in Konya, Miski and I rode a morning train back to Istanbul. As the dusty plains flashed by, I wondered aloud: If someone wanted to experience the taste of silphion, how would they go about cooking the root?

"Keep it in the shade, in a ventilated area, to dry it out," Miski told me. "Then peel off the bark. In the lab, we always slice the root, vertically. Or you could try grinding it. Then add the powdered root to your cooking."

I was already thinking about which Roman recipe I'd tackle first. I'd take a pass on the parrot and flamingo, but a silphion-root-stuffed sausage made with spiny lobster, squid, and cuttlefish, or a fillet of branzino with a silphion and fines herbes sauce? Those sounded pretty tempting.

BACK IN ISTANBUL, I took a stroll through the domed corridors of the Misir Çarsisi, a covered market on the European side of the Golden Horn. Known in the guidebooks as the Spice Bazaar, its name translates as "Egyptian Bazaar," from the days it received its income from taxes levied on grain from Egypt. Since 1657, it's been the end point for one of the great transcontinental spice routes. Pepper, cinnamon, and turmeric left from Sri Lanka and India's Malabar Coast, crossed the Arabian Sea to the port of Basra, and were then transported by caravan across the river valleys of Mesopotamia and the oases of Syria to the Bosphorus Strait. Since my first visit twenty years earlier, many spice vendors seemed to have been elbowed out by merchants retailing snow globes, smartphone covers, and Turkish delight to cruise-ship passengers. I was glad to see there were still a few hole-in-the-wall shops with bins piled high with oxblood-hued sumac, isot chile flakes, cardamom pods, dried rosebuds, and peppercorns.

These days, of course, you can find a similar range of spices at just about any supermarket in the world. An ancient Roman gourmand or Venetian merchant would be shocked at the low status, and low prices, now assigned to the once precious and exotic commodities of pepper, nutmeg, and cinnamon. It occurred to me, as I paused to sample slices of walnut *sujuk*, eggplant jam, and some of the lushest figs and dates possible, that I wasn't exactly sure what made a food qualify as a "spice."

It turns out that spices are, by definition, exotic. The word derives from the Latin *species*, which describes a commodity—indeed any living thing—deemed special. The *Oxford English Dictionary* defines *spices* as "strongly flavoured or aromatic substances of vegetable origin, obtained from tropical plants, commonly used as condiments." In practice, spices are flavorings obtained from the bark, root, flower bud, resin, seed, fruit, or stigma of plants. While herbs may share the same racks as spices, they typically come from the herbaceous green parts of plants. Oregano and basil, which can grow in any old garden or window box, are herbs. A spice, viewed from a Eurocentric perspective, comes from afar—usually somewhere hot, humid, and exotic. The ancients recognized that herbs, fruits, and vegetables could be transplanted over great distances, but for them spices were, as the name suggested, *special*.

Evidence for long-distance trade in spices goes far back in history. Peppercorns were stuffed up the nostrils of Ramses II, as part of the mummification process, in 1213 BCE; the pepper could only have come from faraway India. A handful of cloves has been found in Terqa, Syria, in a home incinerated in a fire dated—by the presence of well-baked clay tablets—to 1721 BCE. At the time, the clove tree grew on only five tiny volcanic islands in the Indonesian archipelago. It seems that the spice routes that linked the Far East to the Mediterranean are ancient indeed.

From Bronze Age proto-cities through the courts of the Middle Ages until their loss of prestige in the seventeenth century, spices—which have almost no intrinsic nutritional value—were partly about the display of wealth through their conspicuous consumption at table.* The "Spice Race" between European powers contributed to the

---

* One thing spices were not about was covering up the taste of rotten fish or meat. While spices were added to make sour wine and bad ale palatable in medieval Europe, and salt was used to preserve fish and meat over the winter, there is almost no evidence that, before refrigeration, spices were commonly used as a preservative or adulterant. Medieval food, which was almost always locally produced, may have been fresher than food today, and spices were simply too expensive to be thrown away on rancid meat.

rise of Venice and other city-states, built independent merchant fortunes that drove the transition from feudalism to capitalism, and was directly responsible for launching the age of exploration. Columbus sailed west from Andalucía in search of a shortcut to the Spice Islands, and his men asked every native Caribbean they met if they knew where to find pepper or cloves. Samuel de Champlain and Henry Hudson searched, in vain, for nutmeg in the snowy forests of Canada.

Portuguese navigators sailed in the opposite direction, circumnavigating the globe in search of pepper, nutmeg, mace, and cloves. Along the way, they established the first of Europe's colonial enterprises, the Estado da Índia, also known as the "Pepper Empire," centered in Goa, which would endure for half a millennium. Eventually the Dutch and English came to dominate the spice trade, wresting the profits from the Genoese, Venetian, and Muslim merchants who had established long-term relationships with Indigenous Peoples in Asia who knew exactly where the spices grew.

Spices, I'd argue, were about something even more elusive than flavor, luxury, or the display of wealth. They brought *wonder* to the dinner table. Because they come from afar, spices activate the imagination, which might be the most underrated ingredient in all of gastronomy. To be served a meal spiced with the unripe flower buds from a tree that only grows in the Moluccas (cloves), or peppered with the fig-sized pods of a West African shrub (grains of paradise)—imagine that! It's a sad irony that, in this age when trade has become efficient enough to courier us the freshest of spices, from just about any corner of the world, we've lost the capacity to appreciate this readily available miracle. Spice's loss of value is, in part, a failure of our imaginations.

No spice was ever more valuable, or wonderful, than silphion. In the Roman cookbook *Apicius*, dozens of recipes call for the plant, in one of three forms: pure gum-resin, referred to as *laser vivum*, resin mixed with flour (*laserpicium*), or the dry root (*laseris radix*) to be cut into pieces and crushed in a mortar and pestle with other seasonings. Interestingly, the book was compiled between the first and fifth centuries, which coincides with silphion's presumed disappearance from Libya. In the absence of hard-to-find "Cyrenaic laser," Apicius recommends using something called "Parthian laser."

I asked Sally Grainger, the British archaeological researcher who had helped me with my *garum* experiments, about her experiences using recipes that call for silphion.

"For ancient food historians," Grainger told me, "finding the original silphion, and experiencing ancient recipes afresh with it, is a kind of holy grail. Even in ancient times, it was a mysterious and elusive spice. When it seemed to become extinct, the loss to ancient culture was immense."

Grainger re-created recipes that call for Cyrenaic laser using the lower-quality substitute mentioned in *Apicius*. "Parthian laser" is believed to be asafoetida, a resin derived from a *Ferula* species that grows in Afghanistan. *Apicius* makes a clear distinction between high-class Libyan laser and its more pungent eastern cousin.

Anybody who knows Indian cooking will have encountered Parthian laser: it's none other than hing, a spice so pungent it's often sold in thick plastic containers that look like pill bottles. I prefer to buy it in the form of gumdrop-sized balls of resin, which is probably the form silphion took in ancient Roman pantries. In German, hing is known as *Teufelsdreck*, or "devil's dung," and to me, its musty odor occupies the same olfactory realm as dirty diapers and overcooked cabbage. (My son Desmond took one whiff and said, "Eww! It smells exactly like a fart!") Sizzle a pea-sized wad in clarified butter or olive oil, though, and it bubbles up and dissolves, imparting a savoriness to dishes halfway between leeks and roasted garlic. A little goes a long way, though; hing is so sulfurous that it can turn a well-balanced dish into something pungent and gag-inducing.

With its thick, grooved stalk, white resin, forking root, and umbrella-like flower clusters, *Ferula asafoetida** closely resembles classical depictions of the Cyrenaic silphion plant. According to Strabo, Alexander the Great's soldiers found the plant growing on their long march through the mountains of the Hindu Kush; starving, they used asafoetida to tenderize and flavor the meat of their dead horses.

Ferula asafoetida still grows in Iran and Afghanistan, where an estimated six hundred tons are harvested per year, mostly for the Indian market. It has never been successfully cultivated; the sap has to be gathered in spring, from wild plants at least four years old. Interestingly, this corresponds to descriptions of the life cycle of not only *asafoetida*'s presumed long-lost cousin, Cyrenaic silphion, but also of *Ferula drudeana*.

After a day wandering the bazaars, I met Miski outside the gates of the University of Istanbul, and we walked to the Faculty of Pharmacy, housed in the former residence of a nineteenth-century Ottoman pasha. In the lobby, we were greeted by a trio of ancient physicians: the Greeks Galen and Hippocrates and the Persian Avicenna, whose busts peered benevolently over potted fig trees. Miski explained that he had been trained in pharmacognosy, the study of plants as the source of useful medicines. The once-flourishing field has lately fallen out of fashion. Pharmaceutical companies have run into intellectual property challenges from Indigenous Peoples, who rightfully question the way the developed world turns traditional plant remedies into patented medicines for profit.

"Big Pharma has no patience," lamented Miski. "They want everything the next day. Synthesizing a plant compound block by block is very time-consuming, very expensive. If it is difficult to make something in huge quantities, they simply drop it."

We made a stop in the faculty's herbarium, where dried plant samples were preserved in dusty folders in rows of tall filing cabinets, and

---

* Asafoetida, a Persian-Latin portmanteau word, means "stinking resin," and hing is derived from the Sanskrit verb han, "to kill."

then walked up a broad marble staircase to the faculty's labs. Over demitasses of sludgy-sweet Turkish coffee, Miski introduced me to the graduate students who had assisted him in isolating *Ferula drudeana*'s secondary metabolites.

One of his students brought a beaker from a fridge, which contained an amber-colored liquid, extracted from the sliced and ground root. Miski explained that it contained all of the potentially interesting medical compounds from the plant's resin; many of them had cancer-fighting, contraceptive, and anti-inflammatory properties. It was especially high in shyobunone, which acts on the brain's $GABA_A$ receptors, and may contribute to the plant's intoxicating smell.

Opening the folder from the herbarium, Miski showed me the samples he'd collected almost forty years earlier. They were attached with brittle tape to a yellowing page, on which the date "14.6.1983" was written in ballpoint pen. The papery fruits resembled the lobes of a Valentine's heart, and the grooved stalk and dried-out flower clusters looked a lot like the images on the ancient coins.

On my last full day in Istanbul, Miski and I went to the Nezahat Gökyiğit Botanical Gardens, which sit among the glass towers of the city's financial district. We rode an electric cart to the Anatolian section, which was shaped like the map of Turkey. Near a mound meant to represent Mount Hasan, Miski showed me plots of soil where *Ferula drudeana* plants had been planted by the staff. Miski inspected the ground, but the basal leaves that announced the appearance of the stalk wouldn't appear until spring.

At a picnic table next to the gardens' greenhouses, Miski confessed that he was still agnostic on the issue of whether the plant was the original silphion. For the time being, he was happy to have identified a species with so many potentially useful disease-fighting compounds.

THE FOLLOWING SPRING, Miski returned to Dikmen, where Mehmet Ata had been monitoring the plants' development. Snowmelt from Mount Hasan had abundantly irrigated the site, and the orchard was a riot of brilliant yellow flowers. At least sixty of the plants were in full bloom, which meant the roots would have been at their most pharmacologically active. As Miski approached the site, he had to chase away several goats, who, attracted by the intoxicating odor, were trying to make a supper of the leaves.

I decided to fly to Istanbul a second time. To satisfy her curiosity about the plant, Sally Grainger had agreed to travel to Turkey from her home in England. We met at the botanical gardens, where, next to an enclosure where a white peacock strutted, we helped employees set up a makeshift outdoor kitchen. Grainger had packed a mortar and pestle and all the spices and condiments needed to re-create recipes from *Apicius*, including sweet wines, bottles of *liquamen*, and herbs such as rue and lovage. As she ground cumin and pepper, and terracotta pots full of lentils stewed over charcoal braziers, Miski showed her a thick, ridged stalk of *Ferula drudeana*, with pearl-colored sap oozing from a fresh cut. She began by dropping a bit of hardened resin into a pan of heated olive oil, the first step in making *laseratum*, a simple silphion-based dressing.

"I'm getting a very great sense of culinary value," said Grainger, as the fumes perfumed the air. "It's intense and delightful. Earthy, I'd say, and mushroom 'green.' When you smell it, your saliva flows."

Enlisting Miski and myself as sous-chefs, Grainger set to work on half a dozen recipes, being sure to make versions flavored with asafoetida for contrast. As picnic tables began to fill with plates of finished Roman dishes, a crowd, which included the botanical gardens' directors and staff and Miski's students, gathered around for samples. A bowl of *aliter lenticulam*, lentils made with honey, vinegar, coriander, leek, and *Ferula drudeana*, was deemed complex and delicious, while the same dish made with pungent asafoetida resin provoked grimaces and was left largely untouched. Squash sautéed with the plant's grated root was also eaten with gusto, as was a delicate dish referred to in *Apicius* as *isicia*, in which prawns are pounded with lovage and cumin and boiled, with the resulting dumplings dipped in the *laseratum* sauce. The biggest success, though, was *ius in ovifero fervens*, a sauce for lamb made with sweet wine and plums spiced with an ample dose of *Ferula drudeana*.

"It's beautiful!" said Grainger. "Even though the sauce is rich and dense, the flavor of the silphion isn't buried by the fruits and spices. It has this intense 'green' flavor that actually brings out the qualities of the other herbs in the sauce." A version made with asafoetida was obnoxiously pungent. Grainger believed *Ferula drudeana* had great gastronomic merit, and was a good candidate for being the long-lost plant of the Greeks and Romans.

"Oh yes," she said. "I'm tasting silphion in a botanical garden in Istanbul! It's a fascinating plant, and I can understand why the Romans craved it. Quite apart from its medicinal qualities, whether it was a soporific or a stimulant, it just tasted great!" She was already thinking of how to use pine nuts or flour, the way the Romans did, to make a little of the precious resin last longer.

I was also impressed by the results. The mildly bitter resin mellowed when cooked, and the medicinal, pine-forest-like smells seemed to play in mysterious ways on the olfactory receptors. We seem to have found another example of *kakushi-aji*, a hidden flavor. That day, it felt like we'd revived another of antiquity's missing ingredients, one whose presence elevated the dishes from *Apicius* to something more subtle, intense, and complex.

Miski seemed pleased with the results of Grainger's experiments and surprised by the flavors, though he confessed he was concerned about what might happen next.

"There are only six hundred individual plants we know of in the whole world," he pointed out. Three hundred of them grow in the wild. An equal number are now being grown from seed in the botanical gardens, though it will take several years before any are mature enough to produce fruiting bodies. "You'd have to grow a thousand times as many plants to produce a commercial supply." For the time being, numbers are so low that *Ferula drudeana* qualifies as a critically endangered species.

"That's what's stressing me out," said Miski, a genuine note of alarm in his voice. "If everyone starts making silphion sauce, wait! We're not going to have enough to go around."

At the end of a long day of cooking and eating, we collapsed into lawn chairs, feeling slightly intoxicated by the rich foods, still trying to understand the strange synergy between the silphion and the other seasonings. Over the shrieks of the peacocks, a sound that had undoubtedly provided the soundtrack to many Roman feasts, I told Miski and Grainger that I was a little uneasy too. I was remembering the concerns I'd raised with the spice hunters back in Montreal, and I was suddenly acutely aware that our own all-too-human curiosity might make us part of the problem. There are only a few plant foods in history that have been eaten to the edge of extinction, and silphion happened to be one of them.

Two thousand years after the original supply was cut off, the legendary herb may have reemerged only to face a threat from its ancient nemesis: human appetite.

8

SAINT-JEAN-SUR-RICHELIEU
Bread Alone

I HADN'T EXPECTED THIS JOURNEY to take me quite so far. A wild impulse to experience the taste of ancient foods had brought me to spots on the globe I'd never imagined going: a windswept barrier island off the coast of Georgia; the aquatic gardens of Mexico City; the flanks of a volcano in the heart of Turkey. And though I've been to more distant places in my life, I've never traveled further back in time. As big as the world is, the past is even bigger, and the beautiful thing is that you don't have to go far to find it: it's all around us, in the soil under our feet, in the canopies of the trees overhead, in the food in our kitchens, and in our memories.

The secret to time travel, it turns out, is that humans today are identical in physique, intelligence, and problem-solving abilities to just about anybody who has lived in the last sixty thousand years. When confronted with a problem—like how to build a shelter or assemble a meal—our prehistoric ancestors drew on the same set of innate capacities that we possess. The challenge, I realized, was seeing the world through their eyes. Once I knew that, the only things I needed to travel in the past were my own curiosity and imagination.

This has changed my day-to-day relationship with food, in ways I hadn't anticipated. Before this journey began, I flattered myself that, with my diet heavy on small fish, vegetables, grains, and pulses, I was one of the world's responsible eaters. My thoughtfulness, though, was limited to my consumer choices—the items I picked off the shelves of local stores and markets. Thinking about the past of food has made me think harder about what I eat in the present, and every trip has changed the way I cook and eat.

Inspired by my trip to the Yorkshire Dales, I tracked down a cheese-maker in Quebec with a commitment to sustainability that rivaled the Hattans. The Fromagerie du Pied-De-Vent, on the Magdalen Islands, uses an endangered breed of cows called Canadiennes, originally brought to New France in the sixteenth century. I'd followed the small reddish-brown cows out to pasture, where they made good use of their large splayed hooves to climb high up seaside hillsides, grazing on salt-crusted grass and wildflowers. Pied-De-Vent's Cheddars, Tommes, and Camembert-style cheeses were easy to find in Montreal, and reliably delicious.

Then I started making my own cheese. I'd already schooled myself in the ancient Turkish art of fermenting milk, restoring the yogurt-maker I'd bought to turn sardines into *garum* to its intended calling. The biggest investment was buying a digital thermometer, and, as with yogurt, the greatest commitment was not letting a pot of milk boil over before it reached 110 degrees Fahrenheit. Mozzarella, pressed paneer, and silky fresh-made ricotta, which is great in pasta sauces, have become staples in our kitchen.

There were times I suspected that, with all this home cookery, I was connecting with atavistic impulses centuries, maybe even millennia, old. My mother's people come from Ireland, a place known for potato-growing, tax-evading, autarchic farms—until a water mold came along and destroyed the monoculture on which many had come to depend for their calories, driving them to new pastures across the Atlantic. My Ukrainian grandparents on my father's side were products of the chernozem, the humus-rich black soil that has made Ukraine the envy, and target, of tyrants from Catherine the Great to Vladimir Putin. Ukrainians are justifiably suspicious of tsars and commissars, and their resistance to power manifests in a penchant for home canning, fermenting, summer kitchens, and keeping their own supply of potatoes, as well as beets, in the fields. With every home food-making skill I acquired, I felt like I was tapping into some deep wellspring of self-sufficiency that connected me to my historic—and even prehistoric—ancestors.

True autarchy, unfortunately, continues to elude me. In the absence of a vegetable garden, a fishing hole, and a ruminant to milk, I've managed to turn myself into a micro-pastoralist. Every morning, I wake up to check on my herds of yeast and bacteria, leading the hungry ones to pasture with feedings of flour, sugar, or milk. Though this sometimes fills our kitchen with overflowing mason jars and sticky globs of starter, I think Erin senses the pleasure I take in keeping them thriving and multiplying, and tolerates the mess.

Disentangling myself from industrial agriculture has had other benefits. I've lost weight; I feel more energetic; and when I'm not recovering from jet lag, I sleep better than ever. Among nutritionists, there is a theory that for optimal health, we're better off eating the foods our ancestors did. Not our Old Stone Age progenitors— our genes adapt too rapidly to local conditions for a Paleo diet to make sense—but those who lived, say, five hundred years ago. In his book *100 Million Years of Food*, biological anthropologist Stephen Le argues that five centuries ago is recent enough for ancestral foodways to have had an impact on our own genomes, but long enough ago that our ancestors wouldn't have been eating industrially processed foods. If you're of Southeast Asian descent, for example, your forebearers' diets didn't include a lot of milk or alcohol but would have been heavy on rice, fish, fermented soybeans, and seaweed, which you should be able to readily digest. As I've diversified my diet, my senses of taste and smell seem to be guiding me back to the foods that allowed my ancestors to survive to pass on their genes.

Anyway, that's what I like to tell myself. Desmond and Victor, who share some of my Ukrainian and Irish genes, have proved resistant to my more extreme culinary adventures. Though they like to pitch in making fettucine and gnocchi, my experiments with kefir, kombucha, kvass, and kimchi—four Ks that have done wonders for my gut microbiome—have so far left them cold.

The one thing Desmond and Victor *do* enjoy is my bread. The first time they asked to stay up past their bedtimes so they could eat my sourdough hot out of the oven, I was proud of myself. I'd started home baking with a cast-iron Dutch oven and the no-knead recipe from Jim Lahey, of New York's Sullivan Street Bakery. The resulting boule was irresistible, especially when it was warm, steamy, and spread with melting butter...

Sorry about that—I did promise I wasn't going to get carried away again. Lockdowns made sourdough baking a pandemic cliché, so I'll spare you further rhapsodies over the miracle of lofting grain with hot air. Besides, my experiments took me down a different road from those striving to achieve an Instagram-worthy crumb. What really interested me was the quest for a secret ingredient that had been lost in the industrialization of bread-making, and whose absence has taken a toll not only on human health but also, I believe, on our happiness: diversity.

It was a way to return where this voyage began: in prehistoric Çatalhöyük, nine thousand years ago. Unlike my other trips, this one was going to start and end in my kitchen, with our oven serving as the time machine. Before I started, though, I had to get my hands on a few pounds of ancient grain.

THE STANDARD FAIRY TALE of the birth of bread begins on the banks of the Nile with, fittingly enough, some neglected bowls of porridge.

"Once upon a time somewhere in ancient Egypt, probably about six thousand years ago, something seemingly miraculous happened to one of these porridges," Michael Pollan wrote in his book *Cooked*. "It was hatching bubbles from its surface and slowly expanding, as if it were alive." Pollan imagines a curious Egyptian heating this enchanted dough in an oven, where "it grew even larger, springing up as it trapped the expanding bubbles in an airy yet stable structure." So, he continues, "was born bread baking, the world's first food-processing industry." Pollan's own engaging adventures in baking lead him to believe that the "story of Western civilization is pretty much the story of bread," which has been nutritionally debased by industry. "To bake the bread I wanted," he concludes, "I needed a whole different civilization."

It's true the ancient Egyptians loved their bread, and the written and archaeological evidence shows they were phenomenal bakers, as well as accomplished brewers.* They baked with ceramic molds, which would have produced bread shaped like pyramids, cones, and craters. There were at least one hundred distinct names for bread—among them *beset*, *hetjat*, and *toot*—and I imagine the ones flavored with dates, figs, and coriander seeds were pretty delicious.

Several hundred examples of well-preserved Egyptian bread are kept by the world's museums. These dried-out loaves were meant to be eaten by royals in the afterlife, so they don't offer much clue about the bread non-elite Egyptians ate. No detailed recipes have been

---

* Beer, of course, is just bread in liquid form. A "beer before bread" school in anthropology holds that people first gathered in settlements to make and consume alcoholic beverages. This is supported by the fact that large fermenting vats, but no grain silos, have been found at such sites as Göbekli Tepe, the hunter-gatherer temple in Turkey that predates Çatalhöyük. I find this plausible, though I've also noticed the main supporters of this hypothesis tend to be people who really, *really* like beer.

found in the hieroglyphics, leaving it up to experimental archaeologists to give us an idea what ancient Egyptian bread tasted like. One theory is that Egyptian bakers scooped yeasty froth off the surface of their fermenting beer to make their bread rise, but this technique is unpredictable and often produces a bitter bread. It is more likely they used a technique called backslopping, which involves using a bit of the previous day's dough, with its active community of bacteria and yeast, to get the morning's bread rising.

The Egyptians weren't the first to bake something more than simple unleavened flatbread. Recently, the origins of bread-making have been pushed back to 14,400 years ago. Amaia Arranz-Otaegui of the University of Copenhagen excavated a circular stone-lined fireplace at a Paleolithic archaeological site known as Shubayqa 1 in the Jordanian desert. After analyzing plant remains, she realized that the site's occupants, herders of goats and gazelles known as the Natufians, were collecting and grinding the seeds from stands of wild grasses, and stocking them in round elevated structures, the first known grain storehouses.

Archaeologists had long known that dense stands of wild wheat could be efficiently harvested; it took agricultural historian Jack Harlan just one hour to gather two pounds of clean grain from wild wheat in Turkey, using scythes with blades of sharpened stone. On that basis, he estimated that it would take a small family three weeks to harvest enough grain to sustain them for an entire year. But until Arranz-Otaegui's work, there had never been any evidence that Paleolithic people processed wild cereals. It turned out the charred plant remains she'd found were the earliest known crumbs of bread.

"This evidence was showing us for the first time that bread was not a product of the Neolithic period," Arranz-Otaegui marveled. "It was invented by hunter-gatherers." In other words, a "civilization" wasn't required to make bread, at least not in the sense of a class-divided society, with specialized labor and a ruling elite. "I believe that we will find even older evidence of bread-making, dating to twenty thousand years ago." The find, which also predates the earliest evidence of beer-making, shows that well before we were farmers, we were bakers.

This was the same conclusion reached by the archaeologists who excavated the later Neolithic settlement at Çatalhöyük: the gathering, storing, and processing of grain didn't mark some irreversible step toward priests and pharaohs, private property, and inequality. I talked to Lara González Carretero, an archaeobotanist at the British Museum, who used a scanning electron microscope to analyze some of the fifteen thousand samples collected from the site over three decades.

"I was able to identify a type of bread dough, a flatbread, a porridge-like material, and another kind of bread—the first naturally leavened bread," González Carretero told me. "We believe that people in this community left the bread dough in the open air to gather some of the wild yeasts floating in the environment. And after three or four hours, they would bake this bread. They ate this bread every day."

She told me that she'd built her own clay oven to re-create the bread, and the results had been excellent. I asked her what kind of grain went into the bread of Çatalhöyük.

It was, she said, almost exclusively *Triticum dicoccum*. The same species that provided almost all the bread in Mesopotamia, ancient Egypt, and the Roman Empire, and was still grown in Turkey under the name *kavilca*. A grain that the modern baking industry has almost completely abandoned, on the grounds that it's too hard to work with.

It took me less than an hour to track down a source in western Canada and place a home-delivery order for five pounds of the little-known—but hardly lost—wheat known as emmer.

IT'S NOT SURPRISING that so many people believe that adopting agriculture—and specifically the cultivation of grains like emmer—was, in historian Jared Diamond's oft-repeated phrase, the "greatest mistake in the history of the human race." The idea that, in domesticating wheat, we allowed wheat to domesticate us is one I confess to swallowing whole. For a while.

The first casualty of the agricultural revolution, this story goes, was human well-being. Studies of skeletal remains in the eastern Mediterranean have shown that after the adoption of farming, life expectancy decreased by over two years, with average male heights dropping from five foot ten to five foot three. Prehistoric hunter-gatherers were stronger, taller, and—if they survived infancy—could expect to live longer, healthier lives. And, as any Paleo dieter will be happy to tell you, early agriculturalists were prone to anemia, tooth decay, and, because their diets typically depended on a single cereal crop, serious vitamin and mineral deficiencies. Women in particular suffered, as shown by the characteristic bent-under toes and deformed knees found in bodies unearthed in agricultural villages on the Nile and in the Fertile Crescent, a testament to the hours spent every day kneeling and rocking back and forth over a quern to grind grain. Food surpluses allowed the lucky few at the top to escape toil and benefit from more abundant food, better health, and longer lives. The rest of us, presumably, swapped our freedom for a loaf of bread and the jugs of mind-numbing ale that helped reconcile us to existences of drudgery and subjugation.

The unprecedented concentration of food and waste in increasingly populous human settlements also attracted commensals, creatures who—invited or not—came to "eat at the same table": sparrows, mice, dogs, pigs, crows, rats. Our sedentary ancestors became a feasting ground for ticks, fleas, mosquitoes, and species-jumping pathogens. The first animal we brought into our Paleolithic camps, the dog, sixteen thousand years ago, had introduced us to giardia, rabies, and noroviruses; sheep and goats made us prone to measles; living alongside camels gave us smallpox, while cows gave us tuberculosis; and our domesticated waterfowl gifted us with influenza. We continue to be prey to zoonotic diseases,* amplified by our concentration in cities, the latest being the civilization-pausing coronavirus pandemic.

There is some evidence that hunter-gatherers do lead better lives than those who opt for agriculture. The contemporary !Kung San people of the Kalahari desert, who geneticists believe may be the closest living relatives of the band of *Homo sapiens* that left Africa as much as seventy thousand years ago, require as little as two hours a day to hunt and forage all the food they need, leaving them ample time for more pleasurable pursuits. When an investigator asked a member of the tribe why he didn't farm, he received one of the more celebrated replies in contemporary anthropology: "Why should we, when there are so many mongongo nuts in the world?" (Or as nomadic "barbarians" like the Scythians might have said, "Why should I till the soil when I can raid the storehouses of those idiotic farmers?") In other words, when the natural world provides you with an ample and varied diet, spending your life in backbreaking labor to stockpile grain doesn't make a lot of sense.

The way this meshes with the Biblical narrative may be part of its unconscious appeal to certain Western anthropologists. According to this story, we were once noble savages (Adam and Eve) living in harmony with the environment (the Garden of Eden), until we made the mistake of taking up the hoe and the plow (our Fall from Grace). In fact, the Judeo-Christian tradition, with its story of the murder of the pastoralist Abel by Cain (a farmer who, according to the Bible, was also responsible for building the first cities and introducing weights and measures), is one of the few origin stories to cast agriculture in a negative light. For the Babylonians and Phoenicians, grain was a holy gift, bestowed by the god Oannes; for the Greeks, it came from

---

* Almost all of the diseases that have terrorized the globe in the last twenty years can be attributed to human appetite and the way our species has spread into the last habitats remaining to wild animals. The outbreaks of Ebola, swine flu, SARS, and COVID-19 were almost certainly transmitted from their wilderness reservoirs via wet markets, factory farms, and the consumption of "bushmeat."

Demeter; the Romans received it from Ceres; and for the Egyptians, it came from Isis, the goddess of fertility, death, and rebirth. The god of the Old Testament is explicit, informing the disobedient Adam, "In the sweat of thy face shalt thou eat bread, till thou return unto the ground."

If there was one place that truly seemed to be cursed by an abundance of bread, it was ancient Egypt, the archetype of the oppressive grain-state. The Egyptians practiced *décrue*, or flood-retreat, agriculture, a low-effort form of farming in which seeds were broadcast in the silt deposited when the floodwaters of the Nile receded in early autumn, a way of using nature as a plow. The rich soil brought security, in the form of vast harvests of wheat and barley, providing the daily bread and beer that allowed the population to grow. But when the crops failed, as they did on a regular basis, devastating famines swept the land. Unlike the Çatalhöyükans, whose crops were also river-fertilized, the Egyptians were dominated by a brutal, self-aggrandizing ruling class. Farmers had to surrender up to half of their grain to priests and pharaohs, and were subjected to corvée labor to raise temples and pyramids to their glory. Under Greco-Roman domination, Egypt was turned into the granary of distant powers, its farmers working to fill the storehouses of Athens and Rome. For Egyptian commoners, the fertility conferred by the Nile was indeed a burden.

But Egypt is an extreme case. There is a gap of about 160 generations between the domestication of cereals and the appearance of the first socially stratified societies. "There was in fact no 'switch' from Paleolithic forager to Neolithic farmer," wrote David Graeber and David Wengrow in *The Dawn of Everything*. "The transition from living mainly on wild resources to a life based on food production took something in the order of 3,000 years."

Egypt's rival grain-civilization, Mesopotamia, in what is now Iraq, has a reputation for being equally obsessed with beer and bread. According to Dorian Fuller, an archaeobotanist at University College London with a distinguished career investigating Neolithic foodways, the latest research shows that leavened bread was consumed in the early cities in the land between the Tigris and Euphrates Rivers.

"Egyptian breads were made in ceramic molds, a tradition they borrowed from Mesopotamia," he told me. "The famous bevel-rimmed bowl, the prototype for what the Egyptians used, is actually a bread mold, and it was produced by the Uruk people." The Uruk period, which began six thousand years ago, is the era that birthed the first cities, the first written recipe—instructions for making beer—and the first known work of literature, the *Epic of Gilgamesh*. "There's a kind of bubble of mold-made bread culture that spreads across the Iranian plateau, all the way to western Pakistan. And they were certainly making leavened bread." At least three hundred kinds of bread are recorded in cuneiform inscriptions, including loaves flavored with oil, milk, and beer.

People first gathered in Mesopotamia nine thousand years ago, because the environment, then an open forested parkland rich in wild foods, offered a varied diet of wild grapes, figs, pears, hackberries, cherries, sour wild plums, yellow hawthorn, capers, and juniper berries. Such diversity offered resiliency to individuals, households, and settlements. Similarly rich wetland, riverine, coastal, and lake-side environments would encourage people to establish permanent settlements along the Yellow River in China, on the shores of Lake Texcoco in the Valley of Mexico, and in the Indus Valley in Pakistan.

Among the foods gathered in the oak parklands of Mesopotamia were grasses with hard, energy-rich seeds. The oldest, and genetically simplest, of them was the wheat we now call einkorn. Half a million years ago, a close relative of einkorn and another species cross-pollinated in the wild, producing emmer, which has twenty-eight chromosomes, twice as many as either of its parent plants. *Einkorn* means "one grain" in German; emmer might then be called *zweikorn*, because it has two seeds on each spikelet, as the flower arrangements of the grass are known. Both emmer and einkorn are hulled wheats, meaning their grains are tightly bound up in a protective layer of scaly bracts, or chaff, that has to be soaked, dried, and thwacked to get to the grain. A mutation in some emmer plants produced thinner hulls, making the nutritious grain easier to get at. The people of Mesopotamia began to save these seeds, plant them, and eventually store them for future use.

For thousands of years, the people of the Near East, including Çatalhöyükans, made emmer part of their diet, without giving up the diversity conferred by their hunter-gatherer ways. Stores of grains allowed people the security against famine to gather in ever-larger settlements. Human numbers increased from four to five million in the first five thousand years after grasses were domesticated, and this population growth gradually initiated a new process.

"Planting and livestock rearing as *dominant* subsistence practices were avoided for as long as possible because of the work they required," wrote historian James C. Scott in *Against the Grain*. But conditions changed—and possibly the climate, too, during a cold snap known as the Younger Dryas—forcing an increased reliance on emmer and other crops. "About the development of agriculture proper," continues Scott, "the jury is in. There was growing population pressure; sedentary hunters and gatherers found it harder to move and were impelled to extract more, at a higher cost of labor, from their surroundings, and most large game was in decline or gone." The disadvantage of relying too much on an easily stored food like emmer is that it can be seized by bandits, nomads, or tax collectors. This is not the case when you draw your dinner from a diverse variety of food chains or, for that matter, from such tubers as potatoes and cassava, which are easily hidden underground.

When most people today think of Mesopotamia, they think of the later ziggurat-raising regimes of such fearsome kings as Sargon, Nebuchadnezzar the Great, and Hammurabi, he of history's first law code. But before them were the Sumerians, who built Uruk, the world's first city. Though it may have been seven times as populous as Çatalhöyük, there is no sign Uruk was administered by a royal elite;

archaeological evidence suggests it was governed by popular rule, through citizen assemblies. Uruk's economy was centered in temples, where cuneiform script—inscribed on clay tablets, which were baked in ovens, like bread—was first employed to keep track of beer, wine, fish, cheese, wool, and leavened bread, which also served as offerings to the gods. The latest research suggests that the later royally ruled cities of Mesopotamia were created by warrior societies that rose up in opposition to the "primitive democracy" of places like Uruk. In other words, when we became too dependent on emmer and other grains, bandit-kings swooped in to seize part of the wealth.

As Wengrow and Graeber put it in *The Dawn of Everything*, "Aristocracies, perhaps monarchy itself, first emerged in opposition to the egalitarian cities of the Mesopotamian plains." Farming cereals provided the semblance of food security that encouraged populations to grow, providing ever-larger masses of ever-less healthy and ever-more oppressed people to carry out the ridiculous building schemes of bandit-kings. If the first five thousand years of the Neolithic were a period of transition from foraging, the next five millennia brought an acceleration in urbanization, and human numbers increased to 100 million. By the first century CE, most people in the world were farmers or city dwellers, and the world's few remaining hunter-gatherers had been pushed to the margins, living on as fisherpeople, pastoralists, and tribal foragers forced to exploit ever-more impoverished environments.

Is farming—and bread, its ultimate symbol—in itself responsible for overpopulation and environmental collapse?

Of course it isn't. But the way we practice agriculture, and what we've turned our bread into, definitely is.

MY EMMER HAD ARRIVED IN THE MAIL: three twenty-six-ounce bags from an organic farm in British Columbia. Now I had to figure out how to turn the whole grains into flour.

I decided to reach out to an expert on reconstructing ancient breads, Seamus Blackley (a fitting name, I thought, for a rogue baker).

In the early months of the pandemic lockdowns, Blackley, a high-energy physicist and jazz musician who also invented the Xbox gaming platform, caused a furor on social media by claiming he'd produced a loaf of Egyptian sourdough using ancient yeast scraped off a piece of Old Kingdom pottery.

When Serena Love, an Egyptologist then at Stanford, suggested on social media that what Blackley had likely gotten was a mix of old dust and whatever yeast was floating around in the museum, he asked her if she would consider helping him out. Love conceded it was possible to extract ancient yeast; it's a single-celled fungus that can go into quiescence for millennia and even survive in the vacuum of space. A team of Israeli scientists had recently succeeded in extracting and reanimating a colony from five-thousand-year-old pottery used to brew beer. Love leaned on her credentials to get Blackley into the basement of the Museum of Fine Arts in Boston, as well as Harvard's Peabody Museum, where they assembled a collection of ceramics thought to have been used to bake bread in Egypt's Old Kingdom.

"The thesis is that the open pores of this low-fired ceramic can absorb microorganisms that then go dormant for thousands of years," Blackley told me over a video call from his home in Pasadena. "We were able to perform a kind of gentle fracking. We injected a type of warm food into the ceramic matrix, let it sit there for five minutes, so the yeast would wake up and loosen its foothold on the pottery. Then we vacuumed it out and propagated it with simple sugars and sent them to a big lab, where an army of grad students sequenced the DNA and RNA. We could actually date the organisms by mutations in their genome."

Blackley selected the isolated samples of yeast that seemed to be the oldest, then inoculated dough made with flour sterilized at high temperatures. After a week of feeding the starter, he baked a loaf using fresh-milled einkorn and Kamut. The resulting loaf looked great: its round crust was scored with the hieroglyphic character representing the sound *T* in ancient Egyptian. "The crumb is light and airy, especially for a 100% ancient grain loaf," wrote Blackley in a social media post. "The aroma and flavor are incredible. I'm emotional." The loaf, which he and his wife polished off for breakfast with apricot jam, had rich notes of caramel and brown sugar. News websites around the world picked up the story, reporting that a self-described "gastroegyptologist" had baked bread using 4,500-year-old yeast.

Blackley, who is nothing if not curious and persistent, showed me a picture of a concave clay pot that he'd convinced a master ceramicist to fire for him. "This is a year-and-a-half-long project, to learn how to make low-fire silt clay vessels to replicate this kind of baking. We've discovered that you have to season them, as you would with a cast-iron pot. You just put animal fat in there, and then put it over the fire for a minute so it seals up the pores in the pottery." In his backyard bakery, Blackley drops the dough into the seasoned pot, covers it with another pot—ancient images show bread being baked in stacked molds—and, to get the temperature right, bakes it over acacia wood, a fuel favored in ancient Egypt, with orange-hot embers.

I told him that I planned to do my own experiments with emmer, which bakers had told me was hard to turn into a leavened loaf because of its low gluten levels. "The reason that you believe that is because of *bullshit*," Blackley said. "Baking emmer was a skill that every society mastered. It was the grain that built the pyramids and fed the Roman centurions. In many ways, I think emmer is the mother of civilizations." When Love and Blackley fed their starter with regular bread wheat, it remained almost inert. When they added emmer, though, it rose quickly. "Emmer makes a magnificent bread with a fabulously open crumb. I add a little roasted coriander seed, which was always present in Old Kingdom bread, and it just turns out super-delicious."

I was encouraged by what Blackley said about emmer, if not as enamored of ancient Egypt as he seemed to be. The more I learned about this prototypical nation-state, whose greatest monuments were built on the backs of millions of toiling grain farmers, the less there seemed to be to admire. But I understood exactly what Blackley got from striving to experience the flavors of the past. "I feel like baking ancient bread is a time-travel experience," he said. "With Egypt, because it has a written language, you can read poems and love stories, you can know people's minds. And now I can share their bread, which was the basis of their society. I find it really poignant."

This was a man after my own heart. After making it clear that he fully approved of my plan to use emmer, Blackley gave me a few tips on grinding the grain, which I filed away for later use.

AROUND THE WORLD, 840,000 square miles of land are planted with wheat. That's equivalent to all the land in Mexico and Southern California combined. Wheat now provides one-fifth of all our calories, and 40 percent of the protein we consume. It goes into our beer, our noodles, our soy sauce, our breakfast cereals, our dumpling wrappers, our empanadas, and is present in some form in almost any kind of processed food you can think of.

Bread is often poetically called "the staff of life," but the label is inaccurate. Wheat could sustain life, except for the fact that it lacks lysine, one of the nine amino acids essential for building the proteins we need to survive. Humans can almost—but not quite—live on bread alone.*

Wheat is a cereal, which simply means it's an edible grass, one of a huge family of flowering plants known as Poaceae, which includes barley, rice, corn, millet, oats, and rye. Cereals grow in such disturbed sunlit habitats as the edges of rivers or forests, and are among the first species to spring up after wildfires. We humans are champion habitat-

---

* We could, however, survive solely on a diet of grilled cheese sandwiches, pizza bianca, or Welsh rarebit; cheese, like eggs, soybeans, and red meat, is an excellent source of lysine.

disturbers, and cereals followed us as we cut down and burned forests during our long spread out of Africa to the Siberian Arctic, Australia, and Tierra del Fuego. Rice was cultivated for the first time ten thousand years ago in the Yangtze River basin, around the same time that two weeds, rye and oats, were domesticated in the Fertile Crescent.

Domesticated wheat spread westward with livestock-raising and other Neolithic farming methods, crossing the straits from Turkey into Europe around 9,500 years ago, and the English Channel to England 3,500 years later. Four thousand years ago, cultivated wheat reached China by way of Iran and India. Wheat found a particularly welcoming habitat in what is now Ukraine, in the chernozem, a richly aerated loam crawling with worms and microorganisms. From the black soil where it thrived north of the Black Sea, wheat was carried to coastal markets along ancient trading routes known as "black paths."

"The black paths, according to Ukrainian legend, were formed by a band of ancient warrior-merchants, predecessors of the Cossacks, called the *chumaki*," wrote historian Scott Reynolds Nelson in *Oceans of Grain*. For centuries, perhaps millennia, the *chumaki* trudged alongside heavily laden carts pulled by pairs of oxen, singing as they brought their wheat to hungry settlements. "Empires rose and fell— Persian, Athenian, Roman, Byzantine, Mongol, Venetian, Genoese, Ottoman—trying to get their hands on *chumaki* grain."

The port of Odessa was founded by Catherine the Great as part of her failed effort to make Russia's fortunes by channeling wheat, grown by landless serfs, to the growing cities of western Europe. After Britain, France, and the Ottomans defeated Russia in the Crimean War, North America took up the role of the world's wheat grower. Nelson argues that the railways of the New World became the new "black paths," conveying western wheat to hungry Europeans. My own grandparents were lured across the ocean from their Ukrainian homeland with the promise of vast tracts of unoccupied chernozem, a soil type also found on the Canadian prairies. They found a land rich enough in black humus—the infamous, tractor-fouling "Red River gumbo" of Manitoba—but also very much occupied by Cree, Dene, Dakota, Métis, and Ojibway.

It was the rediscovery of a technology from classical antiquity that allowed New World grain to supply distant markets. The Romans realized that heating and drying grains, and then sealing them underground, prevented the growth of fungi. This allowed wheat to be stored safely for years. Some classicists argue that the Greek myth of Persephone's banishment to the wintry underworld—which is at the heart of the initiation into the Eleusinian mysteries—can be read at once as an allegory and an explicit step-by-step instruction manual for storing wheat underground, to be replanted in the spring. After the fourth century, "Persephone's secret" was lost, and medieval farmers returned to the practice of drying grain in the open air.

"The French invasion of Italy allowed Napoleon's chemists to investigate what the French called 'Caesar's vaults' to figure out the mystery," wrote Nelson. Excavations showed that sand and dried grass had been piled around the foundations of ancient Roman storehouses, "drying the grain and sealing it without oxygen in a non-porous shell." The French found that Black Sea grain could be kept in suspended animation in containers they called silos. In 1840 the first such silo, known as an elevator in North America, went up in Buffalo. The combination of grain elevators, the building of the railways to the Great Plains, and the financial instrument known as the futures contract turned North American grain into the ultimate commodity, one that would create more fortunes than gold or diamonds.

If wheat built civilizations, lack of wheat could cause regimes to fall and societies to collapse. Bad harvests in France in the 1770s, followed by royal deregulation of the grain market, provoked a series of famines; a decade later, rumors of a plot to destroy wheat to starve the common people led six thousand women to march on Louis xvi's summer residence in Versailles. Chanting *"Pain! Pain! Pain!"* they raided the royal bread stores and, with baguettes brandished on bayonets, marched the king and queen to Paris, where they would be executed by guillotine.

Lack of bread had incited Europe's first modern revolution. Fifty years later, failures in the grain harvest, combined with the potato blight, which starved peasants from Galway to Galicia, led to the liberal revolutions of 1848. The Young Turk revolution of 1908 and the Russian Revolution in 1917 began with calls for bread, as did the Arab Spring of the early 2010s. By temporarily cutting off the "black paths" that carry wheat from the Black Sea, Putin's invasion of Ukraine has provoked famine in the Horn of Africa.

Even more significant than the French and Russian revolutions, arguably, was history's second agricultural revolution, which began about four hundred years ago. Advances in crop rotation techniques, fertilizing with manure, and the selective breeding of livestock increased food production enough to double Britain's population in the eighteenth century. Driven from commonly held agricultural land, peasants moved to cities, providing the workforce that would kickstart the industrial revolution in Britain, Europe, and the Americas. New forms of fertilizer were exploited, supplied by scraping nitrates from the guano-covered rocks off the coast of Chile. Then German industrial chemists pulled off a near-miraculous breakthrough: by using iron, magnesium, and calcium as catalysts, and burning fossil fuels to provide electricity, they were able to synthesize nitrogen-rich fertilizers. The Haber-Bosch process, as it's known, doubled the amount of food the world's farmers could produce, making it possible to "win bread from air."

Another technology behind Agricultural Revolution 2.0, the industrial-age version, was hybridization, the ancient foundation of all agriculture. Varieties of cultivated wheat that have adapted to local climate and soil conditions are known as landraces; they are roughly equivalent to pig breeds or olive cultivars. Crossing landraces of wheat can produce hybrids with seeds that are bigger, tastier, easier to harvest, or more resistant to disease. Beginning in the 1830s, progress-minded British wheat farmers planted their fields with only the highest-performing landraces. But the "hybrid vigor" that allows crossed plants to outperform their parents typically lasts for only a single generation, meaning farmers have to buy new seeds every year if they want to keep up the yields.* The spread of hybrids was encouraged by the Plant Patent Act of 1930, which gave American plant breeders the right to patent living things. Farmers, who had traditionally saved their seeds, became even more dependent on industry. The triumph of commercial hybrids wiped away the genetic diversity embodied in the varied populations that grew in traditional wheat fields.

"The difference between a field of wheat in the eighteenth century and a field that was the result of breeding and selection is striking," wrote soil ecologist Catherine Zabinski in *Amber Waves*. "The yield is much lower in the eighteenth-century field, but the genetic variation is much higher... Landraces are valuable because the variation that breeders got rid of, the smaller, scraggly, less productive individuals, may also hold the genes for greater tolerance to abnormal rainfall or late frost or fungal pathogens."

After the first commercially successful wheat hybrids, Victor and Little Joss, were released in 1906, the old landraces began to vanish from the fields. High-gluten hybrids, ideal for pasta or bread-baking, came to dominate, among them Marquis, a cross between Red Fife and Red Calcutta, which by 1920 accounted for nine-tenths of the wheat harvested in Canada.

Wheat is an annual, completing its life cycle in a single year. If a pathogen gets the number of a commercial hybrid, it can cause the

---

* In biology, hybridization can occur between two species, as when a mare who mates with a donkey gives birth to a mule, or between two members of a population, which is more often the case when plants are crossed. Hybrids are often, but not always, sterile. "Crop wild relatives," a crucial reservoir of largely unexplored genetic diversity, are closely related to, or ancestors of, cultivated plants. A stand of wild grass growing on the edge of a parking lot, for example, might be a crop wild relative to wheat.

failure of an entire year's harvest. Wheat's nemesis is stem rust, a fungal disease so ancient that the Romans had a rust god, Robigus, whom they propitiated with sacrifices of red foxes and roan-colored cattle. In the nineteenth century, famines, most caused by crop diseases, killed 100 million people, or 8 percent of the global population.

"In North America we managed to plant a carpet of wheat from northern Mexico well into the prairie provinces of Canada," Jack Harlan observed in *The Living Fields*. Stem rust infection begins every year south of the Rio Grande as trillions of black spores are blown northward, and wheat stalks become covered with brick-red blisters and die. "We have, in effect, provided a substrate like an agar plate"— the nutrients on a petri dish that allow microbes to multiply—"ready to receive and propagate the several kinds of rust." In 1916, stem rust took out one-third of North America's wheat harvest. In the decades that followed, prairie farmers optimistically planted a succession of hybrid wheat varieties—first Marquis, then Ceres, followed by Thatcher and Hope—only to see each of them taken out as new strains of rust spread north.

One man's heroic effort to solve the ancient problem of stem rust launched Agricultural Revolution 3.0. Norman Borlaug was born on an isolated Iowa farm in 1914, where he witnessed how the coming of an early Ford tractor liberated his family from the drudgery of the corn harvest. The great-grandson of Norwegian immigrants, Borlaug called on ancestral reserves of stamina when the Rockefeller Foundation sent him to an underfunded research station outside of Mexico City. The region was one of the cradles of stem rust, which in Mexico killed up to a fifth of each year's wheat crop. Strapping a plow to his own back, Borlaug turned the soil and planted emmer, durum, and 8,600 varieties of bread wheat. After months spent weeding out those that succumbed to rust, he found that only four varieties remained untouched. He drove these survivors north to Sonora, where he personally planted 140,000 plants, and then sat on a stool painstakingly tweezing the tiny male anthers from each spikelet to prevent the wheat from fertilizing itself. Each of the emasculated spikelets was then pollinated with pollen from one of the other resistant varieties.

By the end of the season, Borlaug had five acres of grain-topped stalks that were unaffected by stem rust. Unfortunately, the plants lodged, or fell over because their stalks were too tall. When a dwarf variety derived from a Japanese wheat known as Norin 10 was crossed with the rust-resistant varieties, it produced a shorter, stouter wheat that could support the heavy grains. By the early 1960s, a Rockefeller Foundation team had developed a semidwarf, rust-resistant, all-purpose hybrid that was also photo-period insensitive; lacking an internal clock, it would start to grow at whatever time of year it was planted. Unlike locally adapted landraces, Borlaug's hybrid wheat would also grow just about *wherever* in the world it was planted— provided it was copiously supplied with fertilizer and water.

Borlaug became a global evangelist for the new hybrids. When the United States cut off shipments of grain to India in the midst of a famine, the Indian government decided to plant Borlaug's hybrids and, aided by above-average monsoon rains, reaped a bumper crop. Borlaug was motivated by a desire to help the poor, but it was the rich who profited most. From the start, his wheat benefited the already prosperous farmers of Sonora, who could afford to fertilize and irrigate hybrid crops, rather than the campesinos outside Mexico City whose struggles with stem rust had first touched him. The green revolution, as it became known, increased yields and fed hungry mouths, but, from the Punjab to the Palouse hills, it also accelerated the industrialization of agriculture, concentrating farmland in the hands of those who could afford the new chemicals and combines.

We all live with the consequences of Agricultural Revolution 3.0. The fertilizer that keeps Borlaug's wheats growing is synthesized by burning fossil fuels, which makes agriculture a leading contributor to global heating. Naturally adapted landraces of wheat thrive without irrigation, watered by rainfall alone. With green revolution hybrid wheats, fertilizer only really works when it's accompanied by extravagant inputs of water. The result is a global accumulation of depleted soil and, as I saw on the sinkhole-ridden Konya Plain in Turkey, the draining of aquifers that took thousands of years to fill. The degraded rural environment has broken agrarian communities, driving the poor to gather in the outskirts of Mexico City, Mumbai, Manila, and the other megacities of an ever-more urbanized world.

Until his death in 2009, Borlaug maintained that, in spite of such harms, the green revolution was justified by all the hungry mouths it had fed. By some estimates, a billion people have been spared death by starvation thanks to disease-resistant hybrid wheat.

That's one way of looking at it. Another is to consider the fact that 3.5 billion people alive on Earth today wouldn't have been born at all if it weren't for the synthetic fertilizers created by the Haber-Bosch process, and that another billion wouldn't exist if it weren't for Borlaug's green revolution. Human life is precious, of course, and no one life is more valuable than another. But thanks to a fossil-fuel-driven glut of cheap, ever-less nutritious food, there may be too many people for this equally precious planet to support.

"The green revolution has bought twenty to twenty-five years," Borlaug said when he became the first agricultural scientist to win the Nobel Peace Prize in 1970. He predicted humanity had a single generation to bring the population problem under control—and he was right. Since 1986, population has been growing faster than crop yields, while the total area of wheat harvested has been falling. After declining for a few decades, hunger is once again on the rise. In 2022, 829 million people were considered seriously undernourished, a total that had increased by 150 million people over the previous three years.

"Greater food production didn't mean that the poor had more to eat," wrote geomorphologist David R. Montgomery in *Dirt*. "It usually meant more people to feed." Montgomery was writing of how the spread of rice paddies boosted population, but also hunger, in

Asia. His observation also sums up the consequences of Agricultural Revolution 3.0.

There may soon be ten billion of us on the planet, and that is a problem. Evidence of soil degradation and ecosystem collapse is growing more obvious every day, but there is no Agricultural Revolution 4.0 visible on the horizon.

DIVERSITY WAS THE FIRST VICTIM of the green revolution. This is ironic, because Borlaug was only able to develop his hybrid wheat because he had access to thousands of different landraces that farmers had preserved in their fields for centuries.

Today 95 percent of all wheat in the world is *Triticum aestivum*, the species known as bread or common wheat. (Almost all the rest is *Triticum durum*, which goes to make couscous and pasta.) In 2018, the genome of bread wheat was decoded, and it was found to be the largest of any crop: it has as many as 334,000 genes, eleven times more than humans do. Bread wheat is the result of the hybridization of emmer and a cereal known as goat grass, which happened eight thousand years ago in the Fertile Crescent; scientists debate whether the cross was natural or the product of human tinkering. Bread wheat is particularly rich in gluten, the complex of proteins that forms an elastic network that traps gas and allows dough to swell into a dome without collapsing, bringing loft to a baked loaf. This accounts for its popularity: *Triticum aestivum* gives much of the world its daily bread.

Since the green revolution, a few mega-varieties of hybrid bread wheat, with names like Attila, Siete Cerros, and Redeemer, have come to dominate the world market, pushing landraces out of farmers' fields. To make sure landraces don't disappear entirely, eleven major gene banks around the world store seeds of rice, cassava, potatoes, corn, peas, and a dozen other important crops. Wheat biodiversity is backed up in banks in North Africa, Australia, Mexico, and Kansas, which together hold over half a million wheat landraces and crop wild relatives. The "backup of the backups" is the Svalbard

Global Seed Vault, located north of the Arctic Circle on an island halfway between the Norwegian mainland and the North Pole. Svalbard stores seeds of a thousand different crops, and 213,000 wheat varieties, in a setting where the average winter lows hover around −4 degrees Fahrenheit. Keeping seeds on ice in Svalbard and the other gene banks may lead some to believe humanity has an iron-clad insurance policy against species loss, and that we can carry on farming without changing our ways.

I asked Ahmed Amri, who runs the International Center for Agricultural Research in the Dry Areas (ICARDA) in Morocco, known for its huge collection of wheat landraces, about the strengths and weaknesses of gene banks. "The best example of their value," he told me, "is how they help with diseases. In Uganda, a very virulent race of rust has emerged." One hundred percent of plants affected by the fungus known as Ug99 will die, and nine in ten varieties of wheat worldwide are vulnerable. "Everyone was afraid it will reach them. When they screened the accessions at ICARDA, they found many resistant varieties. Now those varieties are in the hands of farmers." Gene banks work like public libraries: anybody, apart from developers of medicines and biofuels, can request seeds, and the gene bank is obliged to send them, free of charge. "Whenever there is a challenge, we find the solution within the gene bank."

There is a problem, pointed out Amri. Seeds can't remain inert indefinitely; they have to be removed from cold storage on a regular basis and allowed to germinate. When a new pathogen emerges, growing a resistant variety from seeds in a bank takes a minimum of five years. "When we collect a landrace for conservation, we take a small sample. It doesn't represent the whole diversity of the landrace. I don't think we can rely on gene banks unless we support efforts to preserve biodiversity hotspots. We have to work with and support farmers who are growing those landraces in the field to improve their incomes." This is known as conservation through use, and before Agricultural Revolution 2.0 (the industrial version), this was how all crops were grown.

Amri reckoned that since the green revolution, the number of wheat landraces in the world has diminished by a factor of ten. Fewer than a thousand are now preserved in farmers' fields. Another issue is that gene banks are poorly stocked with crop wild relatives, the kinds of plants from which cultivated varieties emerged in the first place. "You still find large populations of wild emmer in Syria, Lebanon, Iraq, and growing in very harsh environments, like the deserts of Jordan. And we're finding that they are very useful, because they have high tolerance to drought and heat, and great resistance to disease. Though wheat's wild relatives are the least affected by climate change, their existence is still threatened by soil depletion and the degradation of land."

Another problem with gene banks is that, like nuclear power plants, they are especially vulnerable to calamities and tend to become targets in times of war. Prolonged power outages have wiped out some of the smaller gene banks; melting permafrost recently flooded the entrance of the Svalbard gene bank, though fortunately the collections weren't affected. Amri used to live in Aleppo, where ICARDA was located for thirty-four years. When the war in Syria began, more than twenty thousand crop varieties in the bank hadn't been duplicated in other collections. Working quietly, they sent half to Lebanon; another half were driven across the border to Turkey. A skeleton staff, amazingly enough, managed to keep the power on through four years of fighting.

Before saying goodbye to Amri, I asked him whether the collection was still intact. "No," he said, sighing deeply. "The latest news is that it's been completely destroyed. I think it was looted."

A few weeks after we talked, Russian shelling in Kharkiv damaged the National Gene Bank of Plants of Ukraine, which was founded in 1908 and stored 160,000 crop varieties. Some suspected it was a deliberate attempt to undermine the country's agricultural economy. But I was inclined to take the long view—something I have a hunch the history-haunted leader of Russia also does. The assault on Ukraine's library of plants was the rage of the sterile: protracted revenge for Catherine the Great's failure to possess the secret of the fertility of the chernozem, the ancient black soil of the steppes.

WHEN I WAS A KID, baking seemed like a magical feat, like speaking Cantonese or flying a Cessna, something only the most accomplished adults were capable of. As an adult, I baked my first loaf of bread because I was curious to see if I could pull it off.

The second loaf was slightly better than the first, so I baked a third one. I kept on going, and got pretty good at making picturesque boules, complete with fish-eyes (those blisters on the glossy crust) and eyeliner (the thin strip of blackened char on the scored "ears" on the top of the loaf). But I was still using white flour and instant yeast, meaning my homemade bread wasn't much more nutritious than a plastic-wrapped loaf of sliced Wonder.

I decided I needed to rise to the occasion and bake something healthier. The first couple of times I tried to get a sourdough starter going, nothing happened. But after three days on our dining room cabinet, a jar of whole wheat flour and filtered water began to show unmistakable signs of life. After chucking half, and refeeding the mixture every twelve hours for another five days, the mess had doubled in size and began to push up gauzy bubbles. I had a viable starter. Something circulating in the air of our apartment, and probably on our skins, had colonized the lifeless slurry. A typical starter is a community of ten distinct species of bacteria and three of yeast, which collaborate to turn glucose and maltose into carbon dioxide and alcohol. It lives on in a jar in our fridge today, its suspended animation maintained with weekly feedings.

The first time I baked a sourdough loaf, using just salt, water, flour, and my starter, I felt liberated. I no longer needed lab-produced commercial yeast to nourish myself. I didn't realize it at the time, but I'd taken a first step in deindustrializing my diet. By baking sourdough, I was traveling in time, scrolling through Agricultural Revolutions 3.0 and 2.0, all the way back to 1.0, the Neolithic.

For ten thousand years, all leavened bread was sourdough. Each had its own unique starter, which meant the bread in every settlement—and every baking household—would have tasted a little different. This was a function of the grain used and of the yeasts and bacteria in the starter, which can make a loaf that's buttery, sweetly sour, or pleasantly gooey. Microbial diversity remains the essence of traditional bread-baking; there's even a global gene bank for such microorganisms. The sourdough library at the headquarters of Puratos, a baking supply company in Belgium, keeps 130 starters from 23 countries in its refrigerators. One sourdough has been alive since a gold miner brought it to the Klondike in 1898, while Japan's Kimuraya bakery claims to have been using the same starter since 1875. About twenty new accessions are added to the collection every year.

Commercial yeast became widely available in the 1860s, when it was sold in the form of cakes by the Fleischmann brothers, Hungarian-Jewish immigrants in Cincinnati. The shelf-stable granules in commercial yeast are always the same fungus: *Saccharomyces cerevisiae*, also known as brewers' yeast. When commercial yeast is mixed into dough, it rises quickly, sometimes in minutes. Because sourdough fermentation takes much longer, it breaks gluten proteins into smaller peptides, making them more digestible. My sourdough is naturally mold-resistant and is still edible—in the form of toast, anyway—up to ten days after coming out of the oven.

My next challenge was weaning myself off white flour. My white sourdough rose beautifully and had a kind of easy, elemental appeal; my boys gobbled it up, especially when it was hot out of the oven. Unfortunately, it wasn't particularly good for us. A food's glycemic index is a measure of how high it causes blood glucose to spike, with pure sugar assigned the maximum value, 100. Whole-grain bread scores 51. Because pasta is made with harder durum wheat, which slows down the transport of glucose, it can score as low as 25, especially when cooked al dente. White bread scores 72, just a notch down from high-fructose corn syrup.

By using white flour, I might as well have been spooning sugar into my boys' mouths. I started mixing in whole wheat bread and rye flour, slowly diminishing the proportion of white. This took some tinkering: the bread didn't rise as high, and my boys balked at an all-brown loaf. Salvation came when Nick, a home baker in my neighborhood, gave us a loaf made with the ancient grain khorasan.* Desmond and Victor liked his boule better than my rye-and-whole-wheat, and after I got over my hurt feelings, I started using khorasan, which has a glycemic index of 40, in place of white. I continue to bake with it: it makes a buttery and chewy loaf, nothing like the wholesome particle-board texture I remember from whole-grain bread of the 1970s.

Refined white flour's triumph in the nineteenth century was the equivalent of the flood of cheap, empty calories provided by the green revolution in the twentieth. Whole wheat flour tends to go rancid in a matter of weeks. White flour, from which the fiber- and micronutrient-rich germ and bran has been removed, remains shelf-stable for months, a quality that allowed it to be shipped from the Canadian prairies and the Great Plains to Europe. In the nineteenth century, Europeans got up to 60 percent of their calories from bread. The problem is that white flour is so nutritionally void that, by the First World War, many conscripts in Britain and North America who had grown up on store-bought bread couldn't meet the minimal fitness requirements for soldiering. Ever since, national laws have required packaged loaves be supplemented with synthetic vitamins.

---

* Kamut, the trade name for khorasan, was originally marketed as "King Tut wheat" by a biochemist from Montana who claimed the ancient grain had been discovered in a pharaoh's tomb.

Industry found another ingenious way to make bread cheaper, more profitable, and less nutritious. The Do-Maker process, developed in the United States in 1953, involved adding ready-made liquid ferment of yeast and nutrients to dough, producing loaves of fast-rising "no-time" bread that fermented for a grand total of twenty minutes. Many nutritionists believe the recent outbreak of self-reported gluten intolerance is a reaction to Do-Maker and its British equivalent, the Chorleywood bread process; because of the short fermentation, gluten proteins don't have time to break down into digestible peptides.* Many people who self-report as gluten intolerant find they have no problem digesting long-fermented sourdough.

As a lover of good bread, I counted myself lucky to live in Montreal, a city that built its fortunes on processing and shipping grain to foreign markets (diverting some of it to make into Seagram's rye whisky and Molson's beer). My go-to flour for baking comes from La Milanaise, which produces a range of all-organic flours, from einkorn to Red Fife. It turned out my friend Herbie knew the founder, so one day we headed for the mill, near the town of Saint-Jean-sur-Richelieu, about an hour's drive outside the city.

Robert Beauchemin, an affable man in his seventies, welcomed us into his office. Fifty years ago, he explained, he'd bought a small farm, raising fifty acres of wheat near the flyspeck village of Milan, a dozen miles north of the border with Vermont. "Everybody was telling me, wheat doesn't grow in Quebec," Beauchemin told us. In fact, in the seventeenth century, the fertile soil of New France was famous for producing bumper crops of grain. Except when the winter was bad, that is, as it often is in Quebec. "They'd have three very good years, then they'd have some years where they had to eat bark. In 1705, an agronomist brought some seed from Sweden, from a more Nordic area. It worked well here, and they started to develop landraces, increasing the yield while reducing the agronomic risks."

---

* For what it's worth, three-quarters of people who claim to have a medical intolerance to wheat show no symptoms of real distress in double-blind tests.

Beauchemin decided there was more future in grinding wheat than in growing it, and he's slowly turned Milanaise into Canada's largest organic mill. He now buys three-quarters of the wheat grown in Quebec and grinds it in his three mills. In the process, he's helped launch a grain renaissance: he works with 350 farmers, with properties that range in size from 20 to 6,000 acres. Milanaise produces eighty thousand tons of flour a year, most of which goes to industrial bakeries. This is small beer compared to the million or so tons milled in Montreal annually, but nobody expected Beauchemin to get this far.

"Even ten years ago, we were a laughing stock. Now I've got General Mills coming up for a look at our mill because they want to do more organic." Organic staple foods have a bright future, for a number of reasons. Corn and soybeans, almost all of which are genetically modified, contain the DNA of a bacterium, first discovered in a California waste pond, that allows them to be sprayed with glyphosate, the powerful weed killer sold under the name Roundup. Transgenic corn and soybean plants survive the assault, while everything else around them dies. Nobody really knows how much harm glyphosate, which is a product of Second World War bioweapons research, is doing to ecosystems and human health. It has been found to kill wildflowers and devastate pollinators, destroying the microbiome in the guts of bees and causing colonies to collapse. Indigenous elders in northern Ontario have begun sounding the alarm about the spraying of Roundup, saying that it's killing birds, mammals, and edible plants on their traditional territories. In the United States, a recent Centers for Disease Control and Prevention study found glyphosate in the urine of 80 percent of the children and adults sampled. Glyphosate was recognized by the World Health Organization's cancer research agency in 2015 as being "probably carcinogenic to humans."

Wheat grown in the Americas—with the exception of Argentina—is still not genetically modified. This is mostly because important markets, including the European Union, Australia, and Japan, ban the import of transgenic wheat. But almost all of the wheat grown on the Canadian prairies is sprayed with glyphosate, and for a very stupid reason: when wheat is shocked to death by a herbicide right before harvest, combine harvesters can move through the fields at double their normal pace. Italy recently enacted a ban on Canadian wheat over concerns about high levels of glyphosate. That's why I'm willing to pay fifty cents a pound more for Milanaise's flour. I want as little glyphosate in my body as possible, and I suspect, as time goes on, fewer people will want to participate in a massive industrial experiment that uses their children as guinea pigs. Of the many insults industry has inflicted on the bread we eat, putting a "probable carcinogen" in the package has got to be one of the worst.

Beauchemin explained that because the legal definition of flour includes a long list of additives, nonorganic millers can sell their product as white flour without listing the other ingredients. "They can put enzymes in there, bleaching agents, correctors, a whole cocktail of products. Because these are 'processing aids,' they don't need to be declared. The only thing that we add is vitamins, and that's only because the regulations require us to fortify the flour. But it's a minuscule amount, like forty grams per ton."

Herbie, Robert, and I donned smocks, hairnets, and rubber boots, and took a walk through the mill. If I'd been expecting a Dickensian bedlam of conveyor belts, clouds of flour, and scurrying rodents, I was disappointed. Beauchemin said that when construction was completed in 2016, it was the first new mill built in North America in twenty-five years. All the machinery had been shipped from Turkey in containers, and assembled by a team that worked seven days a week—Ramadan and other Muslim holidays excepted—for over a year. The result was a soaring cathedral of stainless steel and glass, crisscrossed by cat's cradles of vacuum tubing. The tubes lofted the grain five stories up, then returned it to the ground floor; before being completely milled into flour, the grain would complete sixty up-and-down circuits. Montreal's oldest flour mills crawl with mechanics trying to keep the aging machines running. Milanaise,

which can operate twenty-four hours a day, is run by a single techni-
cian working in front of screens from a glassed-in control room.

I was eager to see the heart of the operation. The roller mills
were housed in metal cylinders on the building's second floor. They
looked like a fleet of small beige submarines in dry dock. "There's
twenty-four sets of rollers inside," explained Beauchemin. "In each
set, there's one roller on top, one on the bottom. The one on the
top goes two and half times as fast as the one on the bottom, which
spins in the opposite direction." After the first break, the slower
roller on the bottom holds the grain, while the upper roller, turning at three hundred revolutions per minute, strips away the germ,
the protein-and-vitamin-rich embryo from which a new plant grows.
"There's grooves in the rollers that cut the grain, so there's cutting and
compression at the same time. We can adjust the gap between the
rollers electronically." What remains is the endosperm, the energy-
filled starchy food for the embryo that gets ground into white flour.
Multiple passes through reduction rollers turn it into various grades
of flour. "If we're making whole wheat flour, we take the bran and
the germ that's been removed and recombine it with the white flour."
All the action happened inside those beige submarines: the only part
of the rollers visible was a rectangle of metal behind a strip of glass.

Beauchemin brought us to the end of the line. Some of the flour
was packaged for retail sale, but most poured in a stream from a
hatch into waiting semitrucks, which could be filled with forty tons
of flour in just under half an hour.

Since Neolithic times, wheat was ground between stones, first
by hand on saddle querns, then by millstones driven by livestock or
water power. In the industrial era, this became a disadvantage: the
harder high-protein winter wheats grown in North America didn't
respond well to millstone grinding. Legend has it that the idea for
the roller mill came when a man named Müller visited his dentist in
Switzerland in 1830, and wondered whether wheat could be milled
by rolling and crushing it at the same time, like a kernel of grain

between molars. A Swiss engineer named Jacob Sulzberger ran with the idea, setting up corrugated iron rollers, powered by steam, that reduced whole grain to fine white flour. He set up a mill in Hungary, substituting iron with more durable grooved steel. The Austro-Hungarian Empire monopolized the technology until 1880, when an industrial spy brought the secret to the United States. The largest flour mill in the world, Washburn A, was opened in Minnesota, eventually becoming General Mills. From the massive mills of Minneapolis and Montreal, a powdery stream of white flour flowed to the bakeries of the world.

The roller mill kicked off the democratization of bread; commercial yeast, along with the Do-Maker and Chorleywood processes, finished the job. Together they've combined to make bread cheap, widely available, and almost devoid of nutrition.

On the drive home, I told Herbie I was happy to see where my flour came from, and to know that it was safe to feed to my family. But I confessed I was surprised to learn that the organic whole wheat we ate was also a reconstituted, blended product of industry. The mill, gleaming and impressive as it was, was an enormous machine for reducing a seed into its component parts. As the steel rollers reduced the grain to flour, the bran and germ were stripped off and then recombined with the purified white flour. In theory, that meant nothing had been removed: the rich store of antioxidants, vitamins, fiber, minerals, and amino acids had been restored. The problem was there's a synergy that occurs when the grain is kept whole, as it is with stone mills, rather than being separated into its constituent parts. Scientists haven't been able to pin down the mechanism, which may involve the enzymatic reactions that occur when the germ and endosperm are crushed together, but there seems to be a difference in the bioavailability of nutrients when grain is stone milled. A really *big* difference: it turns out that people who eat flour made from whole grains, especially stone-milled flour, rather than white flour significantly lower their risk of cardiovascular disease, and lengthen their healthy life-spans.

If there was one secret that was older than Persephone's, it was surely this: that the germ, the bran, and the starch in a seed should never be rent asunder. The closer you can eat them to their natural state, the better. Milanaise's flour, milled from wheat grown in the fields of Quebec, made bread that my family and I loved, but it was still very much a product of industry, of Agricultural Revolution 2.0.

By the time this journey was over, I realized, I was going to have to find a way back to the early Neolithic, by stone-milling whole emmer. And for that, I was going to have to use my own muscles.

Before getting ready for my next trip, one that would take me back to the place that had formed my vision of the world, I got back on the computer. After a lot of searching, I placed an order for the tool I hoped would help me turn all the emmer in my kitchen cupboard into something that would really nourish my family.

9

MI'WER'LA

The Cooked and the Raw

I GREW UP IN ILLAHEE CHUK, which, in Chinook, the old trade jargon of the Northwest Coast, means the "place where the land meets the water." (On maps of Canada, it's still labeled as the province of British Columbia.) On this visit, I was staying with my parents, who live on an island in the North Pacific, a short ferry ride from K'emk'emeláy. (The city of Vancouver, as it's better known, is referred to by the Sḵwx̱wú7mesh People as the "place of many maple trees"—the big-leaf kind, *Acer macrophyllum*, as opposed to the dainty-leafed sugar maples that abound on the other side of the Continental Divide, where I now live.)

This is the biome of my youth, and whenever I'm here, my heart soars. From the deck of my parents' house, I can look out toward the pair of snow-capped Coast Mountain peaks known as Ch'ich'iyúy Elxwíkn, the "Twin Sisters." (I grew up calling them the Lions, though the only big cats I'd ever heard of on the coast were cougars.) There's a bald-eagle nest on a flat-topped fir tree just down the slope, and below it, the wings of floatplanes cast dancing shadows over the log booms being towed by slow-moving tugs toward the Salish Sea. (The traditional maritime homeland of the Coast Salish people is still known as the Strait of Georgia, after the English sovereign George III.)

Earlier in the day, I went for a swim in the Pacific; when I clambered back up on the pier, some excited boys asked if I'd seen the dorsal fin of the juvenile orca breaking the surface next to me. (Many coastal Indigenous Peoples believe that great hunters come back as killer whales—members of the "side-by-side tribe"—and are drawn into the shore by the sound of children's laughter.)

The British Crown recognized Aboriginal title to the land that's now Canada in 1763. In much of the eastern part of the country and the prairies, treaties were duly negotiated and signed, ceding vast swaths of land—often fraudulently obtained, and always on unfair terms—to the newcomers. But when the colony of British Columbia joined the Dominion of Canada in 1871, only a handful of treaties had been signed with its inhabitants.* This means that in the vast majority of Illahee Chuk, Aboriginal title has never been extinguished, and all subsequent colonization has been illegal. Everything I could see from my parents' deck, including the high-rise towers of the city now known as Vancouver, was the traditional, unceded land of the Coast Salish Peoples.

I spent my childhood on stolen land, though few of the grown-ups in my life saw it that way. We'd come from the slushy, sprawling suburbs of Toronto, and to me, the West Coast felt like some freshly minted evergreen paradise. In one of the last places on Earth to be mapped by explorers, European settlement went back barely a century. There was an Indian reserve—to this day that's what they're called on maps—about a mile from where we lived, on the north shore of the Fraser River, but we rarely saw members of the thousand-strong xʷməθkʷəy̓əm (Musqueam) band in local stores or

---

* In Canada, the Indigenous population, which is the youngest and fastest-growing in the country, is set to nearly double to 3.2 million in the next twenty years. Almost a third of Canada's 634 First Nations and bands are located in British Columbia. Since 1998, when the Nisga'a signed the first modern treaty covering eight hundred square miles of the Nass River Valley, a number of First Nations have begun to negotiate agreements with the provincial and federal governments.

parks. The impression I had, as a child, was of a landscape of fathomless, inexhaustible bounty, one strikingly empty of humans. We could hike in old-growth rainforest that bristled with edible fungi, pick blackberries on the banks of streams that ran red and silver with spawning salmon, and gather clams and mussels from the tide pools at Jericho Beach. In this land of plenty, there seemed to be more than enough resources to go around.

Of course, what we actually ate, most days of the week, didn't come from the forest or seashore, but from Stong's supermarket up on Dunbar Street. My mother kept a kitchen garden and prided herself on serving healthy, home-cooked meals, but our staples were straight out of the standard Western diet: white flour and white sugar, bacon and burgers, potatoes and Parkay margarine. We may have eaten more salmon and seafood than most North American families, but that was mostly because my father loved Asian food, and enjoyed taking us out for sushi and black-bean cod.

I remember going to exactly one restaurant that purported to serve Coast Salish food. Shortly after our visit, the Indigenous staff at Muckamuck in downtown Vancouver unionized, and after three years of picket lines, the non-Indigenous owners decided to close the restaurant's doors forever.

A youth spent in one of the world's last great wildernesses has proven to be both a boon and a burden. I was privileged to experience nature in a place where the hand of humanity had yet to come down too heavily. But that makes the sadness brought on by the catastrophes afflicting my childhood Arcadia even harder to take. In the last couple of years, an entire village was incinerated after an Arabian-style heat wave; forests already decimated by pine beetles have been ravaged by wildfires; atmospheric rivers have turned agricultural communities on the Fraser River back into floodplains. The climate crisis has hit Illahee Chuk with particular violence, and is causing the food webs that once nourished its people to collapse.

I'm writing this as a land acknowledgment, a recognition that I've profited, in ways it's taken me a long time to recognize, from a life spent on land that wasn't mine. And I need to make one thing clear: this story isn't about me. As a European settler, my ancestors' history on Turtle Island, an Indigenous name for North America, goes back no more than 150 years—five generations. I'm the descendant of farming people who were enticed over an ocean by British colonialists with the promise of "free land." This New World terra nullius was, of course, the traditional homeland of Indigenous Peoples. Justice begins when we call things by their proper names. And the Coast Salish, who have lived in Illahee Chuk since the Time of Transformation—geologists call it the late Pleistocene—might justly call me a *hwunitum*.

Hwunitum means the "hungry ones," and it's a label that, given my fellow settlers' appetite for resources—for land, for fish, for freshwater, for the Douglas-firs and western red-cedars whose majestic girth still makes me gasp—I can only accept as fitting and just.

"I CALL IT FOOD WARFARE. It's been used since the beginning. Sieges, scorched earth. They're all ways to remove people's food, to win them over. When the Europeans arrived here, they moved tribes to reserves where there was no food, away from places where Indians had worked for generations so they could have food. And then they're like, 'Why aren't you living happily?' And we're like, 'Well, our food is over *there*. Where you moved us out of!'"

Qwustenuxun, who also goes by the name Jared Williams, had invited me to meet him on his property on the Cowichan Indian Reserve, an hour's drive south of Nanaimo on the east coast of Vancouver Island. He was wearing a purple dress shirt, cinched with a necktie printed with a stylized Coast Salish image of a killer whale, and above the shaved sides of his head his hair was swept up, in the style of an Iroquois warrior, to form a brush whose tips he'd dyed cardinal red. We were standing in the midst of what looked like a medieval village, with half-timbered houses arranged around a village green. Qwustenuxun explained that he used his property to host a live-action role-playing game. Up to two hundred people gathered here every week to act out scenarios from *Lord of the Rings* and *World of Warcraft*.

I'd been hoping to meet a Coast Salish cook who worked with traditional foods, but until a botanist had given me Qwustenuxun's name, I hadn't had much luck. There are no Indigenous-run restaurants in Victoria, the provincial capital and the largest city on the island. Qwustenuxun graduated from the culinary arts program at Vancouver Island University in Nanaimo, and then went on to work at Rebar Modern Food, a venerable vegetarian restaurant in Victoria. Now in his late thirties, and the father of two young boys, he works as the kitchen manager for the Cowichan Tribes, the largest First Nations band in the province, providing meals to elders.

Qwustenuxun said he wasn't surprised I hadn't been able to track down Indigenous cooks on Vancouver Island. The reasons were many, and complicated. "White people say to us, 'If you don't want to eat our food, why don't you eat your own damn food?' I'll tell you why. They took all the food! When I was a kid, we used to go out and harvest two hundred salmon from the river in one evening. I went out with my young ones last year, and we only harvested ten. *Ten* salmon, not two hundred. There's no fish left." Eating traditionally, he pointed out, is no longer affordable. "I've done the math. A family of six, which is pretty average on the Res, might need two sockeye every day. A single sockeye can cost seventy-five dollars. So it would cost us eighty-five thousand a year, just to eat our sockeye. Whereas it used to be free! Our food has been gentrified. That's why our elders now eat white sugar, white flour, rice, and potatoes. Because they can't afford to eat the other way."

Qwustenuxun was one of the lucky ones. His father, who was Cowichan, was among the few in his generation who'd escaped being sent to residential schools. Under the federal Indian Act, hundreds of thousands of Indigenous children were taken from their families, to be educated in church-run boarding schools where they were prevented from speaking their language or learning their traditions. Thousands died of disease, hunger, or abuse. This isn't something that happened in the distant past. Canada's last residential school shut its doors in 1997.

Qwustenuxun's relatives gave him a rough-and-ready introduction to preparing sea cucumber and sea urchin, dried clams, geoducks and herring roe, and lots of coho, chum, and chinook salmon. "My aunts would say, 'Hurry up, nephew! I need you to cut up that fish. Here's a knife.' I'd say, 'I'm not old enough to use a knife, auntie!' They'd say, 'Ah, bullshit, come here!' And *slit-slit*, I'm cutting. There was no education in the Western way. You learned through osmosis."

Most of the food Qwustenuxun remembered from his childhood is no longer eaten. "We used to make *spa*, fermented salmon eggs. You'd wrap them in skunk cabbage with some salt, and bury them a foot underground for a week or two. Europeans called them 'stink eggs.' Weird foods like that, they're almost all the way gone." Even the shellfish that were a mainstay of the Cowichan diet are hard to find. "Most of our foods, you just can't legally use in a restaurant."

Qwustenuxun walked me through the property, twenty-four acres of grassy fields and forest in the estuary of the Cowichan River. There were originally seven villages in the river valley, the heartland of the Cowichan people, who call themselves the Quw'utsun. The word refers to the low-backed mountain whose evergreen-rimmed ridgeline rises on the other side of the road from which we'd come. "It means to warm your back in the sun. In our legends, the mountain was a giant frog that raised up to save our people during the great flood."

Lately Qwustenuxun has been inviting children onto his property to teach them the names of plants his people use for medicine and food in the Hul'q'umi'num' language. As he stopped to point out chokecherries, cow's parsley, salal, red clover, and other edible plants,

I explained what had brought me to Vancouver Island. I told him I was looking for camas, a tuber that was widely consumed on the Northwest Coast before the Europeans came. Some accounts said that, as a source of calories and an item of trade, camas was second in importance only to smoked salmon. In all my years living on the West Coast, though, I'd never heard of it.

"I've been at a few cookouts where they used camas," said Qwustenuxun. "It's not something you can cook using Western techniques. It has to go into the ground at high heat, and wet heat. The taste is a mix of cauliflower and potato." The problem, he said, was that his people no longer had access to the lands where camas grew. "When it comes to camas, the elders like to say, 'There are plants that live where white people want to live.'" Camas tends to grow in meadows, beneath oak trees, exactly the kinds of places the Europeans coveted. "A meandering grassy meadow—that's where you're going to build your homestead. Big field, nice trees—I'm moving in! If the tribe tried to come back to harvest their camas, they'd be chased out, or shot."

His people were also forbidden from using the techniques that encouraged camas's growth. "White people *really* don't like to light things on fire. And to grow camas, you need to be able to light fires. Prior to Europeans arriving, every year we would light up the camas fields. That would add nutrients to the soil, and allow sunlight to reach the ground. If you did that, every year, there would be more and more camas." There was no genetic design with Coast Salish agriculture, he pointed out; the goal was to increase the yield of a plant without altering it. But, he added, his people were more than foragers. "We looked after the land. The difference is reciprocity. You don't just take blackberries, or salal, or camas. After you've harvested them, you watch them, you light them on fire, you help them to thrive."

When he cooked for Quw'utsun elders, he almost always served potatoes. It was the food they'd grown up with. "When I grow potatoes here, they're wormy. We never had that problem with camas.

Instead of using all the energy we do to grow potatoes, which aren't actually supposed to be here, we could be looking after the environment to increase the yield. Imagine how much camas we'd have!"

As we walked back to his pickup, Qwustenuxun told me he was worried about the future of his property. "For eight generations, we've worked this land. But I married a non-Aboriginal woman." Thanks to the 1876 Indian Act, still the law of the land in Canada, if his sons have children with a non-Indigenous mother, the grandchildren will lose title, and the land will go back to the tribe. "Only Indians can own Indian land. All my work would have been for naught." Shaking my head, I muttered something about the legacy of colonialism.

"Tell me about it," he said, with a rueful chuckle. "Colonialism is my life."

THE FIRST HUNGRY *HWUNITUM* we know of to arrive in Illahee Chuk sailed into Nootka Sound, on the Pacific-facing west coast of Vancouver Island, on March 29, 1778. In his journal, Captain James Cook described the resident Nuu-chah-nulth People, who at that time of the year were busy gathering shellfish, as "indolent," "wild & uncouth," and incapable of agriculture. Cook, foiled by sea ice in his search for the Northwest Passage, made an ill-advised return to Hawaii—on his first visit, he may have been mistaken for the reincarnation of the god Lono—where he was stabbed to death and roasted over a fire.

Four years later, Captain George Vancouver, who had served as midshipman on Cook's voyage, sailed the HMS *Discovery* into the inlet that would later become the main harbor of the city that bears his name. Tasked with mapping the coast north to Alaska, Captain Vancouver was "mortified" to encounter a Spanish ship's crew doing the same, and the Spaniards were in possession of crude charts of the Salish Sea drawn up by an earlier expedition. Even more disturbing were the deserted coastal villages, some littered with skeletons, whose collapsed longhouses slumped into the rainforest. A decade before Vancouver's arrival, smallpox had come overland from the Columbia River region to the communities of the Salish Sea. It had probably been introduced by the Spanish. In the decades that followed, societies that had no history of keeping livestock, and whose immune systems were completely unprepared for malaria, yellow fever, and zoonotic pathogens, were ravaged by Old World diseases. Far to the east, a plague of viral hepatitis brought by the British in 1616 had already wiped out 90 percent of the Indigenous population of coastal New England.

The weakened Coast Salish settlements of southern Vancouver Island were raided by Kwak'wala-speaking tribes from the north, whose relative isolation reduced their exposure to European microbes. In 1862, a man from San Francisco, part of the rush sparked by the discovery of gold on the Thompson River, caused another smallpox outbreak in Fort Victoria. A little over a century after the arrival of the first *hwunitum*, the central Coast Salish population fell from over twenty thousand to barely more than four thousand.

Ancient civilizations were melting away. Before contact, Illahee Chuk was the most densely settled part of the Americas north of the Valley of Mexico and west of the Mississippi, with a population of well over 200,000. At least thirty-four languages were spoken on the territory that is now British Columbia, some as distinct from one another as Cantonese is from Catalan.

Anthropologists have described the people of the Northwest Coast—among them the Haida and the Heiltsuk, the Kwakwaka'wakw and the Gitxsan, the Quw'utsun and the Nuu-chah-nulth—as "fisher kings." During the spring and summer, people set out in small groups, visiting geographically dispersed sites, often by canoe, to tend to clam gardens, gather plants, and harvest marine resources. In winter, they gathered in large waterfront villages, where a rigid hierarchy was observed. Their material culture was centered on the fantastically accomplished working of cedar trees into masks, bentwood boxes, totem poles, war canoes, and multifamily longhouses. Hereditarily enslaved people may have made up a quarter of the population; the *si'em*, or high-class people, relied on these *skwuyum*, who were often war captives, to clean, fillet, and smoke the vast runs of salmon, oolichan, and herring. Midwinter festivals, the most famous of which was the potlatch, were a way to revive the forces of nature through dance and the destruction of surplus property—which sometimes included enslaved war captives.

In school, I was taught the standard version of New World history: around thirteen thousand years ago, as the Ice Age waned, people who had crossed a land bridge between what is now Siberia and Alaska chased big game down a narrow ice-free corridor between ice shields along the continental divide, from there populating every corner of the Americas. From this founding population, a few societies, notably the Aztecs and Inca, arose that were capable of complex social organization and monumental architecture. But for the most part, the natives of the Americas roamed forests, tundra, and plains living lives of nomadic, noble savagery.

"They were supposed to have followed an arduous crossing from Beringia," ironize David Graeber and David Wengrow in *The Dawn of Everything*, "passing south between terrestrial glaciers, over frozen mountains—all because, for some reason, it never occurred to any of them to build a boat and follow the coast." The ice-free-corridor model has also fallen out of fashion. Genetic and cultural similarities between peoples of northeast Asia and the west coast of the Americas offer more support for the Pacific Coast migration model, in which hunter-gatherer-fishers followed a "kelp highway" down the coast, living on shellfish and other readily available marine resources. "They did indeed think to build boats," argue Graeber and Wengrow, "following a coastal route that passed around the Pacific Rim, hopping between offshore islands and patches of kelp forest and ending somewhere on the southern coast of Chile."

As early as seventeen thousand years ago, the retreat of ice from mountainous coastlines would have allowed oceangoing people to move up and down the Pacific Rim with relative ease, entirely at sea level. Haida historians have long spoken of the time of the Great Flood, when Raven caused an island to form in the primeval ocean, from which plants, other animals, and the First People arose. Such origin stories are starting to sound to me like documentary accounts of the changes in sea level that occurred as the coast warmed after the Last Glacial Maximum.

As the ice sheets retreated from the coasts, nutrients from the oceans were brought inland when salmon, which survived the glaciation in coastal refugia, swam up rivers to spawn, often hundreds of miles inland. The great temperate rainforests of the northwest owe their existence to the rotting bodies of fish, which fertilized the barren land with nutrients from the ocean. The cultures of coastal peoples became entangled with forest and fish, and all were caught up in the biomes of Illahee Chuk, where the boundary between ocean and land can be so blurred that sea lions stray up forest paths, and salmon nitrogen can be found in the cells of mountain goats on inland peaks.

Northwest Coast Indigenous people built elaborate heart- and chevron-shaped weirs in estuaries and river mouths that trapped salmon headed for the shallows while allowing undersized fish to escape. In one location off the east coast of Vancouver Island, archaeologists have mapped thousands of barnacle-encrusted wooden stakes, the remains of the largest complex of fish traps yet found in North America. Such fantastically efficient machines allowed catches that would only be matched in volume by the diesel-powered fishing fleets of the twentieth century.

The people of the Northwest Coast have never lived on salmon alone. They practiced mariculture, building clam gardens by rolling massive boulders down to the low-tide line, which allowed cockles, butter clams, and littlenecks to multiply and be selectively harvested; these structures have been dated to 3,500 years ago, though oral traditions suggest mariculture goes back much farther. They placed hemlock branches in the water on which herring deposited their roe, or gathered them from feather boa kelp, producing the crunchy, salty delicacy known as *y'ák'a*. (The lucrative Heiltsuk Nation herring-roe fishery, considered one of the most sustainable in the world, now supplies a Japanese market hungry for Canadian *kazunoko*.) And they continue to catch oolichans—little smelts sometimes called candlefish because they're so oily they can be lit on fire—which are fermented into a flavorful, butter-like grease.

Northwest Coast peoples have used at least a hundred plant species for food. Pacific crabapples are mixed with whipped oolichan grease and served with cranberries; they were traditionally included as dowry items in noble weddings. The thin rhizomes of springbank clover, similar in taste and texture to bean sprouts, are steamed in bundles and served like spaghetti; early settler accounts describe clover roots being piled so high for cooking that water had to be poured through the holes in longhouse roofs.

Unlike the Aztecs, Inca, and Iroquois, however, Northwest Coast peoples did not raise corn, squash, and beans. The apparent lack of tended fields made Europeans jump to a hasty, and very convenient, conclusion. "Of agriculture they are quite ignorant," one nineteenth-century authority asserted. "They have no aboriginal plant which they cultivate." This made them, according to the scholarly consensus, a fascinating anomaly: "a wholly non-planting and non-breeding culture," in the words of the influential American cultural anthropologist Alfred Kroeber, "the most elaborate such culture in the world."

While it's true that these societies didn't raise livestock, they definitely cultivated plants. The first fur traders on Haida territory reported evidence of well-tended plots of tobacco plants, surrounded by crabapple trees. Ethnobotanists have documented countless instances of edible plants being cultivated and transformed in carefully managed plots, which were often "owned" by noble families.

Of all the plant foods consumed by the peoples of the Northwest Coast, none was more important than the tasty bulbs of the flowering plant known as blue camas. Among the Coast Salish of Vancouver Island, it was the principal source of carbohydrates in a fat- and protein-heavy diet. Ethnobotanists estimate a single family might have gathered ten thousand bulbs in a season, and as many as ten million were harvested on the island every year.

Europeans had been aware of the existence of camas since the earliest days of exploration. Meriwether Lewis, who was served it cooked, in the form of a cake, in what is now Idaho in 1805, called it a "sumptuous treat." For the Scottish botanist David Douglas, cooked camas evoked baked pears, though when he made the mistake of eating it raw, he complained of being "blown out by strength of wind." Later, missionary Narcissa Whitman wrote, "It resembles an onion in shape and colour, when cooked is very sweet, tastes like figs. This is the chief food of many tribes during the winter." One Jesuit priest lyrically described it as "the queen root of this clime."

Camas, as I was about to discover, never went away. It still flowers, turning meadows into pools of alpine azure every spring, and its bulbs swell in the shade of oak trees on islands all through the Salish Sea. Like a lot of secrets buried underground—secrets not at all secret to the Coast Salish—it's waiting for the right time to return to the light.

I'D CHOSEN AN ODD, even eerie time to visit Vancouver Island, which in the Kwak'wala language is known as Mi'wer'la, the "Big Island." It's roughly the same size as the main island of Taiwan, but with less than a million people, it's thirty times less populous. Half the population is in the southeastern city of Victoria, where palm trees thrive, snow almost never falls, and summers are generally mild and dry. The provincial capital is known for its Edwardian botanical gardens, goldrush era Chinatown, and the sprawling harborfront Empress hotel. Victorians still take unironic afternoon tea and get their headlines from a daily called the *Times-Colonist*. I grew up thinking of Victoria as the resort of the "newly wed and the nearly dead," a sedate backwater coasting on a reputation as an erstwhile outpost of the British Empire. Lately, though, the fates seemed to have conspired to visit ecological and social crises on this faded postcard of a city.

Illahee Chuk had recently recorded its highest temperature ever, 121.3 degrees Fahrenheit, as a late-June heat dome settled over the province. A month later, much of Mi'wer'la looked like it had been left too long under a broiler. Rotting kelp, shellfish, and seaweed made a trip to the beach feel like a stroll along an open sewer. Marine biologists were estimating that a billion seashore animals had been boiled alive in the heat wave; the shallows of the Salish Sea had become one vast bouillabaisse. All across the province, eyes were watering and children were gasping as smoke from wildfires reddened the skies.

A two-hour drive west of Victoria, helicopters were plucking tree sitters off towering cedars; the Royal Canadian Mounted Police eventually made over a thousand arrests in the watershed of Fairy Creek. Though 97 percent of the province's old-growth forest has already been logged, a company called Teal Cedar was busy felling one of the last stands of easily accessible valley-bottom yellow-cedars, some of them a thousand years old, to satisfy the demand for shingles, decking, and high-end guitar heads.

Across Government Street from the crenellations of the Empress hotel, I walked past a bronze plaque dedicated to "Capt. James Cook, R.N. 1728–1779." It was bolted to a granite pedestal, but the statue that had stood atop it for half a century was nowhere to be seen. Earlier in the summer, ground-penetrating radar had revealed the graves of two hundred children on the grounds of a former residential school in the province's interior. In the months that followed, thousands of unmarked graves on the grounds of the schools, most of them run by Catholics and Anglicans, were discovered across the country. Following the discoveries, people had gathered outside the provincial parliament buildings to protest on the July 1 celebration of Canada's nationhood. Diverted by the police from attacking a statue of Queen Victoria, the protesters, many of them Indigenous, turned their attention to Cook.

Cook's statue was lassoed by the neck and tipped into the harbor. The body of water it ended up in was James Bay, named after James Douglas, a fur trader who became British Columbia's first governor. The Esquimalt and Lekwungen Peoples had long used the tidal mud-flats here, one of the best clamming and crabbing grounds in the Salish Sea, as a source of food. It had been filled over a century ago to make way for the foundations of the Empress.

Douglas, who was the chief factor for the Hudson's Bay Company, was the author of an 1850 agreement with over a hundred Indigenous "heads of families," which sold the area that was now Victoria for the equivalent of £103.14. The actual payment was made in the form of woolen blankets.

"Our village sites and Enclosed Fields are to be left for our own use," read the agreement, which put words in Coast Salish mouths. "It is understood however that the land itself... becomes the Entire property of the White people forever." The fourteen Douglas Treaties, which were a cut-and-paste version of a colonialist project on the other side of the Pacific—the purchase of Māori land in Aotearoa (New Zealand)—were the only historical treaties ever signed between settlers and Indigenous Peoples in what is now British Columbia.

From the start, the treaties were a disaster for Indigenous people. Explorers and fur traders were followed by gold rushers, settlers, coal miners, and administrators—a population explosion of *hwunitum*. "The 'Indian Wars' of British Columbia came nowhere near the wholesale slaughter of aboriginal people in the western United States," acknowledged historian Chris Arnett. "There remains the colonial myth that... the British resettlement of British Columbia was benign, bloodless and law-abiding." That was far from the case. When warriors resisted, they were tried and executed, and Indigenous homes were splintered by naval warships armed with breach-loading cannons that fired forty-pound shells, "the most powerful weaponry," Arnett noted, "ever used against North American indigenous people."

Key to the colonialists' usurpation of the land was the notion that the Indigenous people were ignorant of agriculture.* British ideas on the subject were based on Swiss legal theorist Emer de Vattel's argument that cultivation alone gave the right to hold title to land. "Those who yet hold to the idle mode of life," Vattel wrote of those who hunted and gathered, "cannot complain if other nations, more laborious and too much pent-up, come and occupy a portion of it."

While the notion that cultivation, as defined by Europeans, alone confers a people the right to occupy their land is ridiculous, the camas bulb provides living proof that the Coast Salish had been cultivating plants for millennia. The greatest diversity of camas subspecies is found in southwest Oregon, which is where the plant probably began its northward spread after the retreat of the ice sheets at the end of the Pleistocene.

"The original term in proto-Salish, which was the ancestor of the Coast Salish languages, was *qwlawl*," the distinguished University of Victoria ethnobotanist Nancy Turner told me. "It was a word for edible bulbs, corms, and roots." Turner has spent her life studying the foodways of the Coast Salish, working closely with Indigenous informants. Earth ovens for cooking camas excavated in Oregon's Willamette Valley are 7,800 years old, and charred bulbs have been found on Vancouver Island from 3,500 years ago.

Brenda Beckwith, a former student of Turner who wrote her dissertation on camas, notes that virtually all of the trading posts established in the Pacific Northwest were built on land where camas

---

* Defending this position takes a special brand of audacity. North America's signature holiday commemorates Pilgrims being taught by a Wampanoag person how to plant corn with beans and squash, and fertilize it with fish, a generous imparting of agricultural knowledge celebrated every Thanksgiving. Moreover, the starving Pilgrims survived the winter of 1620–21 by robbing Indigenous burial sites of their underground caches of cultivated corn.

was cultivated. "I looked into the journals of the Hudson's Bay Company," Beckwith told me, "from Fort Vancouver to Fort Langley, and every single one of them talks specifically about putting their forts on an extremely extensive camas field. And then the colonists came in, and they put their farms in places where they didn't have to clear the land. All these beautiful, managed, cultivated fields, which had been tended by women for generations, were doomed from the beginning, because that's exactly where the colonists and the settlers put their farms. If you want to erase a people, you take away their land."

Explorers and traders wondered at a landscape of towering trees and grassy meadows studded with wildflowers. "I could not believe any uncultivated country had ever been discovered exhibiting so rich a picture," wrote Captain Vancouver. With its "stately forests," it was as "enchantingly beautiful as the most elegantly furnished pleasure grounds of England." Marveled Douglas, "The place itself appears a perfect 'Eden,' in the midst of the dreary wilderness of the Northwest coast." Seeking to excite support from their colonial masters, they inevitably reported the presence of oak trees. The oaks in question were, in fact, *Quercus garryana*, the Garry oak. These trees bear little resemblance to the mighty oaks on English estates; they're often stunted, with gnarled trunks and twisted lichen-covered limbs. Garry oak ecosystems play host to over seven hundred different plant species, including the wildflower known as blue camas.

Most of Victoria, in fact, was an enormous camas meadow. "If you went back 150 years," said Beckwith, "you could walk from the University of Victoria to downtown"—a distance of five miles—"without passing under the canopy of a tree. It was all open, managed parkland." The management tool of choice was the controlled burn. The fires encouraged the growth of grasses that provided browse for deer and elk, but also cleared away underbrush that might have fueled larger, and impossible-to-contain, wildfires. By cycling potassium into the soil, controlled burns increased the size of the camas bulbs to be harvested the following year.

Beckwith experimented by planting 270 wild-harvested camas bulbs in a Victoria nursery. "In wild conditions, they're barely the diameter of a nickel. But over five years in a nursery setting, the bulbs grew to the size of a plum. If you treat camas like a cultivated root vegetable, it will absolutely start acting like a cultivated root bulb. The bulbs will divide, and get bigger. Camas has a cultural memory."

It was only by accident, when I went for a jog on Summit Park, that I found a surviving patch of camas. Beneath a hilltop reservoir surrounded by sunbaked blackberry bushes, I realized I was running through a classic Garry oak ecosystem: an enchanting landscape of trees with twisted, bonsai-like limbs. Rectangular plots of camas plants, which in midsummer had been reduced to stalks with papery bell-shaped seedpods, had been roped off to protect them from being trampled. Ninety-five percent of Garry oak ecosystems have been lost; the few that persist are confined to marginal land, like the rocky outcrop of Summit Park. From this viewpoint, it was clear that the camas bulbs that had once nourished thousands were now buried beneath asphalt, balloon-frame houses, and shopping centers.

The day I arrived on Vancouver Island, headlines announced another horrific discovery: unmarked graves had been found on the grounds of the Kuper Island Industrial School. I'd driven past the ferry landing for Kuper Island on my way to Victoria. Operated by Oblate priests until 1975, the institution was known as the Alcatraz of residential schools; students had drowned trying to swim away from its horrors. It was a frontline institution in Canada's policy of "taking the Indian out of the child"; along with the Indian Act, forced relocations, and disenfranchisement, these institutions sought to forever deal with the "Indian problem" by erasing Indigenous Peoples from the body politic.

Yet, though First Nations cultures were devastated, they were never extirpated. And camas, like the bones of the children buried outside residential schools, never actually disappeared. The bulbs remain in the ground, waiting for the time they can return to the light, and their story will be known.

And for this, we *hwunitum* should be grateful. Humanity's survival in the future depends on looking to the past—and for that, we're going to need all the wisdom and guidance we can get.

"CAMAS WAS OUR POTATO," said Earl Claxton Jr. "That's what we ate, camas and salmon. Until the *hwunitum* came, anyway. They introduced potatoes to us, and potatoes were so similar to the way we cultivated our camas, we easily switched over. Now when we talk about eating salmon, it's always with potatoes. That's our good meal to have. A lot of our people don't even know that we used to eat camas."

Claxton had met me outside his house on the Tsawout First Nation on the Saanich Peninsula, north of Victoria, with a lyrically understated Sen̓ćoten language greeting: *"Íy cens tácel."* ("It is good that you've arrived.") He invited me to follow him to the grounds of the tribal school, which includes an elementary school, an adult education center, and a language survival school; he wanted to show me the garden where the Nation was growing traditional plants.

In a small greenhouse, Claxton introduced me to potted plants that had long been valued by his community. There was devil's club, *Oplopanax horridus*, whose wicked-looking spines caused long-lasting burns but whose bark could be used to make black face paint for mask dancers. There was thimbleberry, *Rubus parviflorus*, whose crunchy shoots could be dipped in sugar and enjoyed as an early spring treat. There was Indian consumption plant, *Lomatium nudicaule*, whose seeds people would burn on the stovetop to alleviate tuberculosis symptoms. Outside the greenhouse, he showed me a Garry oak, little more than five feet tall, beneath which camas plants were growing in a rectangular plot. The camas had suffered in the recent heat wave, and the seedpods on its brittle stalks were a papery yellow. The goal, Claxton said, was to grow enough to hold a pit cook for the students at the elementary school. But they weren't there yet.

We sat down in plastic chairs, and Claxton told me about himself in measured tones. "Claxton," he explained, was an anglicized version of *The-THANK-ton*. (He could pronounce the original name, but wasn't sure how it would have been spelled.) His great-great-grandfather, a medicine man, had refused to adopt one of the English surnames, like Smith, Williams, or Henry, now common among the Tsawout. Claxton's grandmother Elsie taught him about cooking and traditional plants. Ethnobotanist Nancy Turner was a frequent visitor to Elsie's kitchen, where she helped fillet salmon while learning about how the Claxton family used edible plants. Much of the food, Claxton said, was no longer eaten in his community; they'd set up this garden in an attempt to keep the old practices alive.

"We used to cook camas in pit cooks, and this converted the starches to good sugars, ones that didn't raise the sugar levels in our system. Because our people ate salmon and camas, they regularly lived to be over one hundred." Claxton was worried about his own health. "I'm prediabetic. All the potatoes and sugar in my diet. I have to watch myself closely."

The question of potatoes is a fraught one in Coast Salish culture. The previous day, I'd had lunch at one of the only Indigenous-run kitchens on Vancouver Island. Songhees Seafood & Steam is a food truck on the traditional territory of the Lekwungen Nation, also known as the Songhees. I ordered a thick fillet of wild sockeye salmon, served with a garlic-rich aioli, which I ate at a picnic table in a parking lot next to a cannabis dispensary. The salmon was served on a bannock bun.* Another menu option was the Bison Indian Taco, a slice of bannock slopped with bison-meat chili, served with a side of fries.

---

* Bannock, which can be deep-fried, baked, or cooked over a campfire, and is popular in Indigenous communities across Canada, is a post-contact food; the name comes from a flat Scottish quick bread. (It's similar to Navajo frybread and Hungarian *lángos*.) Bannock is typically made with white flour and lard, and has been implicated in contributing to many diet-related diseases. Nancy Turner believes people on the Northwest Coast used to make a much healthier form of bannock by cooking, drying, and flattening camas bulbs into cakes or loaves.

Food historians believe that Spanish, and possibly Russian, explorers brought potatoes to the Northwest Coast from their center of origin in the Andes in the late eighteenth century. The first potatoes reached Mi'wer'la by way of Fort Langley, on the mainland, where they had been cultivated since at least 1842. Potatoes were enthusiastically adopted by the Coast Salish, and for good reason. With the exception of calcium and vitamins A and D, they provide all the nutrients required to sustain life; eaten fresh, they're a rich source of vitamin C. A single acre planted with potatoes can provide ten people with nearly all their energy and protein needs for a year. Unlike camas, which grew in the meadows that the colonists had taken over, potatoes could be grown anywhere. They became a staple of Indigenous diets, while camas came to be considered a rare delicacy.

The easily transportable, glucose-rich foods brought by the settlers—white flour, white rice, sugar, alcohol—have led to an explosion of such chronic diet-related diseases as diabetes, cancer, and heart disease. Northwest Coast people, whose seafood-rich diets were high in protein and beneficial fats, may be metabolically ill-adapted to the starches and glucose in potatoes. The main carbohydrate in camas is inulin, which is also present in onions, garlic, and Jerusalem artichokes. When slow-cooked, inulin is converted into more easily digested fructose and fructans, which don't produce the obesity-inducing glycemic spike caused by potatoes.

Claxton, a resident elder in the school system who gives talks to the children of settlers about Coast Salish creation stories, spoke calmly about colonialism. But frustration bubbled up as he described all that has been lost. Pointing up the road from which we came, he said, "That used to be cedar forest there. Where we got the wood for our canoes and longhouses. A settler family came in, and cut down the cedar trees. The elders said, 'They didn't even use the wood. They burnt it.'

"My dad said there used to be so much salmon, you could find them spawning in every stream, every creek." Claxton pointed out a roadside culvert. "Even there, salmon used to spawn in the ditches. Now the sports fishery takes more salmon than all the other users combined."

Claxton was looking forward to the day when there would be enough camas for a proper pit cook. But he figured that was still a year or two off; he promised to send me an invitation when the big day came. He confessed that he had never tasted camas himself. He was glad that, like the Senćoten language and the Tsawout Nation itself, the bulbs had survived to the present day.

"I think the *hwunitum* were really hoping we would have disappeared by now," Claxton mused as I drove him back to his house. He was lost in thought, and seemed to have forgotten that he was talking to a settler—which was all right with me. "That's probably why the treaties were done in the first place. They didn't expect us to be around, so they would never have to live up to their word.

"My grandmother used to call them '*squati hwunitum.*' Crazy white people. They wanted it all. They still do. Their greed is insatiable."

I WAS BEGINNING TO THINK I would never see a camas bulb, let alone taste one. For months, I'd been reaching out to Coast Salish knowledge-holders, asking if I could come along while they harvested camas outdoors. A few had agreed, only to cancel, often at short notice. I didn't push too hard. We were at a low ebb in the pandemic, but people were still very concerned about protecting elders. And I couldn't blame people for being leery about inviting a *hwunitum* to the feast. We had a well-deserved reputation for taking more than our share, and seriously outstaying our welcome.

Before coming to Vancouver Island, I'd met with Leigh Joseph, an ethnobotanist whose supervisor at the University of Victoria was Nancy Turner. As we strolled through the wetlands where the Squamish River flows into the Salish Sea, north of Vancouver, she explained that her mother was Jewish, her father a member of the Sḵwx̱wú7mesh Nation, and that she used the name Styawat, which means "the wind that blows away the clouds and brings the sun." She'd done her research in this estuary on the traditional use of northern riceroot, also known as chocolate lily.

"It's a lily bulb that's made up of a bunch of tiny rice-grain-like bulblets, all attached to a central hollow stem," Styawat explained. "It was cultivated in estuary root gardens up and down the coast. It cooks quite quickly. I've had it in seafood soup. It's like a combination of rice and potatoes. A really pleasant food." Styawat found evidence that rock walls were erected in the estuaries—in a way similar to shorefront clam gardens—to increase the area in which riceroot and another staple, springbank clover, could thrive.

Both plants are now at risk because of development and pollution. As with so many traditional Indigenous foods, they have suffered neglect under colonialism and are now vulnerable to overharvesting.

I said to Styawat that I loved the idea of learning to identify and gather food from the wild, rather than relying on the packaged products of industrial agriculture. I'd been reading *Braiding Sweetgrass* by Robin Wall Kimmerer, a botanist and member of the Citizen Potawatomi Nation, and I shared a quote from the book: "I know we cannot all live as hunter-gatherers—the living world could not bear our weight—but even in a market economy, can we behave 'as if' the living world were a gift?" I told Styawat I was pretty sure that encouraging my fellow *hwunitum* to forage for Indigenous foods wasn't a good idea. There were a lot of us now, and if a market grew for game, berries, and bulbs, the wilds would soon be exhausted.

"There's a huge interest in wild foraging," agreed Styawat, "and I get it. The act of going out and being in relationship with your environment is inspiring and gratifying. But it doesn't scale up, and if you try to, it changes the whole system." Was there anything, I asked, that non-Indigenous people could do to help?

Simply recognizing the presence of Indigenous people, she said, would be a good start. "When I was writing my masters, I came across so many papers in anthropology that talked about the absolute death of knowledge. They talked about us purely in the past tense. It doesn't sit well with me, because I know so many people who have fought so hard to preserve language, ceremony, and knowledge of food systems. Camas never went away. And we're still very much here too."

She told me about settler friends on Vancouver Island who grew camas and then gave bulbs to the local Indigenous community. "If non-Indigenous people want to give back, they could research the significant plants in the ecosystems where they live. But instead of going out to harvest them in the wild, they can grow them in nurseries or gardens. And then ask if there's a community garden, or an elders' program, that might be interested in having the plants."

It sounded like a respectful approach to me, which is why I was happy when I was contacted by Sarah Milne, yet another of Nancy Turner's former students, who said she had plenty of camas on her property, and was hoping First Nations people would want to harvest it. She invited me to come visit, and maybe dig up some bulbs.

Milne lived just south of the mouth of the Cowichan River, where Qwustenuxun held his live-action role-playing games. Her property was on the traditional land of the Quw'utsun, who weren't included in the Douglas Treaties. Milne walked me down to a beach; on the other side of a narrow channel, I could see the cliffs of Salt Spring, the largest of the Gulf Islands. Wild plums, salmonberries, and trailing blackberries grew above the tideline. Before the coming of the *hwunitum*, this would have been a landing spot for the Quw'utsun and other Nations; they came ashore to harvest berries and clams. Clamming, Milne said, was no longer an option here: decades of spills from ships meant that when you dug into the sand, you hit a layer of toxic petrochemicals.

Milne believed people came onshore here in canoes to tend to the camas patches they'd planted over generations. In the spring, her property was a blue sea of camas blossoms. She pointed to a circle of dried camas stalks that rose from the forest floor. She'd invited an Indigenous knowledge-holder to dig up the first bulb, but an hour earlier, he'd phoned to tell us he couldn't make it. So Milne got down on her knees, and after saying *huy ch q'u* ("thank you" in the Hul'q'umi'num' language), she used a trowel to make a circle in the dirt. Following the stalk to its base, she unearthed an onion-like bulb, about the diameter of a one-dollar coin, that was covered, shallot-like, with a papery brown tunic. Her teenage son and one of his friends joined us with trowels and shovels, and soon we'd dug up several dozen bulbs. It was hard work digging into the packed earth, and the rewards for our efforts seemed small. The largest bulb was only as big as a small chestnut.

I poured water onto a bulb, revealing a pearl-white interior beneath its tunic, and took a little exploratory nibble. The crunchy texture reminded me of water chestnut, and I detected a soapy taste, a hint of the natural detergents known as saponins. I was picking at gummy bits of the bulb that stuck to my teeth when a thought occurred to me.

"Did you happen to see any white flowers around here?" I asked Milne.

I remembered that blue camas, *Camassia leichtlinii*, often grew alongside a similar species, *Toxicoscordion venenosum*—also known as death camas—whose flowers are white. A small bulb of death camas carries enough toxin to kill a child. Earl Claxton Jr. had told me a story about a woman who accidentally threw a single death camas bulb into a pot of nodding onion soup; she'd collapsed on her kitchen floor, and it took six months for her to fully recover. Coast Salish people were said to have planted death camas around blue camas to keep their enemies from harvesting the patches they owned. Suddenly the soapy taste in my mouth seemed like a very bad sign.

Milne laughed. "No, as long as I can remember, we've only had blue flowers on this property." The identity of the plants had been corroborated, she added, by another of Turner's students. A relief, as I didn't relish the prospect of having my stomach pumped.

Later that day, I finally had a chance to talk to Turner in person. We sat on a bench in Nanaimo Harbour, near the little ferry that makes the run to her home on Protection Island, and she told me about her life. The daughter of globe-trotting missionaries, who were also scientists, she was born in Berkeley, but spent the first years of her life in Montana, roaming among the ponderosa pine to gather serviceberries, mushrooms, and wild strawberries. When her father, who studied bark beetles, got a job with Canada's federal forestry service, the family relocated to Victoria. Turner took her love of nature to the University of Victoria, where, in the late 1960s, she realized her high-school dream of becoming an ethnobotanist. Over the years, she has turned what she learned from Indigenous informants into dozens of books and almost a hundred peer-reviewed scientific articles.

I showed Turner the sixteen bulbs that Milne had given me and told her how difficult it had been to dig them out of the compacted forest floor. The whole process would have been much easier, she explained, on a patch of ground that was regularly tended. Harvesters would have used a digging stick, fashioned of dense fire-tempered ironwood, which would have been as effective, and as heavy, as a metal shovel.

"A routinely harvested patch will have loose, black, crumbly, prairie-like soil, with grass on top," said Turner. "You dig around the turf at the top with your stick, forming a circle, and then you flip the whole thing over. In the underside of the turf you've turned over, you find one-, two-, and three-year-old bulbs; the youngest will be teardrop shaped, the size of your little finger. In the hole, you'll find rounder larger bulbs that are five to ten years old. These are the ones you harvest. The bulbs actually drill deeper into the ground every year that they grow. You leave the little ones, and replace the turf. Then you give it a quick burn, and all the ash from the burning grass gets washed into the nooks and crannies when the rains come, which helps to fertilize the soil. In three or four years, you come back, and you can do the whole thing over again. It's like a perpetual harvest system."

I gave Turner some presents to thank her for all the help she'd given me introducing me to informants and former students. Everyone I met had paid tribute to her kindness, generosity, and rigor.

"I guess my role in all of this has been a bridge between the elders and the next generations," she said. The knowledge of how to use camas and other Coast Salish foods was on the brink of being lost when Turner, as a master's student in botany, struck up friendships with elders. Few had escaped the residential schools, where children were taught to look at traditional foods as dirty, unsafe, and backward.

"When they came back, they didn't want that food. They didn't want anything to do with the traditional culture, because it had been brainwashed out of them. And many of them *didn't* come back. What I've learned is that nature is amazingly resilient. And people here worked with that resilience in creating their food systems. They pruned the berry bushes; they partially harvested cedar bark so it would grow back; they used fire to make the camas grow bigger."

When they took something, they also gave something back. And they took in moderation, giving thanks for what they'd been given. In so doing, they made the world a richer place for themselves and the other beings they shared it with, rather than impoverishing the land, seas, and rivers.

That's the difference between sustainability and extraction, and that's what the *hwunitum* have yet to learn.

I DIDN'T KNOW WHAT TO EXPECT when I pulled up outside Ogwilow-gwa's home. She lived in a red-roofed bungalow just across the Big Qualicum River—which was tiny, no more than a serpentine stream between the pines—from a shorefront campground, midway up the east coast of Mi'wer'la. Two fearsome statues, each as high as a three-story building, stood sentinel alongside a stand of tall cedars; I later learned they were depictions of figures from the wolf clan of the Pentlatch people. Though they looked ancient, with gaping maws and black fingernails clutching bulging bellies, they were, in fact, built for the 1994 Commonwealth Games in Victoria and were made of polystyrene.

Ogwilowgwa, who also goes by the name Kim Recalma-Clutesi, is an award-winning filmmaker and an old friend of Turner. Hers is a prominent Coast Salish lineage. Her father's side of the family had inherited the chieftainship of the Pentlatch, who once lived in ninety villages north of the Big Qualicum. Among the first to encounter European diseases, all three thousand Pentlatch are thought to have perished; linguists now consider the language to be completely extinct, though First Nations people refer to it, more gently, as "sleeping." Ogwilowgwa's family has operated in the realm of the Kwakwaka'wakw—people I grew up calling the Kwakiutl, who are distinct from the Coast Salish—and she followed her father in the role of elected chief of the Qualicum Band of Indians. ("It was a sub-poena," she told me of her election. "You don't say no.") The position is now occupied by her brother.

From the outside, her house, which was fenced in by wire mesh to keep out the deer, looked like a sprawling ranch-style bungalow. Once inside, I realized it was more like a modern version of a longhouse, with lofty ceilings, a living room decorated with wooden masks and talking sticks, and a dining room whose long wooden table was surrounded by photos of Ogwilowgwa and her late husband, often dressed in full traditional regalia. She invited me to take a seat on a stool in the kitchen, where she was making biscuits.

She apologized about having to delay our first meeting. The community's freezer had conked out, she explained, and in order to save a year's worth of precious salmon, she'd pulled two all-nighters over-seeing a crew as they skinned and filleted over three hundred fish, packing them into sterilized mason jars before they spoiled.

"We can't afford to waste the salmon," she said. "The Big Quali-cum here has spring, coho, and chum salmon, but the water tempera-ture is too high, and the oxygen level is too low. For a century, we've been logging old-growth forests, and mining, and you cannot sustain the river systems without a healthy watershed."

In the living room, she showed me her collection of bentwood boxes, made of red-cedar, one of which was two hundred years old. "You fill it with water, and with clams or whatever you're cooking, and then you use tongs to put in red-hot rocks. The water *instantly* boils. Then you put the lid on, and allow it to steam."

Ogwilowgwa's kitchen was an ethnobotanist's dream. On the counters, glass jars were filled with wild celery, devil's club, juniper, old man's beard, and other medicinal plants she'd gathered from the forest. Tall cabinets were stacked high with preserved elk, deer, and seal meat. Ogwilowgwa's mother was Icelandic—by way of Hecla Island, in Manitoba—a heritage manifest in her high cheekbones, pale complexion, and a certain elfin twinkle in her eyes. As she kneaded the biscuit dough, she responded to my questions about camas with patient good humor.

"Camas doesn't grow north of Campbell River," she told me. "But it was traded up and down the coast. We have a field of camas, in the campsite you passed, but the problem is our elected chief and council want to make money from campers, so they mow it down before it's fully germinated. I harvested camas a few times when I was young, but not often. Honestly, a lot of the things I learned, I learned in secrecy. Growing up in the '50s and '60s, the residential schools were still operating." Her father was a survivor of the Kuper Island Industrial School, where news of unmarked children's graves had recently broken. "It was run by Oblate priests. They had a particularly gruesome form of horror; they were very orderly in their assault and abuse." One of her uncles was beaten to death, at the age of eleven, for speaking his native language at a residential school. The epidemics, the relocations to reserves, the deliberate destruction of traditional knowledge in residential schools created holes in the culture, the language, and the social hierarchies that had guided lives for millennia. "As all of this was unraveling, we didn't have orderliness.

We lost so many of the knowledge-holders. It's like a holocaust—for a century. We were just communities of walking wounded."

On the stove, half-smoked cuts of coho were slowly pinkening in a pot of simmering water. "Salmon is very important to us, but clams are probably more important. They're more of a staple protein. In the times when the salmon runs failed, we also had oolichans. If the oolichan run failed, we had seal oil." It was another example of the way diversity allows for resiliency. "There were always backups for nature collapsing."

I asked her whether her people cultivated plants.

"Sure! Contrary to popular belief, we didn't just sit around with a frying pan waiting for a sockeye to jump in." Ogwilowgwa has personally found direct evidence of long-term cultivation: stinging nettles, used to make rope and a powerful spring tonic, planted in long, straight rows. Clams were dug in March; eelgrass, which tasted like licorice, was harvested in May, as was the marine algae known as red laver. There were concepts of private property, but they applied to ownership of the resources—clam gardens, berry patches—rather than the ground beneath them. The boundaries between the sites that belonged to different families could be as subtle as a crack in a rock.

"We weren't hunter-gatherers," she said. "We returned to the same spots in different seasons to harvest different things." Nancy Turner refers to the Coast Salish as "complex cultivators." Like the Iroquoian growers of maize, squash, and beans on the East Coast, Northwest Coast Peoples practiced a form of agriculture, but preferred not to become dependent on it. Their pre-contact way of life sounded like the Goldilocks spot occupied by the people of Çatalhöyük, perched between the food security offered by cultivation and the sensual pleasures—and thrills—of hunting, foraging, and life outdoors.

I asked Ogwilowgwa about how she'd seen camas being cooked. "You dig a hole, three to four foot deep, and put the camas bulbs between layers of sword fern, salal, and bracken fern. There are little spores in those plants that are powerful medicine. Then you heat rocks, until they're red-hot—you have to find ones that won't shatter—and you cover everything with canvas, to insulate it. Then you pour in about a gallon of water, so it's steamy. So you're cooking, heating, and steaming slowly, for about four hours. In the end, the camas is almost spreadable." She said she'd rather be serving camas tonight, but it just wasn't possible. "I think camas was deliberately replaced by potatoes. It had nothing to do with nutrition. They had to diminish our traditional use of plants, because they wanted the real estate. And then when we wanted to use our traditional foods, we were all treated like creek robbers."

We heard a voice in the living room. "You should be careful, Kimmy! I could just walk in and steal things." William White, an old friend of Ogwilowgwa, had arrived just in time for dinner. White explained they had first met as mature students in a history class at the University of Victoria. "I thought that Kwakwaka'wakw culture was dead. I didn't know Kim was part of a powerful political family." Ogwilowgwa, for her part, was irritated by White, who is Snuneymuxw, a Coast Salish Nation distinct from the Kwakwaka'wakw. "We sat on opposite sides of the class. The poor prof, she didn't know what to do." Gradually, they overcame their antipathy, bonding over discussions of teachers who had a tendency to look upon First Nations students as subjects for study.

We relocated to the dining room. Ogwilowgwa bowed her head and recited in a low voice: "I give thanks for this day and the bounty of beautiful food, and ask that you continue to allow us to receive these gifts, gifts that you have always provided. Help our visitors travel safely, and have an open and kind heart as we speak of these things that have been given to us." Then she looked up, and with a radiant smile said, "Just begin!"

I was beaming, too, as I dug into the feast, slathering the cured coho and the biscuits with lashings of oolichan grease. "It's really good for you," she said. "So rich in omegas. My late husband used to put it in everything, even his coffee. He called it 'vitamin O.'"

Following her lead, I dipped a boiled potato and a slice of onion in the grease, and cleansed my palate with a slice of apple.

There was a conspicuous absence at the table. Not just of camas, which had been replaced by the colonizers' potatoes, but of Ogwilow-gwa's late husband, whose face smiled from the framed photos all around us. Kwaxsistalla, who also used the name Adam Dick, was the chief of the Wolf Clan of the Dzawataineuk Tribe of the Kwakwaka'wakw People. He was born in remote Kingcome Inlet, on the province's mainland, in 1929; his mother had a prophetic dream while carrying him, so from birth he was surrounded by elders who schooled him in traditional knowledge.

"In Kingcome Inlet, in the winter, the Mounties could not come up the river, because it was frozen, so that was when they had their pot-latches. They knew children would be taken away to go to residential school." The infant Kwaxsistalla was bundled up by his grandparents in a dugout canoe and paddled to an island in the Broughton Archipelago. "His old people thought that if you allow the trees to sing to you, they will gift you with intuition." Kwaxsistalla, one of the few of his generation to escape residential school, was raised in a hut on a beach lined with ancient clam gardens. There he was taught the songs, the stories, the values, and the survival skills of his people, becoming a living repository of traditional knowledge.

Kwaxsistalla also became an informant for researchers who wanted to learn more about traditional foodways. When he'd died, three years earlier, the Kwakwaka'wakw people lost not only a hereditary clan chief but also a living link to millennia's worth of knowledge.

Ogwilowgwa clearly felt Kwaxsistalla's absence keenly, but she remained a cheerful host, inviting me to try my hand at preparing a dish I'd often heard about but never tried.

"These are soapberries," she said, passing me a metal bowl full of cranberry-sized berries, along with a bundle of fresh-cut branches. "You gather up as much as you can with the salal leaves, tilt the bowl, and just turn your wrist." As I used the waxy green leaves as a whisk, natural saponins in the berries were whipped into a delicate pink froth. "It doesn't work as well if you use a baker's whisk. There's a dance between the salal and the soapberries."

We used wooden spoons to suck the berry froth in and out of our mouths, further aerating it. Though some people called this "Indian ice cream," it was more bitter than sweet, with a hint of cranberry and citrus that reminded me of a Campari on the rocks.

"The old people loved eating this!" said White.

"I think they just liked to sit around and burp," said Ogwilowgwa, giggling.

Along with the hot biscuits slathered with tart Oregon grape jelly, it made an excellent grown-up dessert. Ogwilowgwa said that soapberries used to grow all around, but now they're overharvested, usually for floral arrangements. She'd gotten these ones from a friend on the mainland. Like camas, soapberries have the misfortune of growing where white people want to live.

"I'm not that old, and I can't find half the things I used to harvest. My brother says, 'We were stewards for ten thousand years; we had really good relations with the land; and it took white people only one hundred years to bugger it all up.'"

After the meal, talk returned to Kwaxsistalla.

"Adam didn't go to school a day in his life," said Ogwilowgwa. "He didn't read or write, but he was highly trained."

"He was a first-hand knowledge-holder," agreed White. "It's a different world now. We don't have any more Kwaxsistallas."

Ogwilowgwa didn't see it that way. "The fact that we're still here is a testimony to the strength of the old people's teachings. I'm really sad, but I think we can pick up the remnants. As Adam used to say, we survived a flood before. He also used to say, 'If you look backwards, you trip, because you can't see where you're going.' That's embedded in all our cultures."

What had been brought forward, preserved, in part through the work of Turner and her students, was knowledge that could benefit all of humanity: a blueprint for food security that was based in sustainability rather than extraction, a philosophy deeply rooted in gratitude. Over the millennia, they had established an equilibrium with the biomes that nourished them, knowledge that the European newcomers only grudgingly acknowledged and could have sorely benefited from.

I sensed the two old friends had some catching up to do, and I was acutely conscious of being a guest in Ogwilowgwa's house, in more ways than one. I brought out some gifts I'd carried from Quebec: maple syrup, berry preserves from Île d'Orléans, and smoked herring from the Magdalen Islands. In spite of my (half-hearted) protests, Ogwilowgwa reciprocated with two precious jars of coho salmon. They would end up in my carry-on, alongside camas bulbs, carefully wrapped in paper towels and freezer bags.

It's always hard for me to leave Illahee Chuk. Hard, of course, to say goodbye to my parents, whose adventurous spirit brought me and my sister here when we were kids. Harder still, though, to see the damage my fellow *hwunitum* have inflicted on this epic wilderness in my lifetime. To see this fragile beauty marred, in ways more evident every time I return, by fire, flood, storms, and the multiple poisons of human greed, tears strips from my heart.

As hard as it is for me, I can only try to imagine the pain of those who have always called this place home, and whose home it will always be.

IT IS NOT TOO LATE for the world at large to benefit from the traditional ecological knowledge (TEK) of the Indigenous Peoples of the Americas. The milpa system of planting squash, corn, and beans, which spread from Mexico to become the Three Sisters method of the Iroquois, keeps fields fertile without the need for fallowing or chemical fertilizers; the chinampas, or floating gardens, of Mexico City, which allow several harvests a year, are already being adapted into raised field systems that are feeding the world's megacities. Soil scientists have recently discovered that several thousand square miles of the Amazon basin, though perhaps many more, contain a layer of dark nutrient-rich earth known as *terra preta do índio*. It is the result of generations of Indigenous farmers stirring charcoal, excrement, broken ceramics, and turtle, fish, and animal bones into the topsoil. Current slash-and-burn techniques exhaust the soil in a few years, but Indigenous Amazonians actually improved the soil; *terra preta*, which can be up to six feet deep, contains twice the nutrients of other tropical soils. (Similar layers of fertile "dark earth," enriched by humans for over seven hundred years, have been found in central West Africa.) The oldest deposits of *terra preta* have been harvested for two thousand years, and possibly much longer.

Perhaps the greatest example of TEK is the controlled burn, which structured the landscape of the Americas before the coming of the Europeans. Without regular burning, the prairies of the Midwest, the grasslands of the Argentine pampas, the hills of Mexico, and the high plains of the Andes would have been invaded by forest; controlled burns created the camas meadows of the Coast Salish, as well as the parklike oak landscape the conquistadors encountered in the American Southeast. (Paleoclimatologists believe that the three-century cold snap known as the Little Ice Age, which began in 1550, happened because the end of controlled burning led North American forests to grow back, drawing carbon dioxide from the air and lowering temperatures globally.) Indigenous groups have been lobbying for permission to use "cultural burns" to clear the landscape of the underbrush and deadfall that fuel ever-more devastating wildfires in western Canada. If done in the spring, when conditions are damp, these burns can easily be kept under control. Proponents have met with approval in principle but denial in practice, and find themselves stymied by a typically Canadian combination of demands for paperwork and dilatory tactics.

Indigenous Peoples, who account for just 5 percent of the world's population, occupy 20 percent of the Earth's land area, which is home to 80 percent of global biodiversity. They are the stewards of life and fertility; they know how to keep the planet alive. Like the Pentlatch language, as well as the bulbs of camas that lie dormant beneath Garry oaks all over Mi'wer'la, this knowledge may be sleeping, but it is far from extinct. The settlers and colonists of the world ignore this knowledge at their peril, for it is the best hope for our future.

IN THE END, I was able to experience the taste of cooked camas. A couple of weeks after my trip, I cleaned those sixteen bulbs under a tap, placed them between layers of corn husks, and clamped the lid on a pressure cooker. After a day of steaming at the lowest possible temperature, the bulbs, which had been as firm as turnips, were reduced to a soft, spreadable consistency.

Before I tried them, I warned my wife, who was using a laptop on the sofa in the living room, to call 911 if I collapsed. I was worried that, in spite of assurances to the contrary, one of those white-flowered death camas bulbs had slipped into the bunch.

As it turned out, there were no convulsions on the kitchen floor. And the camas was, I should say, delicious. It called to my mind a combination of semisweet cocoa, chestnut paste, and mashed potatoes, with a sweetness that came on subtly, at the sides of the tongue, and a density that slightly dried the mouth; it was unlike anything I'd had before. I definitely wanted more. But, of course, there was no more to be had. Not for me.

I had imagined myself eating camas on a Pacific beach, among those for whom it had meaning, rather than standing next to an Instant Pot in my Montreal kitchen. The sterility of the experience, I suppose, was part of the point. The joy of this particular supper had to be lost on me, because—though these bulbs were gifts willingly given—camas was not my food to eat.

Epilogue

I DECIDED I'D TRY ONE LAST TIME to convince my family, and myself, that bugs were the food of the future and deserved a place in our kitchen. The world's largest edible insect farm is located just outside Peterborough, Ontario. Late one summer morning, I pulled up outside a sprawling two-level barn in a rental car, with Desmond in the passenger seat. We were met by Darren Goldin, one of three brothers, originally from South Africa, who run Entomo Farms. Goldin explained that the twenty-thousand-square-foot barn was built for chickens, and that there were two others of equal size, also clad in light-gray siding, elsewhere on the property. Each barn was home to thirty million *Gryllodes sigillatus*, or tropical house crickets.

"In this barn," Goldin pointed out to Desmond, "there's almost as many crickets as there are people in Canada." I could believe it. The din was incredible, an unremitting high-frequency whine. The sound of one cricket stridulating in the dusk is comforting. It turns out a nation-state's worth of chirps is at the limit of the tolerable.

In the place of chicken cages were row upon row of waist-high rectangles of cardboard, topped by boards covered with feed. The crickets were given a mix of corn, soy, flax, and alfalfa; pretty much the same feed, in fact, as the chickens had gotten before them. Crickets like things hot and humid, so they kept the temperature in the barns at a balmy 88 degrees Fahrenheit, and an elaborate webwork of hoses ensured they were well supplied with water.

Goldin lifted one of the rectangular "cricket hotels" up to eye level. He reckoned about four thousand lived in its corrugations. Crickets are less like grasshoppers than I'd remembered, and there was something especially spiderlike about this particular species. Goldin slammed the hotel down on the ground, shaking its guests to the floor. A black mass of crickets boiled up, scrambling over each other, before fleeing to the surrounding hotels. Desmond let out a shriek, but continued recording it with the camera on my phone.

Goldin explained that crickets don't go through larval and pupal stages; instead, they hatch from eggs as miniature adults. Within six weeks, they've reached the end of their life cycle and are dropped into "harvest" buckets, where they're gassed to death with carbon dioxide. We followed Goldin to Entomo's main offices, a ten-minute drive away, where he showed us the kitchen where the crickets are rinsed and roasted with a variety of flavorings in big commercial ovens. They're either left whole, minus the legs, or ground into powder. Entomo bills its cricket powder as the "planet's most sustainable superfood" and has found a big market catering to bodybuilders and athletes focused on protein intake.

Goldin invited us to sit at a picnic table outside the offices, where we were briefly joined by a grasshopper who cast a wary eye on our activities before hopping off to greener pastures. In an effort to sell Desmond on the virtues of entomophagy, our host had brought along a selection of whole-roasted crickets. Won over by curiosity, and the fact that we hadn't had time to stop for lunch, Desmond reacted with a mix of enthusiasm and disgust.

"Actually," said Desmond, "the cinnamon one tastes like candy. But in a more healthy way!" We tried the ranch flavor: they were crunchy and herby, but Dez found them too salty for his taste. The chile-lime and the BBQ both got a thumbs-up. "Okay, now I'm thinking I'm going to eat bugs!"

"We converted you," said Goldin, with a chuckle. But he'd spoken too soon.

"Oh my gosh!" yelped Dez. "They still have eyes!"

"Don't look at them," said Goldin quickly. "Just pretend you're eating the healthiest candy you've ever eaten."

Dez shook his head in disbelief. "I'm eating cricket eyes!"

I pointed out that he'd eaten shrimp before, and they had eyes. "But I didn't eat their heads!" replied Dez, deploying unbeatable logic. I was thankful we hadn't watched *Pinocchio* before coming. The idea of chomping on Jiminy Cricket would have been met with a hard no.

Goldin highlighted the advantages of insect farming: the low inputs of feed and fertilizer; the tiny amounts of water used compared to other forms of livestock; the lack of zoonotic pathogens that can be passed to humans. He also brought up something I hadn't considered. "Farmers around here might slaughter a pig or a cow when they're one year old, and a chicken when it's thirty-five days old. Well, a cow can live for as long as twenty years. With crickets, we let them live out their whole lives, and harvest them at the end of their life cycle." Dez seemed to understand the distinction, but then he yelped again. A part of the cricket's anatomy had gotten stuck between his molars.

"There's a lot of legs to remove," Goldin said in a meditative tone, "and sometimes we miss the odd one."

We thanked Goldin for his generosity and drove off, bags of whole roasted crickets and fat sacks of ground cricket protein powder scattered over the back seat. On the trip home, I caught Dez noshing on the crickets. And, for a while, he became an advocate for insect-eating. I attended a PowerPoint presentation he gave to his class about the field trip his weirdo dad had taken him on. (The clip of the crickets swarming out of their hotel provoked a gratifying chorus of screams.) And most of the kids were willing to try the samples he'd brought—especially the cinnamon-flavored ones.

For a few weeks, I added the cricket powder to my morning smoothies, which seriously boosted their fiber and protein content, even if it did give them a somewhat muddy taste. When my supply ran out, I went to Entomo's website and had a couple more bags delivered. But when I'd worked my way through those, I called it quits. A pound of organic cricket powder cost sixty-five dollars, and that didn't include shipping. The reality is, eating insects on a regular basis, whether it's in the form of Mexican *escamoles* or Canadian crickets, is far from cheap. And that's a problem if we're hoping that entomophagy is going to offer a real solution for feeding a hungry planet.

The other problem was that, while I didn't actually mind the taste, apart from a few delicacies I'd had in Mexico City, I didn't really find bugs *delicious*. And if there's one thing I'd discovered in this exploration of humanity's long relationship with food, from the pursuit of the ultimate cut of ham to the quest for silphion, it was that deliciousness isn't a detail. It really, *really* matters.

THERE WERE TIMES during this voyage that it seemed humanity was driving down an alley toward a brick wall, fast. Catastrophe loomed everywhere I looked: in the dust bowls on the once-fertile plains of central Turkey, in the vanishing lakes of Mexico City, in the fetid cesspools outside the factory farms of North Carolina, in the disease-ravaged olive trees of Puglia, in the rapid wiping away of diverse food webs in every biome. The demographers' scenario, where we'll have to produce 50 percent more food by midcentury to feed a population of ten billion or face famine, sometimes seemed like the only possible outcome.

Except that maybe it wasn't. As food historian Warren Belasco observes in his book *Meals to Come: A History of the Future of Food*, so-called experts have been making predictions like this since the days of economist Thomas Malthus. And they've almost always gotten the dates, the percentages, and the numbers wrong. Population may not plateau in midcentury, but continue to shoot up to a peak of 11.2 billion by 2100—or global war, economic depression, another pandemic, or a sudden rise in sea level could slam the brakes on population growth before we reach 2050. The reality is, when it comes to the course of human history, *anything* can happen, and it usually does.

For the time being, our cunning plan seems to be to wait until the last second and hope an airbag will deploy to cushion us from the final impact. In modern times, there's a long tradition of techno-optimists or cornucopians—science writer Charles Mann calls them "wizards"—telling us that technology will come to our rescue. In the 1930s, Winston Churchill predicted in the pages of a Canadian magazine that future famines would be averted by raising edible bacteria in underground cellars using "artificial radiation." Others saw yeast factories and transcontinental algae pipelines nourishing the domed metropolises of the twenty-first century. The green revolution had undeniable success in squeezing greater yields out of the land, which may explain the current bullishness about the advent of Agricultural Revolution 4.0, and its promise that once a new array of technologies are deployed in "underdeveloped" places like Africa, all our food-supply problems will be solved.

According to the techno-optimists, the gene-editing technique known as CRISPR will allow us to alter the genomes of crops, creating mushrooms and potatoes that won't brown when exposed to oxygen. Hacking photosynthesis, by genetically modifying rubisco, the enzyme found in all plants that turns sunlight and carbon dioxide into starches, proteins, and other nutrients, will allow us to radically increase rice yields in Asia. Growing perennial grasses, rather than annuals like wheat, will permit us to mow the cereals we eat rather than cutting them down whole, thus keeping root systems intact and putting an end to soil degradation. Using robots to milk cows, and drones for the precision irrigation of crops, will save labor costs and conserve water. And growing meat in the lab, from cultured stem cells in bioreactors, will eliminate the need for raising livestock, and all the environmental havoc that goes with it.

A closer look, though, shows that most of these techno-fixes have serious downsides. Perennial wheat, marketed as Kernza, doesn't have enough gluten to make bread or pasta; robot-milking systems don't allow for pasture-feeding, requiring cows to remain in barns year-round for the system to be profitable; and hacking photosynthesis—like self-driving cars—seems to be one of those innovations that will always arrive in five years, ten tops. (In spite of incessant tinkering, nature has solved the photosynthesis problem exactly once in 3.5 billion years.) As for Churchill's plan to raise bacteria in caves, it's back in the form of journalist George Monbiot's plan for curing "agricultural sprawl" and feeding the billions: calories will once again be plucked out of the air, as Scandinavian labs use electricity and "precision fermentation" to transform bacteria into gray protein pancakes.

My response to the techno-optimists and wizards who tell us that we should all subsist on a diet of bacteria, yeast, or algae is: *you go first*. And by that I don't mean, take the first bite. (As an adventurous eater, I'll try anything once.) I mean show me that you can survive and thrive on that diet for five, ten, or twenty years. *Then* I might consider joining you.

I've noticed something about "scientifically improved" foods. To put it bluntly: *nobody wants to eat that shit*. The first approved transgenic vegetable, the slow-ripening, rot-resistant Flavr Savr tomato, engineered with genes from a bacterial parasite, was a commercial flop, losing millions for the company that developed it. Golden rice, engineered to contain higher levels of beta-carotene, and the Arctic Apple, designed not to brown when cut, have also failed to attract farmers and consumers. (While my kids are willing to choke down the occasional veggie dog, they are deeply suspicious of soy-protein burgers, and outright reject sloppy joes made with plant-based hemoglobin.) The problem is, most of us already consume transgenic food, which is slipped into our diets in the seed oils in processed foods, or in the flesh of cows, chickens, and other livestock fattened on genetically modified corn and soybeans.

It turns out what people *do* want to eat, when they're given any kind of choice, is non-GM food. The market for organic food, which has more than doubled in a decade, accounted for $58 billion in sales in 2021 in the United States alone.

If we're really serious about forestalling famine, we need to stop feeding so much grain to livestock, and save the wheat, corn, and rice we grow for human consumption. Edible insects are already being used to feed poultry and farmed fish, but they could also be included in the feed of cattle and pigs. The black soldier fly is an efficient, fast-growing converter of organic waste into protein for animal feed. I interviewed Keiran Olivares Whitaker, the founder of the British company Entocycle, who has succeeded in raising millions of flies in a tiny rented space in the center of London. The entirely automated operation used the waste from breweries to feed the bugs; the black soldier flies can be used to boost the protein content in feed for cattle, poultry, pigs, and farmed fish. This approach makes a lot more sense to me than hoping humans will suddenly acquire a taste for bug burgers.

But raising insects for feed is a patch, not a solution. The Food and Agriculture Organization of the United Nations has made it clear that, for the time being, food producers pump out enough calories to feed everybody on Earth. It's equally clear that the billions of inhabitants of the "Global South" aren't the problem. It's the people of the world's rich nations, as well as the growing middle classes in Asia, Latin America, and Africa, who consume diets high in processed foods and grain-fed meat and dairy, that keep us hurtling toward that brick wall.

The boom in calories produced by the green revolution has led to an artificial, and probably temporary, boom in human numbers. The question is whether we've already exceeded the carrying capacity of our planet and gone beyond the point where this place can nourish all of us.

Because food isn't something to be conjured out of nothing, by running an electrical current through the atmosphere, deftly snipping genes, or precision fermenting yeast or bacteria. Food comes from the oceans, the lakes, and the rivers; most of all, food comes from the soil, a resource we've been diligently depleting and degrading with plows since the Iron Age, and with synthetic fertilizers and other chemicals since the industrial revolution. This thin layer of topsoil, which is naturally renewed at the rate of just an inch every five hundred years, is the only thing standing between us and starvation.

Food is brought to us by fisherpeople, who are the last of the hunter-gatherers. It's brought to us by the gardeners and orchard-keepers, the inheritors of Indigenous horticulturalists. It's brought to us by the rearers of cattle, pigs, and other livestock, whose forerunners were shepherds and pastoralists. Most of all, it's brought to us by the farmers, who have been stewards of the earth for the last ten thousand years, and probably longer.

The fact that so many of us seem to have forgotten they exist—and can't tell you where on earth their last supper came from—should tell us exactly how much we've lost.

THERE HAD BEEN TIMES in my travels when I toyed with the idea that my premodern genes, going back to Irish and Ukrainian peasants, or even farther, were expressing themselves. Surely I'd inherited my congenitally restless legs from the tattooed, horse-riding Scythians, who roamed the parts of what's now Ukraine where horses were originally domesticated.

But who am I kidding? At best, such genealogical narcissism is tedious; at worst, it's the root of ethnic nationalism. Anthropologists point out that, no matter how different we may look, humans are all members of the same species. Sixty thousand or so years ago, we were *all* Africans. We don't even have to go back that far. As geneticist Adam Rutherford wrote in *A Brief History of Everyone Who Ever Lived*, modern Europeans only have to go back six hundred years before the lines of ascent in their family trees cross in a common ancestor. The most recent common ancestor of *everyone* alive today, no matter what their background, lived just 3,600 years ago. Rutherford quotes Yale University statistician Joseph Chang, who wrote the study that established this mathematical certainty:

> Our findings suggest a remarkable proposition: no matter the languages we speak or the color of our skin, we share ancestors who planted rice on the banks of the Yangtze, who

first domesticated horses on the steppes of the Ukraine, who
hunted giant sloths in the forests of North and South America,
and who labored to build the Great Pyramid of Khufu.

And, by extension, who baked flatbread in Neolithic Çatalhöyük.
Going back a few generations, your ancestors' genetics and foodways will indeed have influenced your genome. Beyond that, though,
things—and people, for we are a mobile and promiscuous species—
get too mixed up for it to matter very much. Under our skin, we are
all family. And, as we always have, we share this in common: if not
now, then very soon, we'll be wondering what we're going to have
for our next meal.

EVER SINCE I'D COME BACK FROM TURKEY, there was a meal I'd been
obsessed with. I knew I wouldn't be satisfied until I'd tried to re-create
the Neolithic flatbread that had been baked at Çatalhöyük.

The quern had arrived about a week after I'd placed the order
on Etsy. It had been sent from a store in Oaxaca, Mexico, and came
heavily wrapped in cardboard and duct tape. Before making my
final decision, I'd contacted archaeological museums in search of
model querns, and gone so far as to jump into the dumpster of a
local kitchen countertop supplier to try to scrounge up a suitable un-
polished stone slab. Then Lara González Carretero, the British Museum
archaeobotanist who had studied the bread culture of Çatalhöyük,
suggested that the closest thing to a Neolithic saddle quern—like the
one I'd seen at the museum in Ankara—in North America would be
a metate, which is used in Mexico to grind corn into masa flour for
tortillas. The model I'd chosen had a nine-by-twelve-inch surface, supported by three pudgy legs, and weighed thirty pounds, which made
me confident it would be sturdy enough to get the job done.

First, though, I needed to figure out how to use the thing. I
packed the metate into a backpack, along with an eighteen-ounce
bag of emmer wheat, and pedaled my bike down to the office where

Marc-André Cyr worked. The longtime baker at Olive et Gourmando, a Montreal restaurant well-loved for its pastries, Cyr now gives private baking courses and is known for his adventurous and scholarly approach to grains and bread. Though he'd made flour with hand-powered grinders before, he'd never used a quern and was curious to give it a try.

Cyr poured a handful of whole emmer into his palm. Each of the silky, glistening grains was about the size and shape of a mouse turd. After weighing out half an ounce, he scattered the grains over the grinding surface. The metate came with a mano, a cylindrical grindstone with four beveled edges, intended for rolling over large kernels of corn. In Çatalhöyük, an oval grindstone had been used for crushing.

"The mano's pretty heavy," said Cyr. He grasped each end with his hands and leaned in, pushing from his shoulders. "You don't need that much pressure to make flour." Using a back-and-forth motion seemed to work better than turning the mano like a rolling pin. After a few dozen passes, the center of the metate was stained white, and bits of rough bran accumulated on the sides. The metate was made of basalt, a porous volcanic rock like the andesite used in Çatalhöyük. The wide pores gripped the grains in place, making them easier to crush. Cyr used his hand to sweep the mingled bran and flour into a plastic tub, and repeated the process several more times. After ten minutes or so, a few dozen ounces of flour had accumulated in the tub. Cyr pointed out that there were little flecks of stone in the flour, and suggested that I throw out the first few batches, until the rough patches on the mano and metate had been smoothed out, or risk abrading my tooth enamel. Cyr was sure the flour was fine enough to make bread. A pound and a half of grain, he figured, would produce nine or ten pita-sized breads, enough for a family meal.

The following morning, I threw four teaspoons of grain onto the metate's surface. The first couple of passes didn't seem to do anything, but then the grains began to crack, and a powdery white flour appeared. There was something in the motion that made it feel like the wheat was being ground between giant molars. (It suddenly made sense to me that the invention of the roller mill was inspired by one Swiss man's visit to the dentist.) The grinding process was the first step in predigesting the wheat, whose caloric riches would otherwise have remained locked up in the hard shell of the seed.

I also felt, deeply and in my bones, what hard work grinding was. Each handful of wheat took up to eight minutes to reduce to powder. In the first hour, I managed to process four ounces of grain. In the second hour, my productivity seriously declined. On the theory that grinding grain in Çatalhöyük was a shared family duty, I asked Victor for help. He gave it a try, but after a few minutes, it was obvious he didn't yet have the muscles to crush much of anything. Later that day, I did a second two-hour session; the following day, a third. In the end, six hours of hard labor yielded just a pound and a half of flour. I came away with lower back pain, blisters on the palms of my hands, and random spasms in my upper arms. I had a new respect for the daily grind: Neolithic farmers must have really, really wanted bread.

My next challenge was to bake my bread in a clay oven, like the beehive-shaped ones I'd seen in Çatalhöyük. González Carretero had shared photos of an outdoor oven she'd fashioned from clay, and I considered borrowing a backyard to do the same, but then settled on a compromise. Cyr had suggested I contact the Turkish-born chef Fisun Ercan. During the pandemic, she'd opened Bika, a farm-to-table restaurant, near to La Milanaise, where my organic flour was milled. When I called up Ercan, she told me she'd never baked with emmer, but would love to try. She had a specially built clay-walled oven in her kitchen and offered to fire it up for me.

I showed up at Bika, an hour's drive southeast of Montreal, late in the morning. In Ercan's sunlit kitchen, I placed two bowls of dough on the counter. One was a control batch, made with whole wheat; the other with my hand-ground emmer. I explained I'd sifted out most of the bran, so the bread wouldn't be too grainy, and combined the fine emmer flour with water, but without too much kneading.

González Carretero had made her bread with wild mustard seed, which was found in large quantities in Çatalhöyük's mud-brick dwellings. I'd found the seeds in the spice section of an Iranian grocery store. *Khak-shir*, as it is known in Persian cooking, tastes like mustard without the harsh bite; in Iran, it's used as a refreshing addition to summer drinks. I'd thrown a handful of the tiny brown seeds into the wet sticky dough, which I'd let sit out overnight. By that morning, the dough had collected wild yeasts from the air and had visibly swollen. This was natural leavening at work.

By then, the dome-shaped oven, which had been charged with logs of ash at seven thirty that morning, was radiating a pleasant heat. Ercan told me that she had grown up in a village on the Turkish seacoast, where bread-making was part of the daily routine. With practiced motions, she used a slender wooden roller to flatten balls of the dough into pita-sized circles. Using a metal peel, she slid them onto the hot bricks next to the glowing wood embers in the center of the oven. After a minute, the bread started to balloon upward, like the puffed-up pitas I've been served in restaurants in Istanbul. After two minutes, when patches on the surface were starting to blacken, Ercan pulled them out of the oven. After wishing each other *"afiyet olsun"*—bon appétit in Turkish—we tore in. The bread deflated, releasing a magical little wisp of steam from the pocket-like interior.

"The texture is so nice," said Ercan. She took the first bite, then let out a swoon-like "Oooh!" and did an endearing little dance, a two-step of delight. "That is delicious bread!" It was. Nutty in flavor, it had all the complexity and enzymatic aliveness of bread I've baked from freshly ground wheat. "I don't know how to explain it," mused Ercan. "It feels a little bit like we're eating the grain itself."

She had made sure to bake a few control pitas from bread wheat. These were acceptable, but a little bland. The pitas we'd made with wild mustard were especially delicious; the seeds added a satisfying, poppy-seed-like crunch as well as a slight spiciness, nowhere near as overbearing as the caraway seeds on a kimmel loaf.

Ercan seemed energized by the experience. "I'm going to order some emmer to bake with!" she said. She bought her flour, which she ground from buckwheat and einkorn, from a local wheat farmer, and she thought she might be able to convince him to plant emmer in his field. She liked the idea that she'd be serving a bread whose roots went back to ancient Anatolia and, indeed, deep into human prehistory.

When I got home later that day, leftovers packed in a Ziploc bag, I was excited about how Erin and my boys were going to react. But the bread, supple and aromatic when it had come out of the oven, had stiffened and lost its olfactory appeal. Desmond took a bite or two and gave a "meh" of dismissal. Heating the bread in the oven improved the experience a little, but it remained hard. It suddenly made sense to me that the oven was the center of the dwellings—and much of the culture—of Çatalhöyük. All the effort that went into growing, scything, and grinding grain would have been worth it for the evanescent miracle of hot, aromatic bread. You'd want to be on hand when the day's bread came out of the oven, when it smelled and tasted its best, and to witness that little puff of steam as you tore into it.

The archaeologist responsible for the slow, methodical excavation of Çatalhöyük, Ian Hodder, uses the term *entanglement* to describe the complex of technologies, tools, and plants and animals that come to enmesh people in different societies. I had a hunch that food, in particular grains and bread, was key to the mystery of why the hunter-gatherers of the Konya Plain chose to stay put in one of history's first proto-cities. They were entangled with those stands of emmer that grew nearby, with the obsidian-bladed scythes they used to cut it down, with the volcanic-rock querns next to the hearths, with the clay they fashioned to make the ovens. They were entangled, in other words, with their daily bread, and curious enough to stick around to see what tomorrow's loaf would taste like.

I realized that, in a similar way, I'd become tangled up with my own kitchen cultures. Quite literally, with the yeasts and bacteria that kept our kefir, sourdough, yogurt, kombucha, and kimchi going—communities that nourished my family, but that also relied on me, their hominin shepherd, to keep them alive. The task of tending them didn't feel like a troublesome responsibility, a constraint on my wanderlust and itchy feet, but a rooting: a salutary deepening and entwining of my connection to the domus, to my home and family.

IN THE FINAL MONTHS OF WRITING THIS BOOK, I was lucky enough to spend a few weeks surrounded by wheat fields. I was staying in the foothills of the Jura Mountains, in the canton of Vaud, a part of Switzerland that prides itself on sustainable, organic agriculture. Many of the farms were centuries old. The entire landscape seemed devoted to turning the richness of the soil into fantastically delicious foods. I witnessed the age-old transhumance, in which Simmental, Jersey, and Charolais cows were transported to summer pastures in Alpine meadows, more than four thousand feet in altitude, where they fed on wildflowers and lush grass, to produce the exquisite Gruyère, Tomme, and Vacherin cheeses sold in village *fromageries*.

The hills that rose from the shore of Lac Léman were terraced with grapevines, some of whose roots went back a thousand years. I pedaled my bicycle to farm stands, where people left bottles of syrup and ciders, there for the taking in exchange for a few Swiss francs deposited in a wooden box. This was a thriving, well-populated countryside, full of young people, woven together by railway tracks, bus lines, cycle routes, and foot trails.

I'd arrived in mid-May, just as the reddish-orange poppies were blooming. On daily bike rides, I got to see the spring wheat planted in fields all around me mature from a lustrous green to a sharkskin amber. I recalled the criticism leveled against wheat: that it's one of humanity's most egregious examples of a monocrop. But in the Vaud, the fields were relatively small, a few dozen acres at most, and people were careful to plant fruit- and nut-bearing trees alongside the edges. A local initiative had dotted *jachères*, richly diverse plots of native

294 THE LOST SUPPER

grasses and wildflowers that encouraged birds to nest and insects to gather pollen, in random spots among the wheat fields.

Some afternoons, I'd walk a few paces into a field not far from where I was staying, and watch the wind running its fingers through the wheat, dragging rippling iridescent furrows through stalks heavy with seed. I saw red kites plunging to earth to spear voles and field mice with their talons, heard owls hunting at night, and spotted hawks perched on barns and bales of hay. The fact that pesticides were banned meant that the much-feared insect apocalypse had not befallen these parts: if I didn't keep my mouth shut when I was cycling, I choked on mouthfuls of tiny flies. A million buzzing pollinators were indicators of a healthy, vibrant countryside.

Being in Switzerland was a reminder that agriculture need not be the problem. Done properly, it was the solution to our diversity and sustainability crisis. I'd seen many good examples in my travels: the chinampas and milpas of Mexico; the mixed farms in the American South where Ossabaw hogs were allowed to forage in the forest; the meadows on the Yorkshire Dales that the Hattan family was making live again with its Northern Dairy Shorthorns. There was a world of other great practices out there, sometimes referred to as regenerative farming, biointensive agriculture, agroforestry, or permaculture, like the mixed mountain farming championed by Sepp Holzer, an Austrian advocate of farming on marginal land.

Even if we aren't in a position to grow our own food, there are straightforward ways we can all become more responsible eaters. The American writer Wendell Berry laid out seven simple principles in his influential 1989 essay "The Pleasures of Eating." Prepare your own food; learn where the food you buy comes from; deal directly, whenever possible, with local farmers, gardeners, and orchardists. In self-defense, teach yourself about the economy and technology of food production and how industry adds to and alters food. Learn what is involved in the best farming, as well as in the life histories of food species. First and foremost, participate in food production, even if that means nothing more than growing herbs or tomatoes on a kitchen windowsill.

"Only by growing some food for yourself," emphasizes Berry, "can you become acquainted with the beautiful energy cycle that revolved from soil to seed to flower to fruit to food to offal to decay, and around again."

In Switzerland, I remembered the wheat fields I've known on the Canadian prairies and the Great Plains, which can cover thirty thousand acres, so vast that walking from one edge to the other can take three hours. Planted with dwarf hybrid varieties, sprayed with pesticides, and shocked dead with glyphosate for easier harvesting by combines, this was the kind of landscape the critics of industrial agriculture decry: one devoid of diversity, dead except for the one plant species that happens to be valued by modern humans, wheat. It was a stark contrast with the Swiss countryside, where agriculture was practiced in a way that kept the soil healthy, and the land and air alive with animal, plant, and insect life.

If humans are defined as the species that adapts to new environments, we've fulfilled our destiny, to the extent that we now find ourselves adapting to impoverished environments entirely of our own making. The monocultures of wheat, rice, corn, and soybeans that feed us depend for their success on the elimination of biodiversity. But diversity is what confers resiliency, and by simplifying natural habitats to serve the needs of industrial agriculture, we've left ourselves open to pandemics, supply-chain-disrupting wars, droughts, floods, and new crop and livestock diseases. Our determination to feed everyone on the planet cheaply has already resulted in malnourishment for the masses. If we don't change our ways, it could soon lead to hunger for all.

When my ancestors left Ireland and what is now Ukraine, they were surely dreaming of a land where they could start over, where they could build a fulfilling life on a fertile patch of soil. They may have told themselves that—this time around—they would find a way to live unharassed by tax collectors, army recruiters, priests and palace-builders, tsars and kings. Instead, they repeated the error, because there is no land on this planet that is empty and ready for the taking; we all have to find a way to share its wealth with those already there. Over the years, the dream of finding a patch of land of one's own, to devote to honest toil and a quiet life, was eroded. What remains are mega-farms of chemical-blasted, ever-more-degraded soil, tended by machines rather than humans.

Perhaps there's still time to find a way back to a sustainable, more nourishing past. Deep down, I don't think we've ever lost hold of the first and greatest of all human dreams, that dream whose outlines can be discerned in the mud walls of Çatalhöyük, in the longhouses of the Iroquois Confederacy, in all those places built outside the confines of authoritarian states. Those places where we dreamt of living together in ways that would amplify our collective possibilities, in settlements that would offer us the material security to imagine and create new realities, without seriously limiting any one person's freedom to experience sensual delight in being alive in the world.

Our world, a world that has always been commensurate with our capacity for wonder, if only we had the eyes to see it.

Acknowledgments

THIS IS MY PANDEMIC BOOK. I began working on it in earnest in 2020, so I'd be remiss if I didn't start by acknowledging SARS-COV-2, the coronavirus strain that changed the world. COVID-19 made the process of researching *The Lost Supper* endlessly frustrating and barred me from traveling to East Asia, part of my original plan. It forced me to make more discrete, short-term expeditions than I normally would have; all air travel for this book was balanced with contributions to two highly ranked carbon offset schemes. (Which didn't, of course, prevent my share of carbon from being emitted into the atmosphere.) That said, travel restrictions allowed me to read widely, to research deeply, to write, and to revise. For this unwonted luxury of time, I'm grateful.

Food is love, and the love of food brings with it the privilege and pleasure of getting to know people who love, and live for, food. Among the passionate people who shared their time, and passion, with me at home and on my journeys, I'd like to thank Maurín Arellano, Jessica Vincent, Nicholas Gilman, I. Lehr "Bris" Brisbin, David S. Shields, Robert I. Curtis, Jill Santopietro, Fernando Medrano, Shauna Beharry, Cameron Abery, Filomena "Flo" Tanzarella, Corrado Rodio, Enzo Suma, Paolo Cherubini, Renée Landry and Dominique Arseneau, Serena Love, Colin Khoury, Patricia Michaelson, Megan Ainscow, Tony Morris, Paul Greenberg, Herbert Aronoff, Ian Mosby, Jakub "Kubo" Dzamba and David Waitzer of Third Millennium Farming, Valerie Trouet, Eduardo Moralejo, Luis Rallo and Concepcion Muñoz Díez, Lara González Carretero, Dorian Fuller, and Mike Finnerty, that errant Canadian cheesemonger in London. A special shout-out to Ethné and Philippe de Vienne, Montreal's *chasseurs d'épices,* whose love of food, flavor, and adventure continues to inspire me.

Hospitality is sacred, and I'm especially grateful to the people who went out of their way to welcome me on my way. I'm thinking particularly of Alberto Ruy Sánchez and Margarita De Orellano in Mexico City, Sally and Andrew Hattan in the Yorkshire Dales, Donato Boscia in Puglia, Tim Gutteridge in Cádiz, Fisun Ercan in Saint-Blaise-sur-Richelieu, Eliza MacLean in North Carolina, Ogwilowgwa (Kim Recalma-Clutesi) and William White in Qualicum, Michael Lines in Victoria, Silvestro Silvestri of Awaiting Table in Lecce, Mauro Barreiro in Cádiz, the Buendía-Peralta family in Chimalhuacán, and Donato Petruzzi and his family in Puglia. Big thanks, as ever, to my sister Lara Aydein and her husband, Justin, for offering succor and shelter when my travels took me to Illahee Chuk. I'm grateful to Christine Moravec of Eat Mexico for setting up a tour of Mexico City's La Merced market and to Ariane Ruiz for taking the time to walk me through it, and to Alfredo Francis Lance for being my good-humored, open-hearted, and adventurous interpreter in CDMX.

The quest for silphion was a long adventure, and I want to thank those who helped me interpret the signposts along the way, including Chris Hunt of the Society for Libyan Studies, Sheila Ager at the University of Waterloo, Yiorgo Topalides at the University of Florida, Panayotis League at Florida State University, Alexandra Livarda at the Catalan Institute of Classical Archaeology, Laura Banducci at Carleton, as well as Vera Keller and Kenneth Parejko. I'm especially grateful to Mahmut Miski, a true gentleman and scholar, and Mehmet Ata for guiding us through his property in Cappadocia. I'd like to emphasize my gratitude to the late Prof. Adil Güner, the director of the Nezahat Gökyiğit Botanical Gardens in Istanbul, for welcoming us to the gardens and allowing our cooking experiments with *Ferula drudeana* to go ahead. And special thanks to Kristin Romey, the archaeology editor at *National Geographic,* for her interest and faith in this obscure and challenging subject.

A shout-out to my fellow grainheads for their enthusiasm and baking and grinding advice, among them Nick Amberg, Seth Gabrielse of Boulangerie Automne, Bernard Pilon, Robert Beauchemin, Seamus Blackley, and Marc-Andre Cyr.

On Mi'wer'la, known as Vancouver Island to many, I'd like to thank Nicole Kilburn, Genevieve Singleton, Shanna Baker, J. B. ("The Native Plant Guy") Williams, Sellemah (Joan Morris), Scott Chernoff, and Jennifer Menard, and especially Nancy Turner, an unfailingly patient and graceful gateway to a world of traditional knowledge.

Very special thanks to the generous and enterprising Sally Grainger, author of *The Story of Garum* and *Cooking Apicius*, for her patience and words of wisdom in guiding me through the byways of ancient cookery.

A six-week residency at the fabulous Fondation Jan Michalski in Montricher, Switzerland, allowed me the tranquility to complete two chapters and do important editing work; I'm grateful to Vera Michalski-Hoffmann for introducing me to her world and to the outstanding team at the foundation, including Guillaume Dollmann, Chantal Buffet, Shadi Saad, and Sabine Beaud. (*Un grand merci pour le vélo, Sabine!*) Ted Scheinman was an attentive and demanding editor of my fish-sauce-related prose at *Smithsonian Magazine*. It's my first time working with Paula Ayer, my intensely supportive editor at Greystone, but I suspect it won't be the last; thanks, too, to Crissy Calhoun for some graceful, sharp-eyed copyediting, to Jennifer Stewart for the thorough proofreading, and to Rob Sanders for his courtliness and kind words of encouragement. And thanks to Jess Sullivan for the eye-catching cover, and to Belle Wuthrich for the interior design.

I'm grateful to the Canada Council for the Arts, the Conseil des arts et des lettres du Québec, and the Access Copyright Foundation for providing generous and timely funding, without which *The Lost Supper* could never have been completed. Michelle Tessler, my always professional and optimistic agent, provided crucial guidance, encouragement, editing advice, and support along the way.

To my wife, Erin Churchill, I pledge my never-flagging love and offer my excuses—for my weird preoccupations, my periodic absences, and, this time around, for several years of odd smells and dirty kitchen counters. To my mother, Audrey, thank you for all the interest, encouragement, and forbearance as your wayward son embarked on yet another of his strange, worry-inducing quests; and thanks, too, for inspiring my love of cooking, which began with your guidance in the kitchen on West 22nd Avenue. To my sons, the intrepid Desmond and resolutely neophobic Victor: thank you, boychuks, you were the motivation for this entire endeavor. It goes without saying, but I'll say it again: I love you.

Finally, this is dedicated to my father, Paul Alan George Grescoe, who was often my first reader. You didn't get to read the final draft of this one, Dad, although I knew you wanted to; nor did you get to hold the copy of *The Lost Supper*, hot off the presses, with your name on the dedication page, in your hands. Your generosity, curiosity, talent, and love made the world a better place and me a better person. I miss you, old man.

Selected Bibliography

PROLOGUE

Atalan-Helicke, Nurcan. "'You Can Never Give Up *Siyez* If You Taste It Once': Local Taste, Global Markets, and the Conservation of Einkorn, an Ancient Wheat." *Gastronomica* 18, no. 2 (2018): 33–45.

Atalay, Sonya, and Christine A. Hastorf. "Food, Meals, and Daily Activities: Food Habitus at Neolithic Çatalhöyük." *American Antiquity* 71, no. 2 (2006): 283–319.

Ayala, Gianna, et al. "Paleoenvironmental Reconstruction of the Alluvial Landscape of Neolithic Çatalhöyük, Central Southern Turkey." *Journal of Archaeological Science* 87 (2017): 30–43.

Balter, Michael. *The Goddess and the Bull: Çatalhöyük; An Archaeological Journey to the Dawn of Civilization.* New York: Free Press, 2005.

Bilgic, Hatice, et al. "Ancient DNA From 8400 Year-Old Çatalhöyük Wheat: Implications for the Origin of Neolithic Agriculture." *PLOS ONE* 11, no. 3 (2016): e0151974.

Birpinar, Mehmet Emin. "Effects of Drought in Turkey and Around the World." *Daily Sabah*, Dec. 23, 2021.

Carretero, Lara González, et al. "Disentangling Neolithic Cuisine: Archaeological Evidence for 9,000-Year-Old Food Preparation Practices and Cooking Techniques at Çatalhöyük East." In *Communities at Work: The Making of Çatalhöyük*, edited by Ian Hodder and Christina Tsoraki, 229–41. British Institute at Ankara, 2021.

Carretero, Lara González, et al. "A Methodological Approach to the Study of Archaeological Cereal Meals: A Case Study at Çatalhöyük East." *Vegetation History and Archaeobotany* 26, no. 4 (2017): 415–32.

Diamond, Jared. "The Worst Mistake in the History of the Human Race." *Discover*, May 1987.

Dunn, Rob R., and Mónica Sánchez. *Delicious: The Evolution of Flavor and How It Made Us Human.* Princeton, NJ: Princeton University Press, 2021.

Fraser, Suzan. "Turkey's Second-Largest Lake Dries Up Because of Climate Change, Agricultural Policies." *Globe and Mail*, Oct. 29, 2021.

Graeber, David, and David Wengrow. *The Dawn of Everything: A New History of Humanity.* New York: Farrar, Straus and Giroux, 2021.

Harari, Yuval Noah. *Sapiens: A Brief History of Humankind.* Harper: New York, 2015.

Hodder, Ian. *The Leopard's Tail: Revealing the Histories of Çatalhöyük.* London: Thames & Hudson, 2006.

Karagöz, Alptekin. "Wheat Landraces of Turkey." *Emirates Journal of Food and Agriculture* 26, vol. 2 (2014): 149–56.

Manning, Richard. *Against the Grain: How Agriculture Has Hijacked Civilization*. New York: North Point, 2004.

McKernan, Bethan. "Turkey Drought: Istanbul Could Run Out of Water in 45 Days." *Guardian*, Jan. 13, 2021.

Monbiot, George. "Lab-Grown Food Will Soon Destroy Farming—and Save the Planet." *Guardian*, Jan. 8, 2020.

Montgomery, David. *Dirt: The Erosion of Civilizations*. Berkeley: University of California Press, 2007.

Morgounov, A., et al. "Wheat Landraces Currently Grown in Turkey: Distribution, Diversity, and Use." *Crop Science* 56, no. 6 (2016): 3112–24.

Newitz, Annalee. *Four Lost Cities: A Secret History of the Urban Age*. New York: W. W. Norton, 2021.

Nizam, Derya, and Zafer Yenal. "Seed Politics in Turkey: The Awakening of a Landrace Wheat and Its Prospects." *Journal of Peasant Studies* 487, no. 4 (2020): 741–66.

Sethi, Simran. *Bread, Wine, Chocolate: The Slow Loss of Foods We Love*. New York: HarperCollins, 2016.

Smith, Hannah Lucinda. "Farmers Live in Fear of Next Giant Sinkhole." *Times* (London), Nov. 13, 2021.

Spector, Tim. *Food for Life: The New Science of Eating Well*. London: Jonathan Cape, 2022.

Stringer, Chris. *Lone Survivors: How We Came to Be the Only Humans on Earth*. New York: Times Books, 2012.

United Nations. "Shrinking Biodiversity Poses Major Risk to the Future of Global Food and Agriculture, Landmark UN Report Shows." *UN News*, Feb. 22, 2019.

Wells, Spencer. *Pandora's Seed: Why the Hunter-Gatherer Holds the Key to Our Survival*. New York: Random House, 2010.

Wilson, Bee. *The Way We Eat Now: Strategies for Eating in a World of Change*. London: 4th Estate, 2019.

Wrangham, Richard. *Catching Fire: How Cooking Made Us Human*. London: Profile, 2010.

Zuk, Marlene. *Paleofantasy: What Evolution Really Tells Us About Sex, Diet, and the Way We Live*. New York: W. W. Norton, 2013.

1. MONTREAL: KITCHEN DREAMS

Berry, Wendell. *What I Stand On: The Collected Essays of Wendell Berry*. New York: Library of America, 2019.

Leopold, Aldo. *A Sand County Almanac and Other Writings on Ecology and Conservation*. New York: Library of America, 2013.

Meadows, Donella H. *The Limits to Growth: A Report for the Club of Rome's Project on the Predicament of Mankind*. New York: Universe, 1972.

Raffles, Hugh. *Insectopedia*. New York: Vintage, 2011.

Schumacher, E. F. *Small Is Beautiful: A Study of Economics as if People Mattered*. London: Vintage, 1993.

Waltner-Toews, David. *Eat the Beetles! An Exploration Into Our Conflicted Relationship With Insects*. Toronto: ECW Press, 2017.

2. MEXICO CITY: THE SECRET OF AXAYACATL

Alcocer, J., and W. D. Williams. "Historical and Recent Changes in Lake Texcoco, a Saline Lake in Mexico." *International Journal of Salt Lake Research* 5, no. 1 (1996): 45–61.

Artes de México. *Bestiario culinario de México.* Mexico City: Artes de México, 2018.

Bricker, Darrell, and John Ibbitson. *Empty Planet: The Shock of Global Population Decline.* Toronto: Signal, 2020.

Carrasco, David. *City of Sacrifice: The Aztec Empire and the Role of Violence in Civilization.* Boston: Beacon Press, 1999.

Cohen, Manuel Perló. "Thirsty City on a Lake." *American Scientist*, Sept. 1, 2019.

Costa-Neto, E. M. "Edible Insects in Latin America: Old Challenges, New Opportunities." *Journal of Insects as Food and Feed* 2, no. 1 (2016): 1–2.

Ebel, Roland. "Chinampas: An Urban Farming Model of the Aztecs and a Potential Solution for Modern Megalopolis." *HortTechnology* 30, no. 1 (2020): 13–20.

Ehrlich, Paul. *The Population Bomb.* New York: Ballantine, 1971.

Eulich, Whitney. "Edible Insects Give Mexicans a Taste of History—and Maybe the Future." *Christian Science Monitor*, Apr. 25, 2017.

Figuerora-Sandoval, Benjamín, et al. "Production of the Escamol Ant and Its Habitat in the Potosino-Zacatecano High Plateau, México." *Agricultura, Sociedad, y Desarrollo* 15, no. 2 (2018): 235–45.

Gates, Stefan. *Insects: An Edible Field Guide.* London: Ebury Press, 2017.

Goldman, Francisco. *The Interior Circuit: A Mexico City Chronicle.* New York: Grove, 2014.

González-Santoyo, Sonia, et al. "The 'Mosco' of Lake Cuitzeo: An Unusual Inland Water Fishery." *Limnology* 21 (2020): 119–27.

Goodyear, Dana. "Department of Gastronomy: Grub." *New Yorker*, Aug. 15, 2011.

Grabinsky, Alan. "Axolotls in Crisis: The Fight to Save the 'Water Monster' of Mexico City." *Guardian*, Dec. 4, 2018.

Hernandez, Daniel. *Down & Delirious in Mexico City: The Aztec Metropolis in the Twenty-First Century.* New York: Scribner, 2011.

Holloway, James. "An Old Aztec Tradition Could Help Feed the Megacities of the Future." *New Atlas*, Nov. 7, 2019.

Holt, Vincent M. *Why Not Eat Insects?* Oxford: Thornton's, 1995 [1885].

Holtz, Deborah, and Juan Carlos Mena. *Acridofagia y otros insectos.* Mexico City: Trilce, 2015.

Hurd, Kayla J. "The Cultural Importance of Edible Insects in Oaxaca, Mexico." *Annals of the Entomological Society of America* 112, no. 6 (2019): 552–9.

"Insectos en Mesoamérica." Special issue, *Arqueología Mexicana* 86 (June 2019).

Kandell, Jonathan. *La Capital: The Biography of Mexico City.* New York: Random House, 1988.

Lesnik, Julie J. *Edible Insects and Human Evolution.* Gainesville: University Press of Florida, 2019.

Levy, Buddy. *Conquistador: Hernán Cortés, King Montezuma, and the Last Stand of the Aztecs.* New York: Bantam, 2008.

Lida, David. *First Stop in the New World: Mexico City, the Capital of the 21st Century.* New York: Riverhead, 2008.

Lockwood, Jeffrey Alan. *The Infested Mind: Why Humans Fear, Loathe, and Love Insects.* Oxford: Oxford University Press, 2013.

MacNeal, David. *Bugged: The Insects Who Rule the World and the People Obsessed With Them.* New York: St. Martin's, 2017.

Martin, Daniella. *Edible: An Adventure Into the World of Eating Insects and the Last Great Hope to Save the Planet.* Boston, New York: New Harvest, 2014.

Müller, A., et al. "Entomophagy and Power." *Journal of Insects as Food and Feed* 2, no. 2 (2016): 121–36.

Raffles, Hugh. *Insectopedia.* New York: Vintage, 2011.

Ramos-Elorduy, Julieta. "Threatened Edible Insects in Hidalgo, Mexico and Some Measures to Preserve Them." *Journal of Ethnobiology and Ethnomedicine* 2, no. 2 (2006): 51.

Sorrentino, Joseph. "Can the Chinampas Survive?" *Commonweal*, Sept. 1, 2019.

van Huis, Arnold. *The Insect Cookbook: Food for a Sustainable Planet.* New York: Columbia University Press, 2016.

Villanueva, Paloma. "¡Lleve crujientes manjares!" *Reforma*, June 29, 2013.

Vincent, Jessica. "Mexico's Ancient 'Caviar.'" *BBC Travel*, Sept. 11, 2019.

Waltner-Toews, David. *Eat the Beetles! An Exploration Into Our Conflicted Relationship With Insects.* Toronto: ECW Press, 2017.

Wright, Ronald. *Stolen Continents: The "New World" Through Indian Eyes Since 1492.* Toronto: Viking, 1995.

3. OSSABAW ISLAND: SOME PIG

Addison, Corban. *Wastelands: The True Story of Farm Country on Trial.* New York: Alfred A. Knopf, 2022.

Albarella, Umberto, et al. "The Domestication of the Pig (*Sus Scrofa*): New Challenges and Approaches." In *Documenting Domestication*, edited by Melinda A. Zeder et al., 209–27. Oakland: University of California Press, 2006.

Berry, Wendell. "The Neighborly Art of Hog Killing." In *For the Hog Killing*, edited by Ben Aguilar, 1–8. Lexington: University Press of Kentucky, 2019.

Brisbin, I. Lehr, and Michael S. Sturek. "The Pigs of Ossabaw Island: A Case Study of the Application of Long-Term Data in Management Plan Development." In *Wild Pigs: Biology, Damage, Control Techniques and Management*, edited by John J. Mayer and I. Lehr Brisbin, 365–78. Aiken, SC: Savannah River National Laboratory, 2009.

Clark, Laura. "People Ate Pork in the Middle East Until 1,000 B.C.—What Changed?" *Smithsonian*, Mar. 18, 2015.

Cullen, Art. "Out in Farm Country, We're Getting Fed Up With Hogs Fouling Our Nests." *Washington Post*, June 3, 2021.

Dove, Rick. "I Saw Florence Sending Millions of Gallons of Animal Poop Flooding Across North Carolina." *Washington Post*, Sept. 24, 2018.

Fessenden, Marissa. "Pigs Aren't Quite as Domesticated as People Once Thought." *Smithsonian*, Sept. 1, 2015.

Fishman, Jane. *The Woman Who Saved an Island.* Savannah, GA: Real People Publishing, 2014.

Genoways, Ted. *The Chain: Farm, Factory, and the Fate of Our Food.* New York: Harper, 2014.

Kaminsky, Peter. *Pig Perfect: Encounters With Remarkable Swine and Some Great Ways to Cook Them.* New York: Hyperion, 2005.

Leonard, Christopher. *The Meat Racket: The Secret Takeover of America's Food Business.* New York: Simon & Schuster, 2014.

Lobban, Richard A., Jr. "Pigs and Their Prohibition." *International Journal of Middle East Studies* 26, no. 1 (1994): 57–75.

Redding, Richard W. "The Pig and the Chicken in the Middle East." *Journal of Archaeological Research* 23 (2015): 325–68.

Spry-Marqués, Pía. *Pig/Pork: Archaeology, Zoology and Edibility.* London: Bloomsbury, 2017.

Stoll, Steven. *Larding the Lean Earth: Soil and Society in Nineteenth-Century America.* New York: Hill and Wang, 2002.

Talbott, Charles W., et al. "Enhancing Pork Flavor and Fat Quality With Swine Raised in Sylvan Systems: Potential Niche-Market Application for the Ossabaw Hog." *Renewable Agriculture and Food Systems* 21, no. 3: 183–91.

Tietz, Jeff. "Boss Hog: The Dark Side of America's Top Pork Producer." *Rolling Stone*, Dec. 14, 2006.

University of Oxford. "Ancient Pigs Endured a Complete Genomic Turnover After They Arrived in Europe." *Science Daily*, Aug. 12, 2019.

University of Oxford. "Iberian Pig Genome Remains Unchanged After Five Centuries." *Science Daily*, Sept. 17, 2014.

Weiss, Brad. *Real Pigs: Shifting Values in the Field of Local Pork.* Durham: Duke University Press, 2015.

White, Sam. "From Globalized Pig Breeds to Capitalist Pigs: A Study in Animal Cultures and Evolutionary History." *Environmental History* 16, no. 1 (2011): 94–120.

Wright, Chris. "The Battle for America's Miracle Pig." *Gear Patrol*, Oct. 31, 2016.

4. CÁDIZ: THE QUINTESSENCE OF PUTRESCENCE

Abulafia, David. *The Great Sea: A Human History of the Mediterranean.* London: Penguin Books, 2014.

Banducci, Laura M. "Tastes of Roman Italy: Early Roman Expansion and Taste Articulation." In *Taste and the Ancient Senses*, edited by Kelli C. Rudolph, 120–37. London: Routledge, 2018.

Beard, Mary. *SPQR: A History of Ancient Rome.* New York: W. W. Norton, 2015.

Beresford, James. *The Ancient Sailing Season.* Leiden: Brill, 2013.

Bernal-Casasola, Darío, and Daniela Cottica. "Produzione e vendita di pesce sotto sale e suoi derivati a Pompei nel 79 d.C." In *L'exploitation des ressources maritimes de l'antiquité*, edited by Ricardo González et al., 235–52. Antibes: Éditions APDCA, 2017.

Bernal-Casasola, Darío, and Antonio Sáez Romero. "Fish-Salting Plants and Amphorae Production in the Bay of Cadiz (Baetica, Hispania): Patterns of Settlement From the Punic Era to Late Antiquity." In *Thinking About Space*, edited by H. Vanhaverbeke et al., 45–113. Lovaina: Universidad de Lovaina, 2008.

Carannante, Alfredo. "The Last Garum of Pompeii: Archaeozoological Analyses on Fish Remains From the 'Garum Shop' and Related Ecological Inferences." *International Journal of Osteoarchaeology* 29 (2019): 377–86.

Curtis, Robert I. "Umami and the Foods of Classical Antiquity." *American Journal of Clinical Nutrition* (2009): 712S–18S.

Davidson, James. *Courtesans and Fishcakes: The Consuming Passions of Classical Athens.* New York: St. Martin's, 1997.

Downie, David. "A Roman Anchovy's Tale." *Gastronomica* 3, no. 2 (2003): 25–28.

Faas, Patrick. *Around the Roman Table.* London: Macmillan, 2003.

Forsythe, Gary. *A Critical History of Early Rome, From Prehistory to the First Punic War.* Berkeley: University of California Press, 2005.

García-Vargas, Enrique, et al. "*Confectio Gari Pompeiani:* Experimental Procedure for the Preparation of Roman Fish Sauces." *SPAL* 23 (Jan. 2014): 65–82.

Grainger, Sally. *Cooking Apicius: Roman Recipes for Today.* Totnes, UK: Prospect Books, 2006.

Grainger, Sally. "Garum and Liquamen: What's in a Name?" *Journal of Maritime Archaeology* 13 (2018): 247–61.

Grainger, Sally. *The Story of Garum: Fermented Fish Sauce and Salted Fish in the Ancient World.* Oxford: Routledge, 2021.

Grainger, Sally. "Towards an Authentic Roman Sauce." In *Authenticity in the Kitchen,* edited by Richard Hosking. Proceedings of the Oxford Symposium on Food and Cookery, 2005.

Grant, Mark. *Roman Cookery: Ancient Recipes for Modern Kitchens.* London: Serif, 1999.

Greenberg, Paul. *The Omega Principle: Seafood and the Quest for a Long Life and a Healthier Planet.* New York: Penguin, 2018.

Hall, Christopher. "Homage to the Anchovy Coast." *Smithsonian,* May 2005, 98–104.

Horden, Peregrine, and Nicholas Purcell. *The Corrupting Sea: A Study of Mediterranean History.* Malden, MA: Blackwell Publishing, 2015.

James, Bruce R., et al. "Bread and Soil in Ancient Rome: A Vision of Abundance and an Ideal of Order Based on Wheat, Grapes, and Olives." In *The Soil Underfoot: Infinite Possibilities for a Finite Resource,* edited by G. Jock Churchman. Boca Raton, FL: CRC Press, 2014.

Malo de Molina, Julio. *Cádiz: A Journey.* Cádiz: Ediciones Mayi, 2013.

Malvarez, G., et al. "Environmental Control on Roman Time Coastal Industrial Settlements at the Confluence of the Atlantic and Mediterranean." *Journal of Coastal Research* (2020): 870–74.

Marchetti, Silvia. "Did Fish Sauce in Vietnam Come From Ancient Rome via the Silk Road?" *South China Morning Post,* July 28, 2020.

Marzano, Annalisa. "Fish and Fishing in the Roman World." *Journal of Maritime Archaeology* 13 (2018): 437–47.

Mata, Diego Ruiz. "Gadir, Its Plural Structure: A Way to Look at the Phoenician Foundation in Space and in Time." *Revista Onoba* 6 (2018): 249–88.

Miles, Richard. *Carthage Must Be Destroyed: The Rise and Fall of an Ancient Civilization.* London: Viking, 2011.

Mitchell, Piers D. "Human Parasites in the Roman World: Health Consequences of Conquering an Empire." *Parasitology* 144, no. 1 (Jan. 2017): 48–58.

Purcell, Nicholas. "Eating Fish: The Paradoxes of Seafood." In *Food in Antiquity,* edited by John Wilkins. Exeter: University of Exeter, 1995.

Quinn, Josephine Crawley. *In Search of the Phoenicians.* Princeton: Princeton University Press, 2018.

Rodríguez-Alcántara, Álvara. "New Technological Contributions to Roman Garum Elaboration From Chemical Analysis of Archaeological Fish Remains From the 'Garum Shop' at Pompeii (1.12.8)." *Zephyrus* (July–Dec. 2018): 149–63.

Santopietro, Jill. "Menaica Anchovies." Master's thesis, Boston University, 2014.

Schuster, Ruth. "Ancient Roman Garum Factory Found in Israel, Suitably Far Away From Town." *Haaretz*, Dec. 16, 2019.

Shaw, Brent D. "'Eaters of Flesh, Drinkers of Milk': The Ancient Mediterranean Ideology of the Pastoral Nomad." *Ancient Society* 13–14 (1982–83): 5–31.

Tammuz, Oded. "*Mare Clausum*? Sailing Seasons in the Mediterranean in Early Antiquity." *Mediterranean Historical Review* 20, no. 2 (2005): 145–62.

5. YORKSHIRE DALES: HARD CHEESE

Calvert, T. C. *The Story of Wensleydale Cheese*. Redditch, UK: Read Books, 2016.

Curry, Andrew. "The Milk Revolution." *Nature*, Aug. 2013, 20–22.

Donnelly, Catherine W., ed. *Cheese and Microbes*. Washington, DC: ASM Press, 2014.

Gamble, Don, ed. *Hay Time in the Yorkshire Dales*. Yorkshire Dales Millennium Trust, n.d.

Gasquet, Francis Aidan. *The Greater Abbeys of England*. London: Chatto & Windus, 1908.

Handwerk, Brian. "How Cheese, Wheat, and Alcohol Shaped Human Evolution." *Smithsonian*, Mar. 13, 2018.

Hartley, Marie, and Joan Ingilby. *Making Cheese and Butter*. Otley, UK: Smith Settle, 1988.

Kinstedt, Paul S. *Cheese and Culture: A History of Cheese and Its Place in Western Civilization*. White River Junction, VT: Chelsea Green Publishing, 2012.

Lang, Tim. *Feeding Britain: Our Food Problems and How to Fix Them*. London: Pelican, 2020.

Mason, Kate. "Yorkshire Cheese-Making." *Folk Life* 6, no. 1 (Jan. 1968): 7–16.

"Nidderdale Couple Embrace Endangered Cattle to Forge a New Farm Future in Cheese Production." *Yorkshire Post*, Aug. 11, 2018.

Orwell, George. "In Defence of English Cooking." *Evening Standard*, Dec. 15, 1945.

Palmer, Ned. *A Cheesemonger's History of the British Isles*. London: Profile, 2019.

Paxson, Heather. *The Life of Cheese: Crafting Food and Value in America*. Berkeley: University of California Press, 2013.

Percival, Bronwen, and Francis Percival. *Reinventing the Wheel: Milk, Microbes, and the Fight for Real Cheese*. Oakland: University of California Press, 2017.

Pye-Smith, Charlie. *Land of Plenty: A Journey Through the Fields and Foods of Modern Britain*. London: Elliott and Thompson, 2017.

Salque, Mélanie, et al. "Earliest Evidence for Cheese Making in the Sixth Millennium BC in Northern Europe." *Nature*, Jan. 24, 2013, 522–25.

Santogade, Elena R. *The Beginner's Guide to Cheesemaking*. Berkeley, CA: Rockridge Press, 2017.

Walker-Tisdale, C. W., and Walter E. Woodnutt. *Practical Cheesemaking: A General Guide to the Manufacture of Cheese*. London: Headley Bros., 1917.

Walling, Philip. *Counting Sheep: A Celebration of the Pastoral Heritage of Britain*. London: Profile, 2014.

Wolfe, Benjamin E., et al. "Cheese Rind Communities Provide Tractable Systems for In Situ and In Vitro Studies of Microbial Diversity." *Cell* 158 (July 17, 2014): 422–33.

6. PUGLIA: THE DEATH OF THE IMMORTALS

Abulafia, David. *The Great Sea: A Human History of the Mediterranean*. London: Penguin, 2014.

Angus, Julie. *Olive Odyssey: Searching for the Secrets of the Fruit That Seduced the World*. Vancouver: Greystone, 2014.

Besnard, G., et al. "The Complex History of the Olive Tree: From Late Quaternary Diversification of Mediterranean Lineages to Primary Domestication in the Northern Levant." *Proceedings of the Royal Society B: Biological Sciences* 280, no. 1756 (2013): 20122833.

Boscia, Donato, and Maria Saponari. "*Xylella fastidiosa*: Un batterio venuto da lontano." *Sapere*, Aug. 2021.

Braudel, Fernand. *The Mediterranean and the Mediterranean World in the Age of Philip II*. New York: Harper & Row, 1972.

Camarero, J. Julio, et al. "Demystifying the Age of Old Olive Trees." *Dendochronologia* 65 (Feb. 2021).

Cognoli, Simona, and Luciana Squadrilli. *Olio: Lo straordinario mondo dell'olio extravergine d'oliva*. Milan: Edizioni LSWR, 2017.

Daley, Jason. "This 4,000-Year-Old Jar Contains Italy's Oldest Olive Oil." *Smithsonian*, June 4, 2018.

DeAndreis, Paolo. "Authorities in Italy Envision a Post-*Xylella* Puglia." *Olive Oil Times*, Apr. 28, 2022.

DeAndreis, Paolo. "New Research Reveals Key Role of Olive Oil in Ancient Roman Diets." *Olive Oil Times*, Sept. 16, 2021.

Diéz, Concepción M., et al. "Centennial Olive Trees as a Reservoir of Genetic Diversity." *Annals of Botany* 108, no. 5 (Oct. 2011): 797–807.

Fanelli, Valentina, et al. "Current Status of Biodiversity Assessment and Conservation of Wild Olive." *Plants* 11 (Feb. 2022): 480.

Martella, Stefano. *La morte dei Giganti: Il batterio Xylella e la strage degli ulivi millenari*. Milan: Meltemi Press, 2022.

Mensing, Scott A., et al. "2700 Years of Mediterranean Environmental Change in Central Italy: A Synthesis of Sedimentary and Cultural Records to Interpret Past Impacts of Climate on Society." *Quaternary Science Reviews* 116 (May 2015): 72–94.

Mueller, Tom. *Extra Virginity: The Sublime and Scandalous World of Olive Oil*. New York: W. W. Norton, 2012.

Pavan, Stefano, et al. "Screening of Olive Biodiversity Defines Genotypes Potentially Resistant to *Xylella fastidiosa*." *Frontiers in Plant Science* 12 (Aug. 2021): 723879.

Pecci, Alessandra, and Francesco D'Andria. "Oil Production in Roman Times: Residue Analysis of the Floors of an Installation in Lecce." *Journal of Archaeological Science* 46 (June 2014): 363–71.

Petroni, Agostino. "The Farmer Trying to Save Italy's Ancient Olive Trees." *Atlas Obscura*, Apr. 29, 2021.

Primavera, M., et al. "Environment, Crops and Harvesting Strategies During the II Millennium B.C.: Resilience and Adaptation in Socio-Economic Systems of Bronze Age Communities in Apulia." *Quaternary International* 436 (2017): 83–95.

Rosenblum, Mort. *Olives: The Life and Lore of a Noble Fruit*. New York: North Point, 1998.

Sacchi, Raffaelo. "Oldest Known Bottle of Olive Oil on Display in Naples Museum." *Olive Oil Times*, Oct. 22, 2018.

Saponari, M., et al. *"Xylella fastidiosa* in Olive in Apulia: Where We Stand." *Phytopathology* 109, no. 2 (Feb. 2019): 175–86.

Scortichini, Marco. "The Multi-Millennial Olive Agroecosystem of Salento (Apulia, Italy) Threatened by *Xylella fastidiosa* subsp. *pauca*: A Working Possibility of Restoration." *Sustainability* 12, no. 17 (Aug. 2020): 6700.

Shepherd, Gordon M. *Neurogastronomy: How the Brain Creates Flavor and Why It Matters.* New York: Columbia University Press, 2012.

Sicard, Anne, et al. "Introduction and Adaptation of an Emerging Pathogen to Olive Trees in Italy." *Microbial Genomics* 7, no. 12 (Dec. 2021): 000735.

Trouet, Valerie. *Tree Story: The History of the World Written in Rings.* Baltimore: Johns Hopkins University Press, 2020.

Tyree, E. Loeta, and Evangelia Stefanoudaki. "The Olive Pit and Roman Oil Making." *The Biblical Archaeologist* 59, no. 3 (Sept. 1996): 171–78.

7. CAPPADOCIA: LOST AND FOUND

Amigues, Suzanne. "Le silphium: État de la question." *Journal des savants* 2, no. 1 (2004): 191–226.

Andrews, Alfred C. "The Silphium of the Ancients: A Lesson in Crop Control." *Isis* 33, no. 2 (June 1941): 232–36.

Asciutti, Valentina. "The Silphium Plant: Analysis of Ancient Sources." Master's thesis, Durham University, Sept. 30, 2004.

Briggs, Lisa, and Jens Jakobsson. "Searching for Silphium: An Updated Review." *Heritage* 5, no. 2 (Apr. 2022): 936–55.

Chamoux, François. "Le problème du silphion." *Bulletin de la Société nationale des Antiquaries de France* (1985): 54–59.

Connor, Steve. "Jason and the Argot: Land Where Greek's Ancient Language Survives." *Independent*, Jan. 3, 2011.

Gemmill, Chalmers L. "Silphium." *Bulletin of the History of Medicine* 40, no. 4 (July–Aug. 1966): 295–313.

Grainger, Sally. *Cooking Apicius: Roman Recipes for Today.* Totnes, UK: Prospect Books, 2006.

Grigoriadis, Ioannis N. "Between Citizenship and the Millet: The Greek Minority in Republican Turkey." *Middle Eastern Studies* 57, no. 5 (Apr. 2021): 741–57.

Keller, Vera. "Nero and the Last Stalk of Silphion: Collecting Extinct Nature in Early Modern Europe." *Early Science and Medicine* 19, no. 5 (Nov. 2014): 424–47.

Kiehn, Monika. "Silphion Revisited." *Medicinal Plant Conservation* 13 (2007): 4–8.

Koerper, Henry, and A. L. Kolls. "The Silphium Motif Adorning Ancient Libyan Coinage: Marketing a Medicinal Plant." *Economic Botany* 53, no. 2 (Apr.–June 1999): 133–43.

Kolbert, Elizabeth. *The Sixth Extinction: An Unnatural History.* London: Bloomsbury, 2014.

Miski, Mahmut. "Next Chapter in the Legend of Silphion: Preliminary Morphological, Chemical, Biological and Pharmacological Evaluations, Initial Conservation Studies, and Reassessment of the Regional Extinction Event." *Plants* 10, no. 1 (Jan. 2021): 102.

O'Connell, John. *The Book of Spice: From Anise to Zedoary.* New York: Pegasus, 2016.

Parejko, Ken. "Pliny the Elder's Silphium: First Recorded Species Extinction."
    Conservation Biology 16, no. 3 (June 2003): 925–27.

Pollaro, Paul, and Paul Robertson. "Reassessing the Role of Anthropogenic Climate
    Change in the Extinction of Silphium." *Frontiers in Conservation Science* 2
    (Jan. 2022): 785962.

Riddle, John M. *Eve's Herbs: A History of Contraception and Abortion in the West.*
    Cambridge, MA: Harvard University Press, 1997.

Roques, Denis. "Synésios de Cyrène et le silphion de Cyrénaïque." *Revue des études
    grecques* 97, no. 460–461 (Jan.–June 1984): 218–31.

Totelin, Laurence. "When Foods Became Remedies in Ancient Greece: The Curious
    Case of Garlic and Other Substances." *Journal of Ethnopharmacology* 167
    (June 2015): 30–37.

Turner, Jack. *Spice: The History of a Temptation.* London: Harper, 2005.

Wright, Paul. *Snakes, Sands and Silphium: Travels in Classical Libya.* London: Society
    for Libyan Studies, 2011.

8. SAINT-JEAN-SUR-RICHELIEU: BREAD ALONE

Aranguren, Biancamaria, et al. "Grinding Flour in Upper Palaeolithic Europe
    (25 000 Years bp)." *Antiquity* 81, no. 314 (Dec. 2007): 845–55.

Arranz-Otaguei, Amaia, et al. "Archaeobotanical Evidence Reveals the Origins of Bread
    14,400 Years Ago in Northeastern Jordan." *Proceedings of the National Academy of
    Sciences* 115, no. 31 (July 2018): 7925–30.

Bats, Adeline. "The Production of Bread in Conical Moulds at the Beginning of
    the Egyptian Middle Kingdom." *Journal of Archaeological Science: Reports* 34
    (Dec. 2020): 102631.

Bobrow-Strain, Aaron. *White Bread: A Social History of the Store-Bought Loaf.* Boston:
    Beacon Press, 2012.

Bottéro, Jean. *La plus vieille cuisine du monde.* Paris: Éditions Louis Audibert, 2002.

Boulos, Loutfy, et al. "Grasses in Ancient Egypt." *Kew Bulletin* 62, no. 3 (Jan. 2007): 507–11.

Carrington, Damian. "Glyphosate Weedkiller Damages Wild Bee Colonies, Study
    Reveals." *Guardian*, June 2, 2022.

Harlan, Jack R. *The Living Fields: Our Agricultural Heritage.* Cambridge: Cambridge
    University Press, 1998.

Heiss, Andreas G. "State of the (T)art: Analytical Approaches in the Investigation
    of Components and Production Traits of Archaeological Bread-Like Objects,
    Applied to Two Finds From the Neolithic Lakeshore Settlement Parkhaus Opéra."
    PLOS One 12, no. 8 (Aug. 2017): e0182401.

Jacob, H. E. *Six Thousand Years of Bread: Its Holy and Unholy History.* New York: Skyhorse,
    2007 [1944].

Labignette, Jean-Eric. "La farine dans la Nouvelle-France." *Revue d'histoire de l'Amérique
    française* 17, no. 4 (Mar. 1964): 490–503.

Mann, Charles C. *The Wizard and the Prophet: Two Remarkable Scientists and Their Dueling
    Visions to Shape Tomorrow's World.* New York: Vintage, 2018.

Nelson, Scott Reynolds. *Oceans of Grain: How American Wheat Remade the World*. New York: Basic Books, 2022.

Pollan, Michael. *Cooked: A Natural History of Transformation*. London: Penguin, 2013.

Ramirez-Villegas, Julian, et al. "State of Ex Situ Conservation of Landrace Groups of 25 Major Crops." *Nature Plants* 8, no. 5 (May 2022): 491–99.

Revedin, Anna, et al. "Thirty Thousand-Year-Old Evidence of Plant Processing." *PNAS* 107, no. 44 (Nov. 2010): 18815–19.

Richter, Tobias, and Amaia Arranz-Otaegui. "Following a New Trail of Crumbs to Agriculture's Origins." *Sapiens*, July 16, 2018.

Rubel, William. *Bread: A Global History*. London: Reaktion, 2011.

Samuel, Delwen. "Bread in Archaeology." *Pains, fours et foyers des temps passés* 49, no. 1–2 (2002): 27–36.

Samuel, Delwen. "Brewing and Baking." In *Ancient Egyptian Materials and Technology*, edited by P. T. Nicholson, 537–76. Cambridge: Cambridge University Press, 2000.

Scott, James C. *Against the Grain: A Deep History of the Earliest States*. New Haven: Yale University Press, 2017.

Wilkinson, Toby. *The Rise and Fall of Ancient Egypt*. New York: Random House, 2010.

Wood, Ed, and Jean Wood. *Classic Sourdoughs: A Home Baker's Manual*. Berkeley: Ten Speed, 2001.

Yafa, Stephen. *Grain of Truth: Why Eating Wheat Can Improve Your Health*. New York: Penguin, 2015.

Zabinski, Catherine. *Amber Waves: The Extraordinary Biography of Wheat, From Wild Grass to World Megacrop*. Chicago: University of Chicago Press, 2020.

Zaharieva, Maria, et al. "Cultivated Emmer Wheat (*Triticum dicoccon* Schrank), an Old Crop With a Promising Future." *Genetic Resource Crop Evolution* 57 (June 2010): 937–62.

9. MI'WER'LA: THE COOKED AND THE RAW

Arnett, Chris. *The Terror of the Coast: Land Alienation and Colonial War on Vancouver Island and the Gulf Islands, 1849–1863*. Victoria: Talonbooks, 1999.

Baker, Shanna. "Coastal Oakscapes." *Hakai*, Apr. 24, 2018.

Beckwith, Brenda Raye. "'The Queen Root of This Clime': Ethnoecological Investigations of Blue Camas." Doctoral thesis, University of Victoria, 2004.

Berglund, Berndt, and Clare E. Bolsby. *The Edible Wild: A Complete Cookbook and Guide to Edible Wild Plants in Canada and Eastern North America*. Toronto: Pagurian, 1978.

Carney, Molly, et al. "Harvesting Strategies as Evidence for 4000 Years of Camas (*Camassia quamash*) Management in the North American Columbia Plateau." *R. Soc. Open Sci.* 8, no. 4 (Apr. 2021): 202213.

Crosby, Alfred W. *Ecological Imperialism: The Biological Expansion of Europe, 900–1900*. Cambridge: Cambridge University Press, 2015.

Earle, Rebecca. *Feeding the People: The Politics of the Potato*. Cambridge: Cambridge University Press, 2020.

Genest, Miche. "Eulachon, Oolichan, Hooligan: A Fish by Any Other Name Is Just as Oily." *Yukon News*, May 24, 2017.

Gill, Ian. "Of Roe, Rights, and Reconciliation." *Hakai*, Aug. 27, 2018.

Glavin, Terry. *The Last Great Sea: A Voyage Through the Human and Natural History of the North Pacific Ocean.* Vancouver: Greystone, 2000.

Graeber, David, and David Wengrow. *The Dawn of Everything: A New History of Humanity.* New York: Farrar, Straus and Giroux, 2021.

Gritzner, Janet H. "Native-American Camas Production and Trade in the Pacific Northwest and Northern Rocky Mountains." *Journal of Cultural Geography* 14, no. 2 (1994): 33–50.

Joseph, Bob. *21 Things You May Not Know About the Indian Act: Helping Canadians Make Reconciliation With Indigenous Peoples a Reality.* Port Coquitlam, BC: Indigenous Relations Press, 2018.

Kimmerer, Robin Wall. *Braiding Sweetgrass: Indigenous Wisdom, Scientific Knowledge, and the Teachings of Plants.* Minneapolis: Milkweed, 2014.

King, Thomas. *The Inconvenient Indian: A Curious Account of Native People in North America.* Toronto: Doubleday, 2012.

Kirkup, Kristy. "Canada's Indigenous Population Growing 4 Times Faster Than the Rest of the Country." Canadian Press, Oct. 25, 2017.

Labbé, Stefan. "Cultural Burning: Could More Fires Be the Solution to B.C.'s Wildfire Problem?" *Times-Colonist*, Aug. 8, 2021.

Mann, Charles C. *1491: New Revelations of the Americas Before Columbus.* New York: Knopf, 2012.

Ostrander, Madeline. "The Local-Carb Diet." *Hakai*, Apr. 17, 2018.

Payton, Brian. "The Ingenious Ancient Technology Concealed in the Shallows." *Hakai*, Aug. 3, 2021.

Penn, Briony. "Restoring Camas and Culture to Lekwungen and Victoria: An Interview With Lekwungen Cheryl Bryce." *Focus*, June 2006.

Pringle, Heather. "In the Land of Lost Gardens." *Hakai*, June 6, 2017.

Pynn, Larry. "Clam Digging Through 3,500 Years of Indigenous History." *Hakai*, Feb. 27, 2019.

Raff, Jennifer. *Origin: A Genetic History of the Americas.* New York: Hachette, 2022.

Sioui, Georges E. *For an Amerindian Autohistory: An Essay on the Foundations of a Social Ethic.* Montreal: McGill-Queen's, 1992.

Steeves, Paulette. *The Indigenous Paleolithic of the Western Hemisphere.* Lincoln: University of Nebraska Press, 2021.

TallBear, Kimberly. *Native American DNA: Tribal Belonging and the False Promise of Genetic Science.* Minneapolis: University of Minnesota Press, 2013.

Turner, Nancy J. "'That Was Our Candy!' Sweet Foods in Indigenous Peoples' Traditional Diets in Northwestern North America." *Journal of Ethnobotany* 40, no. 3 (Sept. 2020): 305–28.

Turner, Nancy J., and Harriet V. Kuhnlein. "Camas (*Camassia* spp.) and Riceroot (*Fritillaria* spp.): Two Liliaceous 'Root' Foods of the Northwest Coast Indians." *Ecology of Food and Nutrition* 13, no. 4 (1983): 199–219.

Turner, Nancy J., Kim Recalma-Clutesi, and Douglas Deur. "Back to the Clam Gardens." *Ecotrust Magazine* (2013).

Turner, Nancy J., and Katherine L. Turner. "'Where Our Women Used to Get the Food': Cumulative Effects and Loss of Ethnobotanical Knowledge and Practice; Case Study From Coastal British Columbia." *Botany* 86, no. 2 (Feb. 2008): 103–15.

Wild, Sarah. "Scientists Find First Evidence of Humans Cooking Starches." *Sapiens*, June 21, 2019.

Will, Joanne. "Hunting the Elusive Wapato." *Tyee*, Jan. 14, 2010.

Zuckerman, Larry. *The Potato: How the Humble Spud Rescued the Western World*. Boston: Faber & Faber, 1998.

EPILOGUE

Belasco, Warren James. *Meals to Come: A History of the Future of Food*. Berkeley: University of California Press, 2006.

Berry, Wendell. "The Pleasures of Eating." In *The Art of the Commonplace: The Agrarian Essays of Wendell Berry*, edited by Norman Wirzba. Washington, DC: Counterpoint, 2002.

Dunn, Robb. *Never Out of Season: How Having the Food We Want When We Want It Threatens Our Food Supply and Our Future*. New York: Little, Brown and Co., 2017.

Gérard, Mathilde. "Pourquoi notre système alimentaire est intenable." *Le Monde*, June 2, 2022.

Gillam, Carey. "'Disturbing': Weedkiller Ingredient Tied to Cancer Found in 80% of US Urine Samples." *Guardian*, July 9, 2022.

Holzer, Sepp. *Sepp Holzer's Permaculture: A Practical Guide to Small-Scale, Integrative Farming and Gardening*. White River Junction, VT: Chelsea Green Publishing, 2010.

Le Page, Michael. "Tackling the Global Food Crisis." *New Scientist*, May 28, 2022.

Little, Amanda. *The Fate of Food: What We'll Eat in a Bigger, Hotter, Smarter World*. London: Oneworld, 2019.

Monbiot, George. "Lab-Grown Food Will Soon Destroy Farming—and Save the Planet." *Guardian*, Jan. 8, 2020.

Montgomery, David. *Dirt: The Erosion of Civilizations*. Berkeley: University of California Press, 2007.

Mosby, Ian, Sarah Rotz, and Evan D. G. Fraser. *Uncertain Harvest: The Future of Food on a Warming Planet*. Regina: University of Regina Press, 2020.

Rutherford, Adam. *A Brief History of Everyone Who Ever Lived: The Human Story Retold Through Our Genes*. New York: The Experiment, 2017.

Smil, Vaclav. *Growth: From Microorganisms to Megacities*. Cambridge, MA: MIT Press, 2022.

Further Reading

Bourne, Joel K. *The End of Plenty: The Race to Feed a Crowded Planet.* New York: W. W. Norton, 2015.

Brillat-Savarin, Jean Anthelme. *Physiologie du goût.* Paris: Flammarion, 2017.

Buchanan, David. *Taste, Memory: Forgotten Foods, Lost Flavors, and Why They Matter.* White River Junction, VT: Chelsea Green Publishing, 2012.

Cutright, Robyn. *The Story of Food in the Human Past: How What We Ate Made Us Who We Are.* Tuscaloosa: University of Alabama Press, 2021.

Freedman, Paul, ed. *Food: The History of Taste.* Berkeley: University of California Press, 2002.

Genoways, Ted. *This Blessed Earth: A Year in the Life of an American Farm.* New York: W. W. Norton, 2018.

Mann, Charles. *1493: Uncovering the New World Columbus Created.* New York: Vintage, 2011.

McGee, Harold. *Nose Dive: A Field Guide to the World's Smells.* New York: Penguin Random House, 2020.

McGee, Harold. *On Food and Cooking: The Science and Lore of the Kitchen.* New York: Scribner, 2004.

McGovern, Patrick E. *Ancient Brews: Rediscovered and Re-Created.* New York: W. W. Norton, 2017.

Morizot, Baptiste. *Ways of Being Alive.* Medford, OR: Polity, 2022.

Mouritsen, Ole G., and Klavs Styrbaek. *Mouthfeel: How Texture Makes Taste.* New York: Columbia University Press, 2018.

Newman, Lenore. *Lost Feast: Culinary Extinction and the Future of Food.* Toronto: ECW Press, 2019.

Parcak, Sarah. *Archaeology From Space: How the Future Shapes Our Past.* New York: Henry Holt, 2019.

Simmonds, Peter Lund. *The Curiosities of Food.* Berkeley: Ten Speed Press, 2001 [1859].

Slingerland, Edward. *Drunk: How We Sipped, Danced, and Stumbled Our Way to Civilization.* New York: Little, Brown Spark, 2021.

Tannahill, Reay. *Food in History.* London: Penguin, 1988.

Tattersall, Ian. *Masters of the Planet: The Search for Our Human Origins.* New York: St. Martin's Press, 2012.

Index

A

acociles (tiny river shrimp), 45
Addison, Corban: *Wastelands*, 83
African Americans, 57–58, 63, 70–71.
  See also Gullah/Geechee Nation
agave, 46
agriculture: animal husbandry, 85–86;
  Biblical and other origin stories, 217–
  18; blamed for ills of civilization, 5,
  6, 8, 215–17; at Çatalhöyük, 3, 4; chinampas (floating gardens) of Mexico
  City, 38, 39–41, 277; colonialism and,
  259, 259n; controlled burns, 76, 260,
  278; in Egypt, 218; environmental
  degradation from, 86, 230–32, 295–
  96; farmers in crisis, 149; fertilizer,
  86, 227, 230–31; genetically modified
  and transgenic foods, 12, 20, 239,
  284–85; green revolution, 230–32, 284,
  286; hybridization, 227–28, 228n, 230;
  milpa system ("Three Sisters" farming),
  36–37, 277; Monbiot against, 6, 129,
  134, 142, 143, 285; by Northwest
  Coast Peoples, 250, 273; plowing,
  197–98; population growth and, 8;
  restoration vs. rewilding, 142–43;
  Spanish conquistadors and, 29;
  sustainable approaches to, 5–6, 285–
  87, 294, 296; techno-optimists on,
  284–85; *terra preta*, 277–78; transition to, 220–21; Turkish crisis, 6–9;
  warnings against industrialization,
  18–19. *See also* cattle; cheese; grain;
  industrial agriculture; pork
agrobiodiversity, 9. *See also* species
  extinction

ahuautle, 25, 32–33, 42–46, 50, 51–52, 53
alcohol. *See* beer
Alexander the Great, 204
alpha-linolenic acid, 27. *See also* linolenic
  acid
Alpini, Prospero, 184
amaranth, 42
Amigues, Suzanne, 184
Amri, Ahmed, 233–34
Anaheim disease, 158. See also *Xylella
  fastidiosa*
anchovies, 90–91, 108, 116, 117. See also *garum*
andaliman, 186
animal husbandry, 85–86. *See also* cattle;
  sheep
antioxidants, 12, 173. *See also*
  polyphenols
ants, 27, 32, 33, 45, 48–49
Apicius (De re coquinaria), 112–14, 202–3,
  206–7
apples, 163, 285
Ark of Taste (Slow Food), 19n
Arnett, Chris, 258–59
Arranz-Otaegui, Amaia, 214–15
asafoetida (Parthian laser, hing), 203–4, 204
Ata, Mehmet, 190–91, 192, 205
Australian finger lime (*Citrus australasica*), 180
Australopithecus, 10
autolysis, 100, 116
axayacatl (water boatman), 25, 31, 32,
  42–43, 43n, 51–52. See also *ahuautle*
axolotl, 40, 41–42
Ayllón, Lucas Vázquez de, 77
Aztecs, 28–31, 34, 35–36, 37–39, 40, 42,
  46, 52–53

B

Babylonians, 5, 217
backslopping, 214
Baelo Claudia, 102–3, 105, 106–7
Bali, 14
bannock, 263n
barbecue, 69–71, 84
Bardines, Hilda, 45–46
barley, 5, 37, 124, 193, 197, 218
BASF, 10
Battiad dynasty, 193
Bayer, 10
Beauchemin, Robert, 238–39, 240, 241
Beckwith, Brenda, 259–61
beer, 213n
bees, 15, 27, 33, 239
beetle grubs, 27
Béjar, Manuel, 97–98, 99
Belasco, Warren, 283
bentwood boxes, 272
Bernal-Casasola, Darío, 108–9
Berry, Wendell, 18, 88, 294–95
Bible, 217–18
Blackley, Seamus, 221–24
black soldier fly, 286
blue camas. See camas
bluefin tuna, 106–7, 108, 111n
bonito flakes, 91
Borlaug, Norman, 229–30, 231, 232
Boscia, Donato, 157, 158–59, 160–61, 163, 176, 179
bracken, 143
Braudel, Fernand, 152
bread: author's home baking, 212, 235–37, 288–92; beer and, 213n; Blackley's reconstruction of ancient breads, 221–24; at Çatalhöyük, 5, 15, 215; commercial yeast and, 132, 236; in Egypt, 213–14, 219; entanglement with, 292; industrialized, 237–38, 242; in Mesopotamia, 218–19; nutritional value, 224, 237; origins of, 213–15; Paleolithic people and, 214–15; regime collapse from lack of, 226–27; sourdough, 132, 212, 235–36, 238; in Turkey, 12–13; white vs. whole wheat flour, 236–37. See also flour; grain; wheat
Brisbin, Lehr, 78–79, 86
Britain. See United Kingdom
British Columbia (Illahee Chuk), 244–46, 257–60, 277. See also Northwest Coast Peoples
Brock, Sean, 62
Buendía, Rosario, 50–51
Buendía Peralta, Samuel, 50–51
burns, controlled, 76, 260, 278

C

Cádiz, 93–94, 95–96, 96–98, 100–102
Cajun cooking, 92
Calvert, T. C. "Kit," 148
camas (*Camassia leichtlinii*): cooking, 250, 256, 263, 273–74, 279; cultivation, 250, 260–61; vs. death camas, 268; harvesting, 267–68, 269; importance for Northwest Coast Peoples, 256; loss to colonialism, 250–51, 259–60, 262, 272; nutritional value, 264; survival of, 265
Canada, 228, 245, 245n
Canadian prairies, 225–26, 240, 295
Canadienne cattle, 210
Cane Creek Farm, 85–87
canola oil, 172–73
Carthage, 95, 95n, 96, 164, 193
Carver, Mathew: Pick & Cheese (London), 119–21, 122
casein, 126
Çatalhöyük: about, 1–2, 8; agricultural and egalitarian lifestyle, 3–4, 14, 215, 220, 273; artifacts from, 13–14; bread and bread-making, 4–5, 15, 215, 288, 289, 290, 291, 292; diet, 11; entanglement and, 292; lactase persistence and, 124
Cato the Elder: *On Agriculture*, 170
cattle: Canadienne, 210; environmental value of, 142, 143; Galloway, 140; Holstein-Friesian, 10, 138–39, 138, 140, 143; Northern Dairy Shorthorn, 140–41, 143–44, 148, 294; Red Devon, 85; transhumance, 293

caviar lime (*Citrus australasica*), 180
cereals, 224–25. *See also* grain
Champlain, Samuel de, 202
champoloco (maguey worm), 46–47
Chang, Joseph, 287–88
Chapman, Edward, 147
chapulines (cornfield grasshoppers), 21, 22, 35
Cheddar cheese, 131, 132, 133, 148
cheese: associations and symbolism, 121, 128–29; author's homemade cheeses, 210; Britain and, 121, 127–28, 129, 130–31, 132, 133; cheese-making process, 144–45; diversity of, 120; farmhouse cheese, 123, 127, 133–34, 148–50; France and, 128, 132–33; Fromagerie du Pied-De-Vent, 210; history of, 125–26, 127–28; industrialized, 128, 130–33, 147–48; lactose and, 124, 124n; lysine and, 224n; at Mathew Carver's Pick & Cheese, 119–21, 122; nutritional value, 126–27; Romans and, 127; Wensleydale, 121–23, 136, 141, 144–45, 145–46, 147–48. *See also* milk
chicatanas (flying ants), 32, 33, 45
chicken, 67–68
chimpanzees, 10, 11, 26–27
China, 68, 80–81, 83–84, 124
chinampas (floating gardens), 38, 39–41, 277
chocolate lily (northern riceroot), 266
Chorleywood bread process, 238
chumaki, 225
Churchill, Winston, 284, 285
Cistercians, 116, 135–36
clams, 254, 258, 267, 273
Claxton, Earl, Jr., 262–63, 264–65, 268
Cleese, John, 121, 130n
climate change, 125, 196–97
cloves, 201, 202
Club of Rome: *Limits to Growth*, 18
Coast Salish, 244, 247, 250, 252, 256, 259, 263–64, 268, 273. *See also* Northwest Coast Peoples
cocopaches, 32, 48

colatura di alici, 116
cold stratification, 190
colonialism, 29, 247, 251, 258–60, 259, 264–65
Columbus, Christopher, 70, 76, 202
Columella, 98, 156, 170
confined animal feeding operations (CAFOS), 82–85, 87
Cook, James, 251
cooking, 10–11
Cordon Bleu, 92, 113
corn, 8, 10, 12, 36, 36n, 37, 239, 295
corn oil, 172–73
Cortés, Hernán, 28–29, 30–31
Corteva, 10
cottonseed oil, 172–73
Cowichan People (Quw'utsun), 248–51. *See also* Northwest Coast Peoples
cows. *See* cattle
Crews, Harry, 65, 66, 84
crickets, 20, 102, 280–82
CRISPR, 284
cypress, Saharan, 196
Cyr, Marc-André, 289, 290
Cyrenaica, 192–93, 196–97

D

Daps (Charleston restaurant), 80
Davidson, James, 93n
death camas (*Toxicoscordion venenosum*), 268
dehesa, 29, 75–76, 77
Deihl, Craig, 62
deliciousness, 14–15, 149–50, 283
De re coquinaria (Apicius), 112–14, 202–3, 206–7
devil's club (*Oplopanax horridus*), 262
Diamond, Jared, 6, 216
Dick, Adam (Kwaxsistalla), 275, 276
Dioscorides, 195
disease, 34, 217, 217n, 252
diversity, 9–10, 11–12, 15–16, 232–34, 273, 295
dogs, 74n, 216
Do-Maker process, 238
Douglas, David, 256
Douglas, James, 258, 260

Douglas Treaties, 258, 267
Dow, 10
DuBose, Elizabeth, 60
Dunn, Rob, 14–15
DuPont, 10, 132
Durrell, Lawrence, 151

E

eelgrass, 273
Egyptians, ancient, 5, 213–14, 218, 219,
    223–24
Ehrlich, Paul R.: *The Population Bomb*,
    23–24, 25, 53
einkorn, 7, 219–20, 222–23, 292
El Cardenal (Mexico City restaurant),
    46–47
El Faro (Cádiz restaurant), 100–102
emmer: author's experience baking
    with, 215, 221, 288–92; bread from,
    13, 223; bread wheat hybridized from,
    232; contemporary cultivation, 7, 9,
    234; domestication, 5, 219–20
entanglement, 292–93
Entocycle, 286
Entomo Farms, 280–82
entomophagy. *See* insects, eating
environment: cattle and, 142, 143; degra-
    dation from industrial agriculture,
    86, 221, 230–32, 295–96; plowing and,
    197–98; sheep and, 139–40
epazote, 47
Ercan, Fisun, 290–92
escamoles, 47–48, 49
ethical eating: farmhouse cheese, 123,
    133–34; meat, 84, 88; spices, 186–87, 208
extinction, species, 9, 76, 182–83, 197

F

farming. *See* agriculture
fat, 27, 172
Felice, Emile de, 79
fenugreek, blue, 186
fertilizer, 86, 227, 230–31
Ferula drudeana, 188–92, 194, 197, 198–
    200, 204–5, 205–8. *See also* silphion
FIG (Charleston restaurant), 79–80

fire: controlled burns, 76, 260, 278;
    cooking and, 15
fish. *See* anchovies; bluefin tuna;
    sardines
fish sauce, 114–15, 116–18. See also *garum*
flour: from La Milanaise, 238–39,
    240–41; milling, 216, 241–42, 290;
    nutritional content, 242–43; white vs.
    whole wheat, 236–37. *See also* bread;
    grain; wheat
fly, black soldier, 286
food: approach to, 6, 14, 19, 294–95;
    author's culinary efforts, 17–18,
    19–20, 210–11, 212; cooking, 10–11;
    deliciousness and, 14–15, 149–50,
    283; diversity and, 9–10, 11–12, 15–16,
    232–34, 273, 295; entanglement with,
    292–93; genetics and ancestral food-
    ways, 211–12; global standard diet, 12;
    health impacts, 172; Mediterranean
    diet, 171–72; organic, 285; Paleo diet,
    14, 28, 211. *See also* agriculture
Food and Agriculture Organization, 88,
    286
foraging, 266
Fox, Robin Lane, 104
France, 128, 132–33, 226–27
Fromagerie du Pied-De-Vent, 210
Fuller, Dorian, 218–19
Future Consumer Lab, 49

G

Galloway cattle, 140
Gargilius Martialis, 99
Garry oak, 260, 261, 262
garum: alternative fish sauces to, 115–18;
    archaeological finds, 97–98, 99, 105–6;
    attempts to recreate *haimation*, 107–8,
    111n; author's homemade attempts, 111–
    12, 118; author's use in home cooking,
    109–10, 114; contemporary disgust with,
    92; deliciousness of, 98–99, 101–2; from
    fermented crickets, 102; Garum Lusita-
    no's recreation, 111, 111n; history of, 96,
    107, 110–11; as *kakushi-aji* (hidden taste),
    92–93, 114; *liquamen* recreated in Cádiz,

99–100, 108–9, 111; nutritional value, 114–15; Romans and, 92–93, 96, 104–7, 110, 113, 114, 115

Garum Lusitano, 111, 111n

General Mills, 239, 242

genes: ancestral foodways and, 211–12; gene banks, 176–77, 232–35; gene editing, 284; genetically modified and transgenic foods, 12, 20, 239, 284–85

Genesis Project, 56

Genoways, Ted, 82

Geoponica (Byzantine-Greek agricultural manual), 107–8

Georgia, barrier islands, 56, 58–59. *See also* Ossabaw feral hogs; Ossabaw Island

Ghazanfar, Shahina, 199

global standard diet, 12

Gloucester cheese, 121, 129

glutamic acid, 91, 100

gluten and gluten intolerance, 223, 228, 232, 236, 238, 238n, 284

glyphosate, 239–40, 295

goat grass, 232

Göbekli Tepe, 3, 213n

Goldin, Darren, 280–82

González Carretero, Lara, 215, 288, 290, 291

Graeber, David, 4, 218, 221, 253

grafting, 164

grain, 5, 215–18, 220–21, 224–25. *See also* barley; bread; einkorn; emmer; flour; khorasan (Kamut); rice; wheat

Grainger, Sally, 110–12, 111n, 113, 114, 116, 117–18, 203, 206–7

grains of paradise, 185, 187, 202

grapes, 152, 158

grasshoppers, 21, 33, 35

Great Britain. *See* United Kingdom

Great Rift Valley, 11, 27–28

Greeks, ancient, 8, 103, 110, 183, 217–18

Green, Bill, 64–65, 66

Greenberg, Paul, 173

green revolution, 230–32, 284, 286

Grillo, Beppe, 160

Gullah/Geechee Nation, 63–65, 66

Gunn, Robin, 56, 57, 58

H

Haber-Bosch process, 227, 231

Hansen, Christian, 131

Harari, Yuval Noah: *Sapiens*, 6

Harlan, Jack, 214, 229

Hattan, Andrew, 137–41, 142–45, 146, 148

Heiltsuk Nation, 252, 255. *See also* Northwest Coast Peoples

Helicobacter pylori, 132

Heliogabalus (Roman emperor), 92

herbs, 201

Herculaneum, 165

herring, 90–91, 106, 249, 253, 255

hing (asafoetida, Parthian laser), 203–4, 204n

Hippocrates, 189

Hobbes, Thomas, 4

Hodder, Ian, 14, 292

Hodgson, Randolph, 130

hogs. *See* Ossabaw feral hogs; pork

Holstein-Friesian cattle, 10, 138–39, 138n, 140, 143

Holzer, Sepp, 294

Homo antecessor, 74

Homo erectus, 10

Homo sapiens, 2–3, 10n

Horace, 104

Howard, Albert: *An Agricultural Testament*, 86

Hudson, Henry, 202

humans: agriculture blamed for ills of civilization, 5, 6, 8, 215–17; common ancestors of all, 287–88; extinctions caused by, 9, 76, 182–83, 197; genetics and ancestral foodways, 211–12; historic food diversity, 10–12; longevity, 171–72, 171n; origins of, 10n; population growth and overpopulation fears, 8, 18, 23–24, 220, 221, 231, 283; protein requirements, 88; seeing through our ancestors' eyes, 209–10

hwunitum (hungry ones), 247

hybridization, 227–28, 228n, 230

I

immune system, 132, 174
India, 23, 24, 68, 201, 202, 230
Indian consumption plant (*Lomatium nudicaule*), 262
Indigenous Peoples, 34, 76, 204, 239, 266–67, 277–79. *See also* Aztecs; Northwest Coast Peoples
indigo, 57–58
industrial agriculture: Big Hog, 79, 81–85, 87–88; cheese, 128, 130–33, 147–48; environmental degradation from, 86, 221, 230–32, 295–96; fertilizer, 86, 227, 230–31; flour and bread, 237–38, 241–42; green revolution, 230–32, 284, 286; hybridization, 227–28, 228n, 230; olives, 174–75; warnings about, 18–19
insects, eating: advocacy for and awakening curiosity, 49–50; *ahuautle*, 25, 32–33, 42–46, 50, 51–52, 53; in animal feed, 286; arguments for and barriers against, 20–22, 54, 282–83; Aztecs and, 31, 42; *champoloco* (maguey worm), 46–47; *chapulines* (cornfield grasshoppers), 21, 22, 35; *chicatanas* (flying ants), 32, 33, 45; crickets at Entomo Farms, 280–82; cultivation advantages, 282; *escamoles*, 47–48, 49; global "apocalypse," 33; by hominin and primate ancestors, 26–28; irony of, 26; in Mexico, 25, 46–48; nutritional value, 27; sustainable harvesting, 48–49
Institute for Sustainable Plant Protection, 157
International Center for Agricultural Research in the Dry Areas (ICARDA), 233, 234
inulin, 264
invasive species, 41, 58–59, 61
Ireland, 210–11
ishiri, 117–18
Istanbul, 200, 204–5
Italy. *See* olives and olive oil

J

Jackson, Tank, 71–74, 77, 80, 86
jamón ibérico, 65–66, 68–69
Jervaulx Abbey, 134–36
Jiménez, Mario, 101–2
Joseph, Leigh (Styawat), 265–67
Julius Caesar, 183

K

kakushi-aji (hidden taste), 91–92
Kaminsky, Peter, 75–77
Kamut (khorasan), 222–23, 237, 237n
Kernza (perennial wheat), 284
khorasan (Kamut), 222–23, 237, 237n
killer whale (orca), 245
Kimmerer, Robin Wall: *Braiding Sweetgrass*, 266
Kimuraya bakery (Japan), 236
Kingcome Inlet (BC), 275
Korovin, Evgenii, 189
Kroeber, Alfred, 255
!Kung San People, 217
Kuper Island Industrial School, 261, 272
Kwakwaka'wakw People, 252, 271, 274, 275. *See also* Northwest Coast Peoples
Kwaxsistalla (Adam Dick), 275, 276

L

lactase and lactase persistence, 123–24, 125, 126
lactose, 123, 124, 124n
Lahey, Jim, 212
Lake Texcoco, 33, 34, 38, 40, 42, 46, 50, 51–52, 53
Lake Tuz, 7
La Milanaise, 238–39, 240–41
Lancashire cheese, 121, 136, 148
La Notte, Pierfederico, 161–62, 176
Lata, Mike, 79–80
Lazarus taxon, 183
Le, Stephen, 211
leaf-cutter ants, 32, 48–49
Leopold, Aldo, 18
Lesnik, Julie, 26–28
Lewis, Meriwether, 256

Libya, 183–84, 192–93, 195, 196–97
lime, caviar (*Citrus australasica*), 180
linolenic acid, 173. *See also* alpha-
    linolenic acid
Liometopum apiculatum, 48–49
liquamen, 99–100, 108–9, 111, 113, 114,
    117. See also *garum*
Little Ice Age, 278
longevity, 171–72, 171n
lovage, 113
Love, Serena, 222, 223
Low Riggs farm, 137–38, 139, 140–41,
    142–45
lysine, 224, 224n

M

MacLean, Eliza, 85–87
maguey worm (*champoloco*), 46–47
Maillard reaction, 47
Mann, Charles, 284
Manning, Richard: *Against the Grain*, 6
Manunta, Antonio, 184
margarine, 172
mariculture, 254–55
Martell, Charles, 129
Martelli, Giovanni, 158
Martin, Anthony, 60–61
Masseria Brancati, 165–71
McCormick & Company, 187
meat, 15, 84, 88, 224n. *See also* chicken;
    pork
medicinal plants, 189, 204
Mediterranean diet, 171–72
megafauna, 34, 76, 182
Melcarne, Giovanni, 176–77, 178–79
Mercado San Juan Pugibet (Mexico
    City), 31–33
Mesopotamia, 218–19, 220–21
Messapians, 166–67
metates, 288–90
Mexico: Aztec legacy, 52–53; corn, 12,
    36; fertility rate, 53; insect eating, 25,
    46–48; milpa system ("Three Sisters"
    farming), 36–37, 277
Mexico City (Valley of Mexico): *ahuautle*,
    25, 32–33, 42–46, 50, 51–52, 53;

Aztecs, 28–31, 34, 35–36, 37–39, 40,
    42, 46, 52–53; chinampas (floating
    gardens), 38, 39–41, 277; colonial
    impacts, 34, 40–41; history of, 33–34;
    Lake Texcoco, 33, 34, 38, 40, 42, 46,
    50, 51–52, 53; lessons from, 53–54;
    Mercado San Juan Pugibet, 31–33;
    population and size, 24–25, 53
microbiome, 132, 174, 212
milk, 9–10, 126–27, 138, 149, 284. *See also*
    cheese
Miller, Adrian, 70
milling, 164, 216, 241–43, 289–90
Milne, Sarah, 267–68
milpa system ("Three Sisters" farming),
    36–37, 277
mirin, 91
Misir Çarsisi (Spice Bazaar), 200
Miski, Mahmut, 188–92, 194, 197, 198–
    200, 204–5, 205–6, 207–8
monarch butterfly, 33
Monbiot, George, 6, 129, 134, 142, 143, 285
Monsanto, 10, 160
Monte Testaccio (Rome), 165
Montezuma, 30, 42, 43
Montgomery, David R., 8, 197–98,
    231–32
Montreal, 238
moth larvae, 27
Muckamuck (Vancouver restaurant), 246
Mueller, Tom, 164–65, 175
mustard seed, 291
myoglobin, 74

N

National Gene Bank of Plants of
    Ukraine, 234–35
Natufians, 214
Neal's Yard Dairy (London), 122–23,
    129–30, 141
Nelson, Scott Reynolds, 225, 226
Neolithic period, 67, 86, 125, 127, 221,
    225, 241, 290. *See also* Çatalhöyük
Nezahat Gökyiğit Botanical Gardens
    (Istanbul), 205
niacin, 36

Noma (Copenhagen restaurant), 102
North America (Turtle Island), 247. *See also* Northwest Coast Peoples
Northern Dairy Shorthorn cattle, 140–41, 143–44, 148, 294
northern riceroot (chocolate lily), 266
Northwest Coast Peoples: about, 252–54; agriculture and, 250, 273; colonialism against, 245, 251–52, 258–60; mariculture, 254–55; Muckamuck restaurant, 246; on orcas, 245; potatoes and, 250–51, 262, 263–64, 274; residential schools, 248–49, 257, 261, 270, 272–73; sustainable practices of, 270, 276–77; traditional foods and losses to colonialism, 248, 249–51, 255–56, 264–65, 266, 273, 274–76; treaties with, 245, 245n. *See also* camas
Nuu-chah-nulth People, 251, 252. *See also* Northwest Coast Peoples

O

oats, 225
Ogwilowgwa (Kim Recalma-Clutesi), 270–77
oils, cooking, 172–73
Olduvai Gorge, 27–28
oleic acid, 62
olives and olive oil: age of olive trees, 169–70, 169n; associations and symbolism, 151–52, 155; curing process, 163; health benefits and nutritional value, 171–72, 173–74; industrialized, 174–75; at Masseria Brancati, 165–71; in Mexico City, 51; olive quick decline syndrome (*Xylella fastidiosa*), 156–57, 157–63, 170–71, 175–76; origins and domestication, 163–64, 180–81; at Petruzzi farm, 179–80; at Piana degli Ulivi Monumentali (Puglia), 152–57; resistance against *Xylella fastidiosa*, 176–79, 179–80; Romans and, 164–65, 167–68; in Spain, 156; tasting process, 168
omega-3 fatty acids, 10, 12, 91, 115, 127, 173

omega-6 fatty acids, 173
oolichans, 253, 255, 273, 274–75
opsophagos, 93, 93n
orca (killer whale), 245
Orchis mascula, 186
organic food, 285
Orwell, George, 122
Ossabaw feral hogs: attempts to control, 60–61; author's search for, 59–60; breeding, 73–74, 86–87; characteristics and genetics, 72–73, 77–78; cooking and eating, 61–62, 64, 79–80, 88–89; in Gullah culture, 64–65, 66; scholarship on, 78–79. *See also* pork
Ossabaw Island, 55–58, 59–60
ovens, 4–5, 259

P

Pacific Northwest. *See* Northwest Coast Peoples
Palacios, Victor, 97, 99, 100, 107–8
Paleo diet, 14, 28, 211
Paleolithic period, 11, 166, 214–15, 216, 218
Palmer, Ned, 133
pannage, 75
Paoli, Ugo, 92
Parthian laser (asafoetida, hing), 203–4, 204n
pasteurization, 131
pata negra pigs, 29, 59, 75, 77
patents, 18, 228
Pentlatch People, 270–71. *See also* Northwest Coast Peoples
pepper, 201, 202
Peralta Gonzalez, Margarita, 51
Percival, Bronwen, 129–30, 132, 133, 134, 141, 146
perennial wheat (Kernza), 284
Persephone, 226
Petronius: *Satyricon*, 105, 110
Petruzzi, Donato, 179–80
Pham, Cuong, 116–17
pharmacognosy, 204
Phoenicians, 94–96, 95n, 103, 106–7, 164, 217

photosynthesis, hacking, 284–85
Pick & Cheese (London), 119–21, 122
Pierce's disease, 158. See also *Xylella fastidiosa*
pigs. *See* pork
Pilgrims, 259n
Plant Patent Act (1930), 18, 228
Plato, 103, 104
Pliny the Elder, 105, 184, 192, 195–96
plowing, 197–98
Pollan, Michael, 173, 213
polyphenols, 12, 15, 168, 173–74
Pompeii, 99, 106, 109
population, human, 8, 18, 23–24, 220, 221, 231, 283
pork: barbecue, 69–71, 84; curing and smoking, 65–66; domestication, 74–75, 80–81; East Asian breeds, 80–81; feral hogs, 77; global consumption of, 68–69; industrialized, 79, 81–85, 87–88; introduction to North America, 75–78; *jamón ibérico*, 65–66, 68–69; lack of genetic diversity, 10; *pata negra* pigs, 29, 59, 75, 77; prohibitions against, 66–68; in Quebec, 69; in Spanish *dehesa*, 29, 75, 77; swine flu, 87–88; wild boar, 74. *See also* Ossabaw feral hogs
Portugal, 202
potatoes, 210–11, 250–51, 262, 263–64, 274, 284
poultry, 67–68
prairies, Canadian, 225–26, 240, 295
protein, 88
Puglia. *See* olives and olive oil
pulque, 38–39, 46, 47, 53
Puratos, 236
Purgatorius, 26
puttanesca, 90–91, 109

Q

Quebec, 69, 238–39
querns, 216, 288–90
Quw'utsun (Cowichan People), 248–51. *See also* Northwest Coast Peoples
Qwustenuxun (Jared Williams), 247–51

R

Rare Breeds Survival Trust, 140–41
Recalma-Clutesi, Kim (Ogwilowgwa), 270–77
Red Devon cattle, 85
Redding, Richard, 68
red laver, 273
Redon, José Carlos, 48–49, 50
Redzepi, René, 49
rennet, 124, 131
residential schools, 248–49, 257, 261, 270, 272–73
Restaurante Bar Chon (Mexico City), 43–45
rewilding, 6, 129, 134, 142–43, 148
rice, 10, 63, 225, 284, 285, 295
Riddle, John M., 194–95
Rodio, Corrado, 165–71, 177, 179
Rojas, Fortino, 44–45
Romans: agriculture origin story, 218; *Apicius* (*De re coquinaria*) cookbook, 112–14, 202–3, 206–7; cheese and, 127; decline, 8; environmental degradation by, 197–98; *garum* and, 92–93, 96, 104–7, 110, 113, 114, 115; Monte Testaccio (Rome), 165; olive oil and, 164–65, 167–68; Romulus and Remus, 103–4; silphion and, 183–84, 194–95; wheat and, 226, 229
Roquefort cheese, 136, 146
Rowan, Erica, 195, 199
rubisco, 284
rue, 113
Rutherford, Adam, 287
rye, 225, 237

S

sago grubs, 21
Sahagún, Bernardino de, 46
Saharan cypress, 196
salep, 186
salmon, 248, 249, 253, 254, 264–65, 271–72, 273
Sanchez, Monica, 14–15
Saponari, Maria, 158, 160
saponins, 268, 276

sardines, 90–91, 108, 111–12, 118. See also *garum*

Saulnier, Louis: *Répertoire de la Cuisine*, 113

Saunders, Nick, 130

Scaurus, Aulus Umbricius, 106

Schenzel, Jeremiah, 80

Schneider, Joe, 129

Schumacher, E. F.: *Small Is Beautiful*, 18

Scott, James C., 220

Scott, Rodney, 69–70, 71, 80

seal oil, 273

sea urchins, 94, 101, 113, 249

seeds, market for, 10

Seneca, 105

sheep, 136, 139–40

Shields, David S., 61–62, 71

shrimp, 45, 101

Shubayqa 1 (Paleolithic archaeological site), 214

shyobunone, 205

silkworm chrysalids, 21

silphion: attempts to rediscover, 184–85; cooking and eating, 199–200, 202–3, 206–8; depictions of, 193–94; extinction, 183–84, 195–98, 196n; medicinal properties, 194–95; native habitat, 192–93; vs. Parthian laser (asafoetida, hing), 203–4, 204n; potential rediscovery as *Ferula drudeana*, 188–92, 194, 197, 198–200, 204–5, 205–8; Romans and, 183, 194–95

slaughterhouses, 82

Slow Food (organization), 18–19, 19n, 49

Snuneymuxw People, 274. *See also* Northwest Coast Peoples

soapberries, 275–76

Songhees Seafood & Steam, 263

Sophocles, 104

Soto, Hernando de, 76

sourdough bread, 132, 212, 235–36, 238

soybean oil, 172–73

soybeans, 224n, 239, 295

Spain, 29, 75, 77, 156

Spanish conquistadors, 28–31, 38, 40–41, 51, 52, 62, 75–77

species extinction, 9, 76, 182–83, 197

Spice Bazaar (Misir Çarsisi), 200

spices, 186–87, 201–2, 201n, 208. *See also* silphion

spirulina, 31

spittlebug, meadow (*sputacchina*), 159, 160, 161–62

springbank clover, 255, 266

St. Catherines Island, 56, 59, 77

stem rust, 229–30

Stilton cheese, 121, 122, 129, 131

stinging nettles, 273

Strabo, 95, 127, 192–93, 195, 204

Styawat (Leigh Joseph), 265–67

Sulzberger, Jacob, 242

Sumerians, 220–21

sustainability, 5–6, 177–78, 270, 276–77, 285–87, 294–95, 296

Svalbard Global Seed Vault, 232–33, 234

swine flu, 87–88

Swinscoe, Andy, 146–50

Switzerland, 293–94, 295

Syngenta, 10

T

Tanzarella, Filomena, 152–53, 154–55, 156–57

techno-optimists, 284–85

Tenochtitlán, 29–31, 35, 38, 41

teosinte, 36, 36n

Teotihuacán, 37

termites, 26–28

terra preta, 277–78

Tertullian, 198

Theophrastus, 192

thimbleberry (*Rubus parviflorus*), 262

"Three Sisters" farming (milpa system), 36–37, 277

Toltecs, 37

tomato, Flavr Savr, 285

traditional ecological knowledge (TEK), 277–79

transgenic and genetically modified food, 12, 20, 239, 284–85

transhumance, 293

Tsawout First Nation, 262, 263, 265. *See also* Northwest Coast Peoples tuckahoe, 76

tuna, bluefin, 106–7, 108, 111n

Turkey: 1908 revolution, 227; agricultural crisis, 6–9; bread and wheat in, 7, 12–13; *Ferula drudeana* discovery, 188–92, 198–99; Misir Çarsisi (Spice Bazaar), 200; Nezahat Gökyiğit Botanical Gardens, 205. *See also* Çatalhöyük

Turner, Nancy, 259, 263, 263n, 269–70, 273

Turtle Island (North America), 247. *See also* Northwest Coast Peoples

U

Ukraine, 211, 225, 227, 234–35

umami, 91, 99. See also *garum*

United Kingdom: cheese, 121, 127–28, 129, 130–31, 132, 133; fertilizer, 227; granges, 135; Northern Dairy Shorthorns, 140–41, 143–44, 148, 294; sheep, 139–40; Yorkshire Dales, 134–36, 137, 142–43, 145–46, 148–49, 294

United States of America: cheese, 121; dairy industry, 9–10, 138, 138n; feral hogs, 77; flour industry, 242; glyphosate in, 239; life expectancy, 12; organic food market, 285; pork industry, 81–82, 87

Uruk period, 219, 220–21

V

Vancouver (K'emk'emeláy), 244–46

Vancouver, George, 251–52, 260

Vancouver Island (Mi'wer'la), 256, 257–58, 264

Vattel, Emer de, 259

Vaud (Switzerland), 293–94, 295

vegetable oil, 172–73

Victoria (BC), 248, 256–58, 260

Vienne, Philippe and Ethné de, 185–88

voatsiperifery pepper, 186–87

W

walls, drystone, 153–54

water boatman (*axayacatl*), 25, 31, 32, 42–43, 43n, 51–52. See also *ahuautle*

water hyacinth, 41

weaver ants, 27

Wells, Spencer: *Pandora's Seed*, 6

Wengrow, David, 4, 218, 221, 253

Wensleydale cheese, 121–23, 136, 141, 144–45, 145–46, 147–48

West, Eleanor "Sandy" Torrey, 56–57, 59, 61, 78

wheat: bread (common) wheat, 232; domestication, 225–26; flour from La Milanaise, 238–39, 240–41; gene banks, 232–35; glyphosate and, 240; hybridization, 227–28, 232; Mediterranean civilization and, 152; milling, 216, 241–43, 289–90; monocultures, 10, 295; perennial wheat (Kernza), 284; regime collapse from lack of, 226–27; Romans and, 226, 229; stem rust and stem rust-resistant hybrids, 229–30, 231; storage underground, 226; in Turkey, 7, 13; ubiquity of, 224. *See also* einkorn; emmer; grain

Whitaker, Keiran Olivares, 286

White, William, 274, 276

Whitman, Narcissa, 256

Williams, Jared (Qwustenuxun), 247–51

Williams, Jesse, 131

wolves, 61, 74n, 143

Worldwide Olive Germplasm Bank, 176–77

Wright, Ronald, 37–38

X

Xylella fastidiosa, 156–57, 157–63, 170–71, 175–79, 179–80

Y

yaupon holly (*Ilex vomitoria*), 57, 57n

yeast, commercial, 132, 236

Yorkshire Dales, 134–36, 137, 142–43, 145–46, 148–49, 294

Z

Zabinski, Catherine, 228

Zurita, Ricardo Muñoz, 47

DAVID
  SUZUKI
INSTITUTE

The David Suzuki Institute is a companion organization to the David Suzuki Foundation, with a focus on promoting and publishing on important environmental issues in partnership with Greystone Books.

We invite you to support the activities of the Institute. For more information please contact us at:

David Suzuki Institute
219 – 2211 West 4th Avenue
Vancouver, BC, Canada v6K 4S2
info@davidsuzukiinstitute.org
604-742-2899
www.davidsuzukiinstitute.org

Checks can be made payable to The David Suzuki Institute.